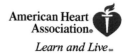

The AHA Clinical Series

SERIES EDITOR ELLIOTT ANTMAN

Metabolic Risk for Cardiovascular Disease

American Heart
Association®

Learn and Live℠
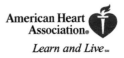

The AHA Clinical Series

SERIES EDITOR ELLIOTT ANTMAN

Metabolic Risk for Cardiovascular Disease

EDITED BY

Robert H. Eckel, MD, FAHA

Professor of Medicine
Division of Endocrinology, Metabolism and Diabetes
Division of Cardiology
Professor of Physiology and Biophysics
Charles A. Boettcher II Chair in Atherosclerosis
Director, Discovery Translation, Colorado Clinical and Translational Sciences Institute
University of Colorado Denver Anschutz Medical Campus
Director Lipid Clinic, University Hospital
Denver, CO, USA

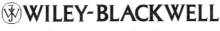

A John Wiley & Sons, Ltd., Publication

Library of Congress Cataloging-in-Publication Data

Metabolic risk for cardiovascular disease / edited by Robert H. Eckel.
    p. ; cm. – (AHA clinical series)
  Includes bibliographical references and index.
  ISBN 978-1-4051-8104-4
  1. Cardiovascular system–Diseases–Risk factors.   2. Metabolic syndrome.   3. Obesity–Complication.
4. Lipids–Metabolism–Disorders–Complication.   5. Diabetes–Complication.   I. Eckel, Robert H.
II. American Heart Association.   III. Series: AHA clinical series.
   [DNLM: 1. Cardiovascular Diseases–etiology.   2. Cardiovascular Diseases–epidemiology.   3. Cardiovascular Diseases–prevention & control.   4. Diabetes Mellitus, Type 2–complications.   5. Metabolic Syndrome X–complications.   6. Risk Factors. WG 120 M587 2010]
   RA645.C34M48 2010
   616.1'071–dc22

                                            2010012034

A catalogue record for this book is available from the British Library.

This book is published in the following electronic formats: ePDF 9781444324792

Set in 9/12 pt Palatino by Aptara® Inc., New Delhi, India

Printed and bound in Singapore by Ho Printing Singapore Pte Ltd

1   2011

Contents

Contributors

Arne V. Astrup, MD, DMSc
Head of Department and Professor
Department of Human Nutrition
Faculty of Life Sciences
University of Copenhagen
Senior Consultant
Department of Clinical Nutrition
Gentofte University Hospital
Hellerup, Denmark

George A. Bray, MD
Boyd Professor
Pennington Center/LSU
Chief of Obesity and Metabolic Syndrome
Pennington Biomedical Research Centre
Louisiana State University
Baton Rouge, LA, USA

John A. Farmer, MD
Professor of Medicine
Baylor College of Medicine
Texas Heart Institute at St. Luke's Episcopal Hospital
Houston, TX, USA

Antonio M. Gotto Jr, MD, DPhil
Stephen and Suzanne Weiss Dean and Professor of Medicine
Weill Cornell Medical College
New York, NY, USA

William L. Haskell, PhD
Professor
Stanford Prevention Research Center
School of Medicine
Stanford University
Stanford, CA, USA

Steven E. Kahn, MB, ChB
Professor of Medicine
University of Washington
Associate Chief of Staff for Research and Development and Staff Physician
VA Puget Sound Health Care System and University of Washington
Seattle, WA, USA

William E. Kraus, MD
Professor of Medicine
Duke University School of Medicine
Medical Director
Cardiac Rehabilitation
Duke University Health System
Director of Clinical Research
Duke Center for Living
Duke University Health System
Durham, NC, USA

Alice H. Lichtenstein, DSc
Gershoff Professor of Nutrition Science and Policy
Tufts University
Director
Cardiovascular Laboratory and Senior Scientist
Tufts University
Boston, MA, USA

Paul Poirier, MD, PhD, FRCPC, FACC, FAHA
Associate Professor in the Faculty of Pharmacy
Laval University, Quebec Canada
Director Cardiac Prevention and Rehabilitation Program
Institut Universitaire de Cardiologie et de Pneumologie de Québec
Québec, QC, Canada

Frank M. Sacks, MD
Professor of Cardiovascular Disease Prevention
Nutrition Department
Harvard School of Public Health
Professor of Medicine
Harvard Medical School
Senior Attending Physician
Hyperlipidemia Clinic
Cardiology Division
Brigham & Women's Hospital
Boston, MA, USA

Jay S. Skyler, MD, MACP
Professor
Division of Endocrinology, Diabetes, & Metabolism
Associate Director
Diabetes Research Institute
University of Miami Miller School of Medicine
Miami, FL, USA

Sidney C. Smith Jr, MD, FACC, FAHA, FESC
Professor of Medicine
Director, Center for Cardiovascular Science and Medicine
University of North Carolina
Chapel Hill, NC, USA

C. Barr Taylor, MD
Professor of Psychiatry
Department of Psychiatry and Behavior Science
Stanford Medical School
Stanford, CA, USA

Mickey Trockel, PhD, MD
Clinical Instructor of Psychiatry and Behavior Science
Department of Psychiatry and Behavior Science
Stanford Medical School
Stanford, CA, USA

Kristina M. Utzschneider, MD
Assistant Professor of Medicine
VA Puget Sound Health Care System and the University of Washington
Seattle, WA, USA

Stan S. Wang, MD, JD, MPH
Director of Legislative Affairs, Austin Heart
Clinical Cardiovascular Disease, Austin Heart South
Assistant Professor of Medicine (Adjunct), University of North Carolina
Chapel Hill, NC, USA

Peter W.F. Wilson, MD
Professor of Medicine and Public Health
Emory University
Atlanta, GA, USA

Foreword

The strategic driving force behind the American Heart Association's mission of reducing disability and death from cardiovascular diseases and stroke is to change practice by providing information and solutions to healthcare professionals. The pillars of this strategy are Knowledge Discovery, Knowledge Processing, and Knowledge Transfer. The books in the AHA Clinical Series, of which *Metabolic Risk for Cardiovascular Disease* is included, focus on high-interest, cutting-edge topics in cardiovascular medicine. This book series is a critical tool that supports the AHA mission of promoting healthy behavior and improved care of patients. Cardiology is a rapidly changing field and practitioners need data to guide their clinical decision making. The AHA Clinical Series serves this need by providing the latest information on the physiology, diagnosis, and management of a broad spectrum of conditions encountered in daily practice.

Rose Marie Robertson, MD, FAHA
Chief Science Officer, American Heart Association
Elliott Antman, MD, FAHA
Director, Samuel A. Levine Cardiac Unit,
Brigham and Women's Hospital

Chapter 1

Insulin action and beta-cell function: role in metabolic regulation

Kristina M. Utzschneider and Steven E. Kahn

Regulation of fuel utilization in health and disease

The normal processing and utilization of fuels is tightly regulated by hormonal, neural, and intracellular mechanisms so that carbohydrates, proteins, and fats supply energy to the brain, muscles, and other tissues, and excess fuel is stored efficiently for use during periods of fasting or increased energy needs. Two key players in the balance of hormones regulating these processes are insulin and glucagon.

Insulin is secreted by the islet beta-cell in response to glucose, amino acids, peptides, and fatty acids and then promotes tissue uptake of glucose and glycogen synthesis. Insulin also acts on lipid metabolism by promoting enzymes involved in *de novo* lipogenesis, while suppressing those enzymes involved in lipid oxidation and lipolysis, resulting in a decrease in circulating free fatty acids (FFAs). The net result is a shift towards utilization of glucose as the primary fuel. Insulin's effects are mainly anabolic as insulin levels increase when nutrient availability is high. During times when insulin levels are low, such as during fasting, these processes reverse and fuel selection shifts to preferentially utilize fat. Insulin also acts centrally in the hypothalamus as a satiety signal by interacting with neural centers that regulate food intake.

In contrast to insulin, the hormone glucagon, which is secreted by the islet alpha-cell, acts as a catabolic hormone, stimulating production of glucose via glycogenolysis and gluconeogenesis, primarily in response to hypoglycemia. Glucagon is also important in the regulation of basal and postprandial glucose levels, with the balance of this hormone with insulin being important. Thus,

Metabolic Risk for Cardiovascular Disease, 1st edition. Edited by R. H. Eckel.
© 2011 American Heart Association. By Blackwell Publishing Ltd.

when insulin levels rise, as occurs after nutrient ingestion, glucagon levels will normally decrease.

In both type 1 and type 2 diabetes, insulin release is reduced, resulting in disruption of normal metabolism. Type 1 diabetes represents the extreme situation in which a near total deficiency of insulin is associated with marked hyperglycemia and the development of ketosis. In type 2 diabetes the deficiency of insulin is less pronounced, but since subjects with this disease are typically insulin resistant, as discussed in greater detail in the next section, the amount of insulin secreted is insufficient to overcome the tissue's reduced responsiveness to insulin, resulting in overall insulin action being diminished.

Insulin sensitivity and beta-cell function: a critical interplay determining glucose tolerance in health and disease

Insulin resistance has long been recognized as a common feature of type 2 diabetes and has been considered by some to be the major underlying feature of the disease. However, it is now clear that it is the interplay between insulin sensitivity and the beta-cell's response which is important. Interpreting the beta-cell's response in the light of concurrent insulin sensitivity is vital and, when doing so, it is apparent that a failure of the beta-cell to release adequate amounts of insulin is the critical determinant of the progression to abnormal glucose tolerance.

Insulin secretion and insulin sensitivity are related in a physiological manner through a feedback loop that ensures maintenance of glucose tolerance. Thus, as insulin sensitivity decreases, insulin secretion increases in a compensatory fashion. The converse is also true so that when insulin sensitivity increases, less insulin is secreted in response to the same stimulus and in this manner hypoglycemia is avoided. This relationship between insulin sensitivity and the acute insulin response to intravenous glucose ($AIR_{glucose}$ or AIR_g) has been shown to be hyperbolic in nature [1] (Figure 1.1a). Based on this hyperbolic relationship, the product of insulin sensitivity and the insulin response should remain constant for any level of glycemia (Figure 1.1b). This product has been termed the disposition index and has been used as a measure of beta-cell function.

Evidence that beta-cell dysfunction is present well before the onset of diabetes has been provided using this approach. In subjects with impaired fasting glucose (IFG; fasting plasma glucose 100–110 mg/dL) compared to those with normal fasting glucose levels (< 100 mg/dL), for any given level of insulin sensitivity, there is a relative decrease in the insulin response, so that the hyperbolic curve for the IFG group is shifted leftward and downward relative to those with normal fasting glucose levels [2] (Figure 1.2a). Furthermore, when subjects were divided into quintiles based on their fasting plasma glucose level and plotted relative to each other, a progressive decrease in beta-cell function can be shown

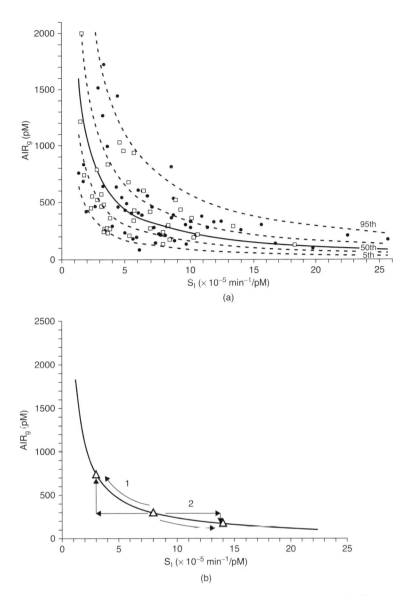

(a)

(b)

Figure 1.1 (a) The hyperbolic relationship between insulin sensitivity index (S_I) and the first-phase (acute) insulin response (AIR_g) in 93 apparently, healthy subjects (55 men [•] and 38 women [□]; log_e regression: $r = -0.62$, $P < 0.001$). The hyperbolic relationship determines that changes in S_I are balanced by reciprocal changes in AIR_g. The cohort has a broad range of insulin sensitivity and insulin responses. The solid line depicts the mean relationship (50th percentile) whereas the broken lines represent the 5th, 25th, 75th, and 95th percentiles. (Reproduced from Kahn et al. [1], with permission from the American Diabetes Association.) (b) Model of the reciprocal changes in insulin sensitivity that is determined by the hyperbolic relationship between S_I and AIR_g. As insulin sensitivity falls (1), a normal adaptive increase in the AIR_g occurs. Similarly, if insulin sensitivity improves (2), the AIR_g will decrease in response to avoid hypoglycemia. (Adapted from Kahn et al. [1], with permission from the American Diabetes Association.)

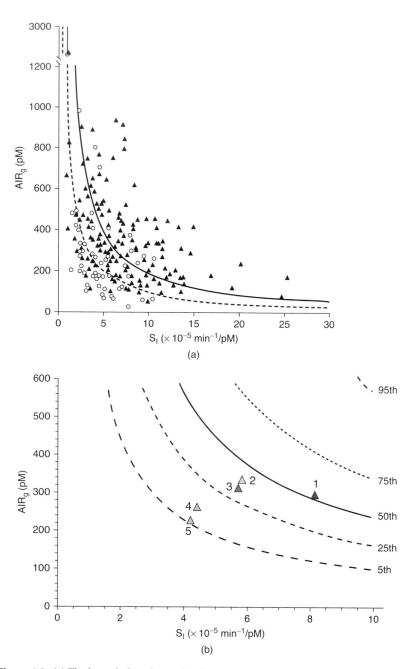

Figure 1.2 (a) The hyperbolic relationship between insulin sensitivity index (S_I) and the first-phase insulin response (AIR_g) in 219 subjects subdivided based on whether they had normal fasting glucose (NFG; fasting plasma glucose < 100 mg/dL, $n = 156$, △ solid line) or impaired fasting glucose (IFG; 100–110 mg/dL, $n = 63$, ○ broken line).

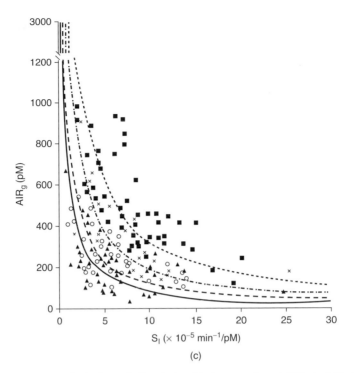

(c)

Figure 1.2 (*Continued*) The hyperbolic relationship between S_I and AIR_g is shifted to the left and downward in subjects with IFG compared to those with normal fasting glucose, indicating poorer beta-cell function in those with IFG. (Reproduced from Utzschneider et al. [2] with permission from the American Diabetes Association.) (b) The relationship between S_I and AIR_g is plotted relative to a normal healthy population (5th to 95th percentiles) for each quintile of fasting glucose for those subjects with fasting glucose < 110 mg/dL. Beta-cell function declines as the fasting plasma glucose concentration increases quintile 1: 80 91 mg/dL, quintile 2: 91–94 mg/dL, quintile 3: 94–98 mg/dL, quintile 4: 98–103 mg/dL, quintile 5: 103–109 mg/dL). (Adapted from Kahn et al. [1] and Utzschneider et al. [2] with permission from the American Diabetes Association.) (c) The hyperbolic relationship between insulin sensitivity index (S_I) and the first-phase insulin response (AIR_g) in 219 subjects subdivided by quartiles of the glucose disappearance constant (K_g). The hyperbolic relationship between S_I and AIR_g is progressively leftward and downward shifted with decreasing intravenous glucose tolerance (lower K_g). (Reproduced from Utzschneider et al. [2] with permission from the American Diabetes Association.)

as fasting glucose increases from below 90 mg/dL to 110 mg/dL [2] (Figure 1.2b). Similarly, division of subjects based on their glucose disappearance constant (K_g), a measure of intravenous glucose tolerance, demonstrated a shift of the curves to the left and downward with decreasing glucose tolerance [2] (Figure 1.2c). Thus, even mild changes in glucose levels may herald early evidence of beta-cell dysfunction and increased metabolic risk.

Groups of subjects who are at increased risk for the development of diabetes also demonstrate decreased beta-cell function using this approach. For example, beta-cell dysfunction has been shown in women with a history of gestational diabetes [3–5] or polycystic ovarian syndrome [6], in older subjects [7,8], and in individuals with a family history of type 2 diabetes [6,9]. Similarly, subjects with pre-diabetes, whether isolated IFG or isolated impaired glucose tolerance (IGT), have defects in beta-cell function. The beta-cell defect in isolated IGT is manifest during both intravenous as well as oral glucose testing. In contrast, the defect in isolated IFG is only manifest during intravenous testing and appears to be compensated for during oral testing by an increased incretin response which would act to enhance glucose-stimulated insulin secretion [10].

Examining the insulin response relative to the degree of insulin sensitivity has also been used to demonstrate that progression to IGT and diabetes over time is associated with decreases in beta-cell function as subjects "fall off" the curve. This was first illustrated in Pima Indians using hyperinsulinemic euglycemic clamp data along with measurement of the acute insulin response to glucose. Over time, all subjects became more insulin resistant, but only those who were unable to adequately increase their insulin response developed diabetes [11] (Figure 1.3). We have made similar observations in subjects with a first-degree relative with type 2 diabetes. In these subjects at increased risk of developing hyperglycemia, the decline in glucose tolerance over time was strongly related to a decline in beta-cell function [12]. The process of loss of beta-cell function appears to be slow with a rapid rise in glucose levels into the diabetic range occurring as a late phenomenon. This was illustrated in a study of women with a previous history of gestational diabetes followed over time. The women who progressed to diabetes demonstrated a slow decline in beta-cell compensation to insulin resistance and this was attended by slowly rising glucose levels, followed by a rapid rise in glucose levels once beta-cell function reached approximately 10% of normal [13]. As discussed later, a similar effect can be observed with data obtained using an oral glucose tolerance test (OGTT).

The approach of interpreting the adequacy of the beta-cell response in relation to the degree of insulin sensitivity has also provided insight into the adequacy of changes in beta-cell function in response to interventions. For example, in older men, 10% weight loss resulted in a 57% improvement in insulin sensitivity, with a consequent 19% decrease in the acute insulin response to intravenous glucose. Adjusting this insulin response for the change in insulin sensitivity demonstrated that overall beta-cell function improved with the weight loss intervention [14]. However, a regular exercise training program alone did not enhance beta-cell function in older subjects despite improvements in insulin sensitivity [15], suggesting that the improvement in insulin sensitivity with weight loss has effects that differ from those observed with exercise training.

Examination of beta-cell function by consideration of the adequacy of the insulin response relative to the degree of insulin sensitivity has also demonstrated

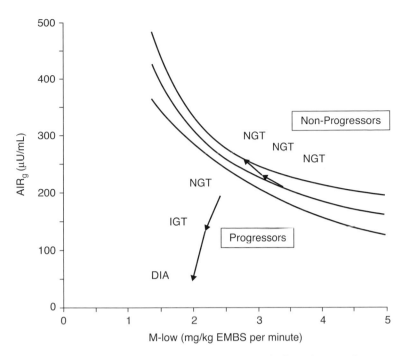

Figure 1.3 Changes in beta-cell function as measured by the first-phase insulin response to glucose (AIR_g) relative to changes in insulin sensitivity as measured by the clamp method at a low insulin concentration (M-low) in 34 Pima Indians studied over several years. Twenty-three subjects maintained normal glucose tolerance (NGT) throughout (non-progressors), and 11 subjects progressed from NGT to impaired glucose tolerance (IGT) and then to diabetes (DIA; progressors). The curvilinear lines represent the mean and upper and lower 95% confidence interval for the regression between AIR_g and M-low based on a population of 277 Pima Indians with NGT. EMBS, estimated metabolic body size. (Reproduced from Weyer et al. [11] with permission from the American Society for Clinical Investigation.)

that beta-cell function can be preserved with the insulin-sensitizing medication, troglitazone. Hispanic women with a previous history of gestational diabetes were administered this thiazolidinedione or placebo in a randomized, double-blinded study. After a median of 30 months on blinded medication, fewer women in the troglitazone arm developed diabetes (12.1% on placebo vs. 5.4% on troglitazone, $P < 0.01$). Protection from progression to diabetes was significantly associated with early improvement in the disposition index at 3 months in the troglitazone group [16].

The series of observations discussed above has made it very clear that the beta-cell is a critical player in determining glucose metabolism and that reductions in the adequacy of insulin release underlie changes in plasma glucose levels even in individuals who are at risk for developing diabetes. However, these analyses have all been based on intravenous testing. As this approach is not practical in epidemiological and large clinical studies, an important issue is whether oral testing provides similar information and can be used in large, clinical research studies.

Insulin sensitivity and beta-cell function: insights from oral testing

Recently, a similar hyperbolic relationship between surrogate measures of insulin sensitivity and the early insulin response derived from an OGTT has been demonstrated [17,18]. When subjects with IFG and/or IGT and diabetes were examined, the curves for these groups were shifted downward and to the left as glucose tolerance declined from normal to IFG and/or IGT and then to diabetes, with those subjects with diabetes demonstrating insulin resistance and a flatter early insulin response. Based on the existence of a hyperbolic relationship, the product of the two variables was calculated to quantify this adjusted insulin response as the oral disposition index. This measure decreased with decreasing glucose tolerance and, importantly, a higher oral disposition index was associated with a decreased relative risk of developing diabetes over a 10-year follow-up period in these subjects [17]. Of further importance, this decrease in beta-cell function with deteriorating glucose tolerance appears to occur similarly in different ethnic groups [19].

Understanding this relationship has highlighted the importance of beta-cell function in determining the magnitude of the glucose excursion during an OGTT. In a large cohort of subjects with varying glucose tolerance, it has been demonstrated that insulin sensitivity is a weak determinant of the magnitude of the glucose excursion during a standard 75-gram OGTT, while beta-cell function was a strong and significant predictor of post-challenge glycemia [19]. Further, data from this analysis demonstrated that while beta-cell function varied tremendously in individuals with normal glucose tolerance, when it was markedly decreased, small changes had dramatic effects on the efficiency of glucose disposal (Figure 1.4) [19].

Using data from OGTTs, subjects with IGT who participated in the Diabetes Prevention Program (DPP) demonstrated improvements in beta-cell function with both the lifestyle intervention (weight loss and increased physical activity) and metformin treatment [20]. From the baseline data in these subjects, the relationship between the measures of insulin sensitivity and insulin release could be plotted as a non-linear function with the mean for all groups being similar. With the two interventions there was a rightward shift which was greater with lifestyle than metformin, while with placebo there was a small change that tended to be to the left of the mean line for the baseline relationship (Figure 1.5). These differences in outcome when examining insulin release and

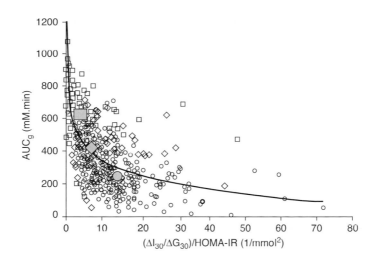

Figure 1.4 Relationship between beta-cell function, as determined by the early insulin response to oral glucose adjusted for the prevailing insulin sensitivity, the latter determined using the homeostasis model (HOMA), and overall glucose tolerance quantified as the incremental area under the glucose curve in response to an oral glucose challenge (AUC_g) in 531 first-degree relatives of patients with type 2 diabetes. The mean value for subjects with normal glucose tolerance (circle, $n = 240$), impaired glucose tolerance (diamond, $n = 191$), and diabetes (square, $n = 100$) are illustrated. As the relationship is non-linear, when beta-cell function is diminished (such as in subjects with IGT and diabetes), small differences in beta-cell function will have a marked effect on the efficiency of glucose disposal compared to similar magnitude differences in subjects with normal glucose tolerance. (Reproduced from Jensen et al. [19] with permission from the American Diabetes Association.)

insulin sensitivity are in keeping with the lifestyle intervention resulting in a 58% decrease in the risk of progression to diabetes, while metformin resulted in a 31% decreased risk [21]. Thus, interventions that improve beta-cell function may explain their ability to delay the progression to diabetes in those at risk.

Effects of insulin resistance and insulin deficiency on regulation of fuel partitioning

One of the major effects of insufficient insulin release in type 2 diabetes is an increase in hepatic glucose production and decreased efficiency of glucose uptake, both resulting in an increase in plasma glucose. This outcome occurs both in the fasting state and following nutrient ingestion when suppression of glucose production is not normal. Insulin, and perhaps other constituents of the beta-cell secretory granule, also acts in a paracrine fashion to suppress glucagon secretion by the alpha-cell; thus, the insulin deficiency in type 2 diabetes is

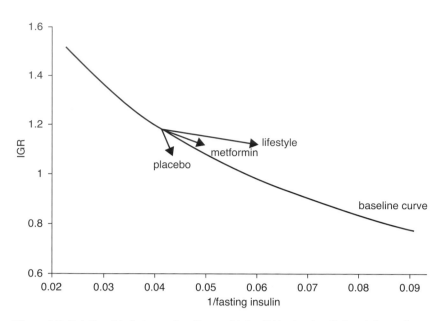

Figure 1.5 Relationship between insulin sensitivity (1/fasting insulin) and the early insulin response (insulinogenic index; IGR) quantified from an oral glucose tolerance test (OGTT) at baseline and after a year by treatment group in subjects with impaired glucose tolerance (IGT) who participated in the Diabetes Prevention Program. Beta-cell function is described by the relationship between insulin release and insulin sensitivity. The curve represents the regression line of the logarithm of estimated insulin release as a linear function of the logarithm of estimated insulin sensitivity for all participants at baseline. The arrows connect the point estimate for median insulin release and median insulin sensitivity at baseline and after a year of the interventions (lifestyle, metformin, placebo). After one year of intervention, subjects who underwent the lifestyle intervention had the greatest improvement in beta-cell function as evidenced by the greatest shift to the right from the baseline curve. In contrast, those in the placebo group had a slight decline in beta-cell function, while those treated with metformin had an intermediate response. These changes in beta-cell function paralleled the positive effects to reduce the rate of development of diabetes by lifestyle and metformin, which were in contrast to that with placebo that had the highest rate of progression from IGT to diabetes. (Reproduced from Kitabchi et al. [20] with permission from the American Diabetes Association.)

associated with a paradoxical increase in postprandial glucagon levels which further raise glucose levels.

The effects of beta-cell dysfunction are not simply confined to abnormalities in glucose levels, but have broader impacts on lipid metabolism and fuel selection. As tissues take up less glucose and there is less insulin to suppress lipid oxidation, fuel selection shifts towards more lipid oxidation. For example, in conditions such as non-alcoholic fatty liver disease (NAFLD), oxidative and non-oxidative glucose metabolism are decreased in response to insulin while lipid oxidation remains elevated compared to body mass index (BMI)-matched controls [22].

Effects of insulin resistance and insulin deficiency on free fatty acids and lipid metabolism

One of the major effects of insulin resistance at the level of the adipocyte is an impaired ability to suppress lipolysis via lipoprotein lipase (LPL), resulting in increased free fatty acid (FFA) levels. High FFA levels have been shown to be detrimental in many ways. Increased FFAs produce insulin resistance by competing with glucose as a substrate for oxidation, resulting in the inhibition of the activities of pyruvate dehydrogenase, phosphofructokinase, and hexokinase II [23]. In addition to this mechanism, it has been suggested that an increase in delivery of FFAs to the cell or a decrease in their metabolism results in an increase in the cell's content of metabolites including diacylglycerol, fatty acyl-coenzyme A (fatty acyl-CoA), and ceramides. The increase in these metabolites leads to serine/threonine phosphorylation of insulin receptor substrate-1 (IRS-1) and insulin receptor substrate-2 (IRS-2), which in turn results in reduced activation of PI-3-kinase and diminished downstream signaling [24]. Finally, elevated FFAs in the setting of hyperglycemia may be "toxic" to the beta-cell, thus contributing to beta-cell dysfunction and inadequate insulin secretion [25]. Any decrease in the relative amount of circulating insulin relative to the prevailing insulin sensitivity will thus exacerbate the process by increasing FFAs and impairing glucose clearance.

The metabolic effect of increased FFAs is also frequently manifested as changes in lipid metabolism. The hypertriglyceridemia seen in subjects with the metabolic syndrome and type 2 diabetes is the result of increased export of available triglycerides as very-low-density lipoprotein (VLDL) particles [26]. This occurs mainly as a result of increased FFA flux to the liver, but insulin stimulation of *de novo* lipogenesis via sterol receptor element binding protein 1-c (SREBP1-c) [27] may also contribute. In patients with type 2 diabetes, hyperglycemia also stimulates *de novo* lipogenesis via the carbohydrate receptor element binding protein (ChREBP) [27]. Insulin resistance further contributes to increased VLDL by decreasing the direct inhibitory effect of insulin on apoB secretion. In subjects with low liver fat, an insulin infusion leads to a rapid drop in VLDL apoB and triacylglycerol secretion, but in subjects with high liver fat, including many with type 2 diabetes, the insulin infusion causes no significant change in VLDL secretion [28]. Finally, insulin resistance can decrease degradation of apoB [29,30]. The generation of excess VLDL particles results in subsequent metabolic abnormalities that are associated with an increase in cardiovascular risk, including generation of more atherogenic small dense low-density lipoprotein (LDL) particles and increased catabolism of high-density lipoprotein (HDL) [31].

Insulin regulation of amino acid metabolism

Insulin also has important effects to regulate protein and amino acid metabolism. In the fasted state, insulin levels are low and amino acids are utilized for gluconeogenesis. Using the insulin clamp technique, it has been demonstrated that in the fasting state insulin decreases whole-body protein degradation [32], but does not stimulate protein synthesis in the absence of hyperaminoacidemia [33]. In the fed state the response depends on the composition of the meal. A high-protein meal both stimulatesecretion of insulin and increases plasma amino acid levels with a net anabolic effect and positive nitrogen balance [34]. A meal consisting of glucose alone would lead to a prompt increase in insulin and a subsequent fall in plasma levels of many amino acids, with a continued net negative whole-body nitrogen balance.

In uncontrolled type 1 diabetes there is a lack of insulin and counter-regulatory hormones are increased with subsequent increased protein degradation and utilization of amino acids for gluconeogenesis. The net result is wasting of lean body mass, often seen in the early presentation of the disease. In contrast, in type 2 diabetes the deficiency in insulin is not as absolute and these dramatic effects on muscle wasting do not occur and protein metabolism is maintained fairly near normal [35].

Role of fat distribution and ectopic fat in insulin resistance

For many years it has been considered that insulin resistance was the result of obesity, as determined simply by body size. While insulin resistance is most often associated with obesity, even lean people have been found to be quite insulin resistant [36]. This finding has been shown to be in part the result of increased intra-abdominal fat (IAF), which may occur in people technically considered lean based on BMI criteria alone. Using computed tomography data to quantify IAF and abdominal subcutaneous fat (SQF), IAF has been most strongly related to insulin sensitivity [36]. In addition to being a determinant of insulin sensitivity, IAF has also been shown to be predictive of the future development of the metabolic syndrome [37], IGT [38], and diabetes [39].

In insulin-resistant states, lipid accumulation frequently occurs at "ectopic" sites including muscle and liver. Fat accumulation in the liver [40] is associated with dyslipidemia [41] and increased risk for cardiovascular disease (CVD) in patients with type 2 diabetes [42]. Further, elevated liver enzymes, as a marker of fatty liver disease in the absence of hepatitis C or excess alcohol intake, have been associated with increased cardiovascular disease [43,44].

Mechanisms for hepatic fat accumulation include (i) dietary excess of fats or carbohydrates such as fructose that are converted into triglycerides in the liver via *de novo* lipogenesis, (ii) hyperinsulinemia stimulating *de novo* lipogenesis, (iii) relative decreased lipid oxidation due to low adiponectin levels and/or high insulin levels, and (iv) increased FFAs delivery from adipose tissue due to impaired suppression of lipolysis by insulin. The latter explanation is supported by the fact that addition of basal insulin treatment to patients with type 2 diabetes already on metformin results in reduced plasma FFA levels, a small but significant reduction in liver fat, as well as improved hepatic insulin sensitivity [45]. Thus, relative insulin deficiency may contribute to development of fatty liver.

Increased intramyocellular lipid (IMCL) has been strongly correlated to skeletal muscle insulin resistance in obesity and type 2 diabetes [46]. Interestingly, endurance trained athletes also have increased IMCL despite being highly insulin sensitive [47] and moderate aerobic exercise training that increases insulin sensitivity and aerobic fitness in previously sedentary, overweight to obese, older subjects was accompanied by increases in IMCL [48]. These latter changes were accompanied by favorable alterations in lipid content, specifically with decreases in diacylglycerol and ceramide [48]. Thus it appears that it is not simply the amount of IMCL, but the quality of lipid within the muscle, that may be important.

Accumulation of excess lipid in the pancreas has also been noted and has been suggested to perhaps contribute to the beta-cell dysfunction seen in type 2 diabetes. *In vivo* studies measuring pancreatic lipid content found it to be increased in subjects with type 2 diabetes relative to non-diabetic controls and to be negatively correlated with beta-cell function parameters by oral glucose testing [49]. Adipocyte infiltration of the exocrine pancreas has also been noted in mice in response to a high-fat diet and human autopsy samples have been shown to have variable degrees of adipocyte infiltration in exocrine tissue [50]. Whether this ectopic fat accumulation in the pancreas really contributes directly to beta-cell dysfunction is not clear.

Insulin resistance, insulin deficiency, and bodyweight regulation

As has been discussed, insulin is an important regulator of metabolism. In recent years there has been a flurry of scientific inquiry examining the role of insulin along with leptin in regulating energy balance and thus bodyweight. Insulin acts in the hypothalamus to regulate bodyweight by modulating food intake. Thus, impaired insulin signaling centrally could contribute to weight gain and thereby impact metabolic homeostasis [51]. Beta-cell dysfunction resulting in a relative reduction in insulin release could result in further decreased insulin action in this critical brain region and could be associated with weight gain and further aggravation of insulin resistance. This concept is supported by data from the Pima Indians showing that insulin secretion was inversely associated with the rate of weight gain and relatively reduced insulin secretion was independently predictive of weight gain and adiposity [52].

Summary

Insulin is the major regulator of metabolic processes, including glucose, protein, and lipid metabolism. Beta-cell dysfunction resulting in a relative deficiency in insulin secretion for the prevailing degree of insulin sensitivity can result in metabolic abnormalities and is a marker for increased risk for the future development of diabetes, with a progressive reduction leading ultimately to clinical hyperglycemia and the diagnosis of diabetes. Thus, it is important for clinicians to continue to promote strategies to improve beta-cell function, including lifestyle intervention with weight loss and medications. The net result should be an improvement, not only in glucose metabolism, but overall metabolic regulation.

Acknowledgments
Supported in part by funds from the Department of Veterans Affairs.

References

1. Kahn SE, Prigeon RL, McCulloch DK, et al. Quantification of the relationship between insulin sensitivity and ß-cell function in human subjects: evidence for a hyperbolic function. *Diabetes* 1993;42:1663–72.
2. Utzschneider KM, Prigeon RL, Carr DB, et al. Impact of differences in fasting glucose and glucose tolerance on the hyperbolic relationship between insulin sensitivity and insulin responses. *Diabetes Care* 2006;29:356–62.
3. Buchanan TA, Xiang AH, Kjos SL, et al. Antepartum predictors of the development of type 2 diabetes in Latino women 11–26 months after pregnancies complicated by gestational diabetes. *Diabetes* 1999;48:2430–6.
4. Ryan EA, Imes S, Liu D, et al. Defects in insulin secretion and action in women with a history of gestational diabetes. *Diabetes* 1995;44:506–12.
5. Ward WK, Johnston CL, Beard JC, et al. Insulin resistance and impaired insulin secretion in subjects with histories of gestational diabetes mellitus. *Diabetes* 1985;34:861–9.
6. Ehrmann DA, Sturis J, Byrne MM, et al. Insulin secretory defects in polycystic ovary syndrome: relationship to insulin sensitivity and family history of non-insulin-dependent diabetes mellitus. *J Clin Invest* 1995;96:520–7.
7. Chen M, Bergman RN, Pacini G, Porte D, Jr. Pathogenesis of age-related glucose intolerance in man: insulin resistance and decreased ß-cell function. *J Clin Endocrinol Metab* 1985;60:13–20.
8. Kahn SE, Larson VG, Schwartz RS, et al. Exercise training delineates the importance of ß-cell dysfunction to the glucose intolerance of human aging. *J Clin Endocrinol Metab* 1992;74:1336–42.

9. Elbein SC, Wegner K, Kahn SE. Reduced ß-cell compensation to the insulin resistance associated with obesity in members of Caucasian familial type 2 diabetic kindreds. *Diabetes Care* 2000;23:221–7.

10. Faerch K, Vaag A, Holst JJ, et al. Impaired fasting glycaemia vs impaired glucose tolerance: similar impairment of pancreatic alpha and beta cell function but differential roles of incretin hormones and insulin action. *Diabetologia* 2008;51:853–61.

11. Weyer C, Bogardus C, Mott DM, Pratley RE. The natural history of insulin secretory dysfunction and insulin resistance in the pathogenesis of type 2 diabetes mellitus. *J Clin Invest* 1999;104:787–94.

12. Cnop M, Vidal J, Hull RL, et al. Progressive loss of ß-cell function leads to worsening glucose tolerance in first-degree relatives of subjects with type 2 diabetes. *Diabetes Care* 2007;30:677–82.

13. Xiang AH, Wang C, Peters RK, et al. Coordinate changes in plasma glucose and pancreatic beta-cell function in Latino women at high risk for type 2 diabetes. *Diabetes* 2006;55:1074–9.

14. Utzschneider KM, Carr DB, Barsness SM, et al. Diet-induced weight loss is associated with an improvement in ß-cell function in older men. *J Clin Endocrinol Metab* 2004;89:2704–10.

15. Kahn SE, Larson VG, Beard JC, et al. Effect of exercise on insulin action, glucose tolerance, and insulin secretion in aging. *Am J Physiol* 1990;258:E937–43.

16. Buchanan TA, Xiang AH, Peters RK, et al. Preservation of pancreatic ß-cell function and prevention of type 2 diabetes by pharmacological treatment of insulin resistance in high-risk Hispanic women. *Diabetes* 2002;51:2796–803.

17. Utzschneider KM, Prigeon RL, Faulenbach MV, et al. Oral disposition index predicts the development of future diabetes above and beyond fasting and 2-h glucose levels. *Diabetes Care* 2009;32:335–41.

18. Retnakaran R, Shen S, Hanley AJ, et al. Hyperbolic relationship between insulin secretion and sensitivity on oral glucose tolerance test. *Obesity (Silver Spring)* 2008;16:1901–7.

19. Jensen CC, Cnop M, Hull RL, et al. ß-cell function is a major contributor to oral glucose tolerance in high-risk relatives of four ethnic groups in the US. *Diabetes* 2002;51:2170–8.

20. Kitabchi AE, Temprosa M, Knowler WC, et al. Role of insulin secretion and sensitivity in the evolution of type 2 diabetes in the diabetes prevention program: effects of lifestyle intervention and metformin. *Diabetes* 2005;54:2404–14.

21. Knowler WC, Barrett-Connor E, Fowler SE, et al. Reduction in the incidence of type 2 diabetes with lifestyle intervention or metformin. *N Engl J Med* 2002;346:393–403.

22. Buganesi E, Gastaldelli A, Vanni E, et al. Insulin resistance in non-diabetic patients with non-alcoholic fatty liver disease: sites and mechanisms. *Diabetologia* 2005;48:634–42.

23. Randle PJ, Garland PB, Newsholme EA, Hales CN. The glucose fatty acid cycle in obesity and maturity onset diabetes mellitus. *Ann N Y Acad Sci* 1965;131:324–33.

24. Shulman GI. Cellular mechanisms of insulin resistance. *J Clin Invest* 2000;106:171–6.

25. Robertson RP, Harmon J, Tran PO, Poitout V. β-cell glucose toxicity, lipotoxicity, and chronic oxidative stress in type 2 diabetes. *Diabetes* 2004;53(Suppl 1):S119–24.

26. Julius U. Influence of plasma free fatty acids on lipoprotein synthesis and diabetic dyslipidemia. *Exp Clin Endocrinol Diabetes* 2003;111:246–50.

27. Browning JD, Horton JD. Molecular mediators of hepatic steatosis and liver injury. *J Clin Invest* 2004;114:147–52.
28. Adiels M, Westerbacka J, Soro-Paavonen A, et al. Acute suppression of VLDL1 secretion rate by insulin is associated with hepatic fat content and insulin resistance. *Diabetologia* 2007;50:2356–65.
29. Duvillard L, Pont F, Florentin E, et al. Metabolic abnormalities of apolipoprotein B-containing lipoproteins in non-insulin-dependent diabetes: a stable isotope kinetic study. *Eur J Clin Invest* 2000;30:685–94.
30. Sumner AE, Falkner B, Diffenderfer MR, et al. A study of the metabolism of apolipoprotein B100 in relation to insulin resistance in African American males. *Proc Soc Exp Biol Med* 1999;221:352–60.
31. Lamarche B, Rashid S, Lewis GF. HDL metabolism in hypertriglyceridemic states: an overview. *Clin Chim Acta* 1999;286:145–61.
32. Tessari P, Trevisan R, Inchiostro S, et al. Dose-response curves of effects of insulin on leucine kinetics in humans. *Am J Physiol* 1986;251:E334–42.
33. Tessari P, Inchiostro S, Biolo G, et al. Differential effects of hyperinsulinemia and hyperaminoacidemia on leucine-carbon metabolism in vivo: evidence for distinct mechanisms in regulation of net amino acid deposition. *J Clin Invest* 1987;79:1062–9.
34. Wahren J, Felig P, Hagenfeldt L. Effect of protein ingestion on splanchnic and leg metabolism in normal man and in patients with diabetes mellitus. *J Clin Invest* 1976;57:987–99.
35. Staten MA, Matthews DE, Bier DM. Leucine metabolism in type II diabetes mellitus. *Diabetes* 1986;35:1249–53.
36. Cnop M, Landchild MJ, Vidal J, et al. The concurrent accumulation of intra-abdominal and subcutaneous fat explains the association between insulin resistance and plasma leptin concentrations: distinct metabolic effects of two fat compartments. *Diabetes* 2002;51:1005–15.
37. Carr DB, Utzschneider KM, Hull RL, et al. Intra-abdominal fat is a major determinant of the National Cholesterol Education Program Adult Treatment Panel III criteria for the metabolic syndrome. *Diabetes* 2004;53:2087–94.
38. Hayashi T, Boyko EJ, Leonetti DL, et al. Visceral adiposity and the risk of impaired glucose tolerance: a prospective study among Japanese Americans. *Diabetes Care* 2003;26:650–5.
39. Boyko EJ, Fujimoto WY, Leonetti DL, Newell-Morris L. Visceral adiposity and risk of type 2 diabetes: a prospective study among Japanese Americans. *Diabetes Care* 2000;23:465–71.
40. Utzschneider KM, Kahn SE. Review: The role of insulin resistance in nonalcoholic fatty liver disease. *J Clin Endocrinol Metab* 2006;91:4753–61.
41. Browning JD, Szczepaniak LS, Dobbins R, et al. Prevalence of hepatic steatosis in an urban population in the United States: impact of ethnicity. *Hepatology* 2004;40:1387–95.
42. Targher G, Bertolini L, Poli F, et al. Nonalcoholic fatty liver disease and risk of future cardiovascular events among type 2 diabetic patients. *Diabetes* 2005;54:3541–6.
43. Ioannou GN, Weiss NS, Boyko EJ, et al. Elevated serum alanine aminotransferase activity and calculated risk of coronary heart disease in the United States. *Hepatology* 2006;43:1145–51.

44. Schindhelm RK, Dekker JM, Nijpels G, et al. Alanine aminotransferase predicts coronary heart disease events: a 10-year follow-up of the Hoorn Study. *Atherosclerosis* 2007;191:391–6.

45. Juurinen L, Tiikkainen M, Hakkinen AM, et al. Effects of insulin therapy on liver fat content and hepatic insulin sensitivity in patients with type 2 diabetes. *Am J Physiol Endocrinol Metab* 2007;292:E829–35.

46. Kelley DE, Goodpaster BH, Storlien L. Muscle triglyceride and insulin resistance. *Annu Rev Nutr* 2002;22:325–46.

47. Goodpaster BH, He J, Watkins S, Kelley DE. Skeletal muscle lipid content and insulin resistance: evidence for a paradox in endurance-trained athletes. *J Clin Endocrinol Metab* 2001;86:5755–61.

48. Dube JJ, Amati F, Stefanovic-Racic M, et al. Exercise-induced alterations in intramyocellular lipids and insulin resistance: the athlete's paradox revisited. *Am J Physiol Endocrinol Metab* 2008;294:E882–8.

49. Tushuizen ME, Bunck MC, Pouwels PJ, et al. Pancreatic fat content and beta-cell function in men with and without type 2 diabetes. *Diabetes Care* 2007;30:2916–21.

50. Pinnick KE, Collins SC, Londos C, et al. Pancreatic ectopic fat is characterized by adipocyte infiltration and altered lipid composition. *Obesity (Silver Spring)* 2008;16:522–30.

51. Schwartz MW, Woods SC, Porte D, Jr., et al. Central nervous system control of food intake. *Nature* 2000;404:661–71.

52. Schwartz MW, Boyko EJ, Kahn SE, et al. Reduced insulin secretion: an independent predictor of body weight gain. *J Clin Endocrinol Metab* 1995;80:1571–6.

Chapter 2

Lipid and lipoprotein metabolism, and risk for cardiovascular disease

Frank M. Sacks

In this chapter, I will describe the lipoproteins, vital transporters of nutrients that participate in life-providing processes of energy delivery and storage, and in cholesterol homeostasis. Lipoproteins are especially important clinically because they cause and protect against atherosclerosis and coronary heart disease (CHD), the most prevalent chronic disease cause of death globally [1]. Keeping to the theme of this book, I will link lipoprotein pathophysiology to CHD. The metabolic pathways in which lipoproteins participate are sensitive and sophisticated sensors of the nutritional and metabolic environments that, like most human biological systems, are multi-layered and redundant in most essential regulatory and effector pathways. The rewards for studying lipoproteins are insight as to how genetics and lifestyle individually and interactively perturb a highly tuned system of nutrient and cholesterol transport; how such perturbations cause atherosclerosis; and how to use this information to evaluate the action of both lifestyle and drug treatments. I also firmly believe that lipoprotein metabolism, so essential to life, has a simplicity and logic that can be conveyed to the non-expert reader, and hope that this chapter fulfills that objective.

A snapshot of lipoproteins and their metabolism

The standard clinical lipid panel used for risk assessment is composed of low-density lipoprotein cholesterol (LDL-C), triglycerides (TG), and high-density lipoprotein cholesterol (HDL-C) [2]. Plasma total cholesterol, included in the lipid panel, is used only to compute LDL cholesterol, and is less informative for risk stratification since the protective HDL-C is included. Abnormal

Metabolic Risk for Cardiovascular Disease, 1st edition. Edited by R. H. Eckel.
© 2011 American Heart Association. By Blackwell Publishing Ltd.

concentrations of the three predict cardiovascular disease (CVD) independently of one another. These three lipids are "representatives" of three principal lipoprotein systems: triglyceride-rich atherogenic lipoproteins (very-low-density lipoprotein (VLDL) in the fasting state and VLDL and chylomicrons in the fed state), cholesterol-rich atherogenic lipoproteins (LDL), and cholesterol-rich protective lipoproteins (HDL). These three lipoprotein systems, TG-rich, LDL, and HDL, are linked by metabolic processes that vary among people, and that are the subject of this chapter.

Lipoproteins are spheres that have triglycerides and cholesterol ester in the core and phospholipid, unesterified cholesterol, and proteins on the surface (Figure 2.1). The surface components are amphipathic to solubilize the very lipophilic, non-polar core lipids for their transport in the circulation. The core lipids are the biological "reason" for lipoproteins to exist. The lipoproteins are defined by their density, for example, very low density (VLDL), low-density (LDL), and high-density (HDL). In this instance, "density" is mostly related to the triglyceride and cholesterol content; the more lipids in a lipoprotein the lower its density, as measured by how readily it floats toward the top of a tube during ultracentrifugation. TG-rich lipoproteins transport an energy source, triglyceride, to muscle and adipose tissue for use and storage. TG-rich lipoproteins also contain cholesterol, and can deliver the cholesterol to peripheral tissues and the arterial wall. LDL is a transporter of primarily cholesterol from the liver to peripheral tissues. HDL also functions to transport cholesterol but in the reverse direction as VLDL and LDL, from peripheral tissues to the liver. Lipoproteins also are required to transport fat-soluble vitamins. Finally, new functions are being discovered for lipoproteins including inflammation, innate immunity, and antioxidation.

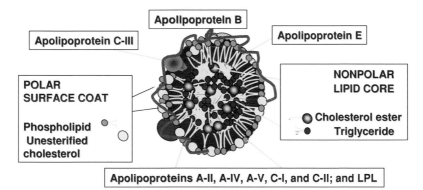

Figure 2.1 Structure of apolipoprotein B lipoproteins: chylomicrons, VLDL, and LDL. One molecule of apoB is associated with one molecule of lipoprotein particle. LpL, lipoprotein lipase.

Triglyceride-rich lipoproteins: chylomicrons and very-low-density lipoprotein

Intestinal triglyceride-rich lipoproteins

The intestine packages into lipoproteins dietary TG, cholesterol from the diet and enterohepatic circulation, and fat-soluble vitamins, and secretes them into the intestinal lymphatic circulation, giving rise to the term chylomicrons [3,4] (Figure 2.2). The intestine makes chylomicrons that have a wide range of size including very large TG-rich chylomicrons, the largest human lipoproteins, and smaller chylomicrons the size of small VLDL and LDL. The intestine also makes

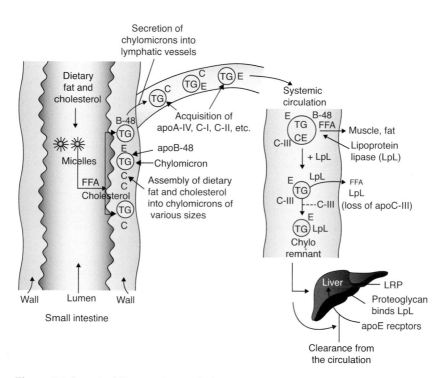

Figure 2.2 Intestinal lipoprotein metabolism. Dietary fat and cholesterol are lipolyzed by pancreatic lipase and solubilized in micelles. Monoglycerides, free fatty acids and cholesterol are transported into the intestinal cell and combined with apolipoprotein B-48 to make a chylomicron. Chylomicrons are secreted into lymphatic vessels, acquire apolipoproteins C and E, and enter the systemic circulation. Chylomicrons encounter lipoprotein lipase at the capillary endothelium of muscle and adipose tissue, releasing free fatty acids, and becoming smaller chylomicron remnants. During this process, chylomicrons lose their apoC-III, and some gain lipoprotein lipase, detach from the endothelium, and are cleared by receptors on the liver. TG = triglycerides; C = cholesterol; CE= cholesterol ester; E = apoE; C-I = apoC-I; C-II - apoC-II; C-III = apoC-III; E = apoE, FFA = free fatty acids.

HDL. The concentration of intestinal lipoproteins comprises just a small portion of the circulating lipoproteins, most of which come from the liver [5,6]. Even after a high-fat meal that stimulates chylomicron production, VLDL, made by the liver, has ten-fold higher concentration than the intestinal chylomicrons [5]. As far as we know from limited information, metabolism of intestinal lipoproteins once in plasma is governed by processes in common with metabolism of hepatic lipoproteins [6]. Although the human lipoprotein system has traditionally been divided into exogenous and endogenous lipoproteins, representing intestinal and hepatic lipoproteins, I will deal with them together as TG-rich lipoproteins (chylomicrons and VLDL), LDL (including LDL-size intestinal lipoproteins), and HDL. For convenience, I will often use the term VLDL to include the intestinal counterparts.

Clinical application: fasting vs. postprandial lipoprotein measurements
Conventionally the lipid profile is obtained in the fasting state [2]. This is to standardize metabolic conditions and reduce biological variation, in order to improve precision of risk prediction and measuring response to treatment. Fasting TG is required for the standard calculation of LDL-C discussed later. After eating, the intestine and liver secrete chylomicrons and VLDL beginning at about 1–2 hours and peaking on average at 4–5 hours. The amount of fat eaten affects the peak TG level, and carbohydrate which is usually eaten with fat stimulates the liver to secrete more VLDL [7]. There is a high correlation between fasting and postprandial TG levels. Since it is established that fasting TG predicts CHD [8], it is not surprising that postprandial TG levels, random [8,9], peak [9], or area under the TG curve [10], predict CHD.

A rather ancient but still relevant hypothesis in the lipid field is that postprandial apoB lipoproteins have some especially atherogenic property [11]. This has been difficult to prove either mechanistically or epidemiologically for human lipoproteins. In some studies people who have insulin resistance or type 2 diabetes have a delayed return of postprandial TG-rich lipoprotein levels to fasting baseline [12]. However, it has not been proven that these lipoproteins that stay in plasma are more atherogenic than those in the fasting state in the same people. A meta-analysis showed that non-fasting and fasting TG predicted CVD similarly [8]. However, in most of the component studies, non-fasting TG was measured at random rather than at a specified interval after a specified meal. One recent study of a large US male population found that non-fasting TG measured 2 to 4 hours after the last meal predicted CVD significantly better than fasting TG in the same population [9]. This could provide support for the postprandial atherogenesis theory; or it could be a marker for people who eat atherogenic diets that raise postprandial TG; or it could reflect a greater lipoprotein response to a meal rather than more atherogenic lipoproteins. People vary in their TG response to a fat-rich meal, some showing nearly no increase and others doubling or tripling. At this point one can confidently say that non-fasting TG is informative in predicting risk, as much so as fasting, but clinicians do not have guidelines for cutpoints for non-fasting TG. If the non-fasting TG is high, then just for evaluation of cutpoints a fasting TG should be obtained.

Very-low-density lipoprotein

Synthesis and secretion of apoB lipoproteins

The liver and intestine secrete TG-rich lipoproteins for the purpose of supplying muscle, adipose tissue, and other peripheral organs with energy-dense lipids. The key feature of VLDL and LDL, and their intestinal counterparts, is the presence of one molecule of apolipoprotein B, a very large protein that is required structurally for the assembly of these lipoproteins. For this reason, VLDL and LDL (and chylomicrons) are called apoB lipoproteins. ApoB is constitutively expressed in the intestine and liver. When there is a supply of TG and other lipids in the intestine or liver, apoB is lipidated in the endoplasmic reticulum, preserving it from degradation. The complex of apoB and lipid undergoes additional lipidation there and in the Golgi to form VLDL or LDL, and the lipoproteins are secreted into the circulation [3,13].

ApoB may be visualized as a belt around a spherical particle that holds a core of fat in the form of triglycerides and cholesterol ester (Figure 2.1). These hydrophobic lipids pack together in a lipoprotein like a droplet of oil. This spherical structure is how very water-insoluble molecules are efficiently packaged and transported through a hydrophilic medium, i.e., blood. The surface of the lipoprotein also has amphipathic phospholipids that are necessary to solubilize the lipoproteins, unesterified cholesterol, and other apolipoproteins that affect the metabolism and clearance from plasma of the lipoproteins. The intestine and the liver make apoB in two distinct sizes. Although both organs transcribe the full-length apoB gene, the intestinal cell has an RNA-editing enzyme that inserts a stop codon into the mRNA at approximately the halfway point. The intestinal apoB protein that is synthesized is 48% of the molecular weight of what the full-length apoB would have been, and is called apoB-48. The hepatocyte does not have this mRNA-editing enzyme and it makes the full apoB, apoB-100. Both apoB-48 and apoB-100 serve their basic structural purposes similarly, although apoB48 may confer to the chylomicron a larger potential for TG packing and a larger size [4]. The hepatic form of apoB has a critical protein sequence, beyond the halfway point, that binds to LDL receptors and is required for normal metabolism of LDL.

Some apoB lipoproteins are secreted with a small apolipoprotein, apoC-III. apoC-III secretion on VLDL is associated with the VLDL production rate, TG-rich VLDL, and hypertriglyceridemia [14,15]. Very recently it has been shown that apoC-III facilitates the accumulation of TG by a newly forming VLDL in the hepatocyte and its progression through the secretory pathway [16].

Clinical application: defects in production of TG-rich lipoproteins and therapeutic potential

Genetic defects illustrate the vital role of apoB in lipoprotein formation [17]. People who lack the essential lipidator of apoB in the intestine and liver, called MTP (microsomal triglyceride transfer protein), cannot make chylomicrons, VLDL or LDL. Heterozygotes have low concentrations of these lipoproteins and are protected against atherosclerosis. Defects in the apoB gene that make a short protein inadequate for lipoprotein formation confer the same phenotype. This is a clear demonstration of how production of VLDL and LDL strongly affects their plasma concentration. Homozygotes for defects in MTP or apoB are rare and have little if any apoB lipoproteins in circulation. Their phenotype is fat-soluble vitamin deficiency and malabsorption of dietary fat. MTP inhibitors are being tested clinically for treatment of hypercholesterolemia and hypertriglyceridemia.

Metabolism of very-low-density lipoprotein in plasma

Once secreted into the circulation, chylomicrons and VLDL soon encounter an enzyme, lipoprotein lipase, sitting on the luminal surface of capillaries [18]. Lipoprotein lipase hydrolyzes the TG that is in TG-rich lipoproteins into free fatty acids. Apolipoprotein C-II, present on some TG-rich lipoproteins, is a required cofactor for lipoprotein lipase. The fatty acids pass through the capillaries to their destinations where they are used for energy via beta oxidation such as by muscle or resynthesized into TG and stored for future use, by muscle and fat. Much depleted of TG, the lipoproteins, now called "remnants," detach from lipoprotein lipase and the vascular endothelium, and re-enter the circulation. A VLDL can probably undergo several episodes of lipolysis at different spots in the capillary circulation during its several-hour vascular sojourn. Lipolysis gradually exposes the epitope on apoB-100 on VLDL that binds to LDL receptors on hepatocytes [19]. VLDL can be cleared from the circulation at any point in the process of lipolytic metabolism [15]. A newly secreted VLDL may be removed from the circulation in an hour; or as a smaller-size VLDL after a few hours; or survive to form its terminal long-lived lipoprotein, LDL, retaining most of its cholesterol content and having lost most of its TG. It is well established that chylomicron remnants and VLDL are present in atherosclerosis [20], and this is one reason why the VLDL concentration (and its surrogate TG concentration) is associated with clinical atherosclerosis and CHD.

Clinical application: severe hypertriglyceridemia and pancreatitis

Lipoprotein lipase and apoC-II are absolutely essential to the normal metabolism of chylomicrons and VLDL and a healthy life. Without the function of these two proteins, chylomicrons and VLDL remain stuck in the circulation. TG levels rise to extremely high levels, 2000–5000 mg/dL, spurred by any fat intake. Absence or no functionality of these proteins is a rare condition, and it is not associated with atherosclerosis as far as is known. However, this is a dreadful condition causing chronic abdominal pain and potentially fatal pancreatitis [21]. Mutations that mildly impair the function of lipoprotein lipase are less rare and are associated with milder hypertriglyceridemia and CHD [22].

Lipoprotein lipase itself can serve the function of an apolipoprotein on chylomicrons and VLDL that accelerates their clearance from plasma [23]. After an encounter with lipoprotein lipase in its active homodimeric form on the endothelium, some chylomicrons and VLDL detach with the enzyme, now either in its homodimeric or monomeric form. Lipoprotein lipase assists the lipoprotein to bind to proteoglycan on hepatocytes, facilitating their removal from the circulation. This does not involve the lipolytic function and is probably an auxiliary mechanism to the high-affinity apoE when it is defective in function or low in concentration.

Apolipoprotein E and apoC-III are by far the two apolipoproteins most strongly linked to the metabolism of apoB lipoproteins, and they function as antagonists [15,24] (Figure 2.3). VLDL is secreted into the circulation in several "phenotypes," containing both apoE and C-III, just apoC-III, or neither. A

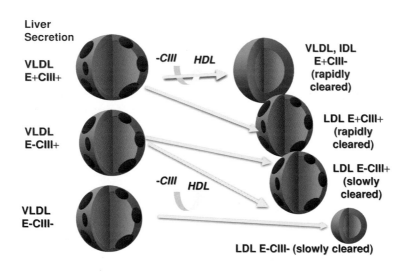

Figure 2.3 ApoE and apoC-III determine the metabolic fate of VLDL. The liver secretes a variety of types of VLDL and LDL. Those VLDL with apoE are cleared rapidly and most are not converted to LDL. Those without apoE, especially those with apoC-III, are rapidly lipolyzed to LDL.VLDL E+CIII+ = VLDL that contains both apoE and apoC-III; VLDL E-CIII+ = VLDL that does not contain apoE but does contain apoC-III; VLDL E-CIII− = VLDL that does not contain apoE or apoC-III; CIII = apoC-III; IDL = intermediate density lipoproteins.

VLDL that has apoE and apoC-III has many molecules of each. About 30–70% of VLDL particles have apoE or apoC-III, and about half of VLDL that contains apoC-III also has apoE. ApoE is a high-affinity ligand for the LDL receptor, even stronger than apoB-100, and it also binds to a secondary receptor on the liver called LRP [25]. Apoc-III impairs the clearance of VLDL from the circulation by blocking the binding of apoE and apoB-100 to these receptors. The presence of apoC-III on VLDL channels it to formation of LDL rather than to clearance from plasma [15,26]. Persistence of VLDL in the circulation is a function of the relative contents of these two metabolic antagonists. Apoc-III comes off VLDL as it is lipolyzed by lipoprotein lipase and it is picked up by HDL. This "disinhibits" the clearance mechanisms, apoE and apoB-100, for VLDL.

ApoC-III is a non-competitive inhibitor of lipoprotein lipase, functional at least in vitro at high concentrations [27]. When apoC-III is absent due to genetic defects, lipolytic conversion of VLDL to LDL is greatly accelerated [28]. However, aside from genetic deficiency of apoC-III, VLDL that has apoC-III is rapidly channeled down the lipolytic cascade of smaller particles to small dense LDL [26]. This raises the question of how important in vivo is the potential antilipolytic property of apoC-III. VLDL rich in apoC-III is lipolyzed normally by lipoprotein lipase in vitro [24]. One can speculate that apoC-III, by inhibiting the early rapid clearance of VLDL, spreads out over several hours after eating energy distribution to peripheral tissues. If there were no apoC-III, TG-rich VLDL and chylomicrons would very quickly be taken up by liver because of their apoE. In summary, the balance between apoE and apoC-III is crucial to control the metabolism of apoB lipoproteins.

Hypertriglyceridemia: metabolic disturbance linked to clinical disease

Triglyceride, as one of the tripartite members of the standard panel of lipid risk factors, is established as an independent predictor of CHD [8]. Since atherosclerosis does not feature TG loading of macrophages, and TG as a molecule has not been shown to stimulate atherogenic or inflammatory processes in vascular cells, it is fair to consider the TG level a marker for the lipoproteins that transport it, chylomicrons, chylomicron remnants, VLDL, and their smaller-size remnants (see Figure 2.4). Hypertriglyceridemia commonly occurs in conjunction with overweight or insulin resistance, and develops during adult life as these causes emerge and worsen [2]. No one mechanism has been proven to dominate to cause hypertriglyceridemia. High secretion into plasma by the liver of large TG-rich VLDL that contains apoC-III is commonly found [14,15]. High production of apoC-III by hepatocytes may be involved in the formation of TG-rich VLDL in hypertriglyceridemia [16] (see Figure 2.5). Since insulin normally decreases apoB and VLDL formation in the liver, hepatic insulin resistance may be responsible for the high production rate of VLDL in insulin-resistant patients [29]. Insulin resistance is moderately associated with TG concentrations [30]. However, a counterargument is based on the finding of similar levels of VLDL in patients with widely

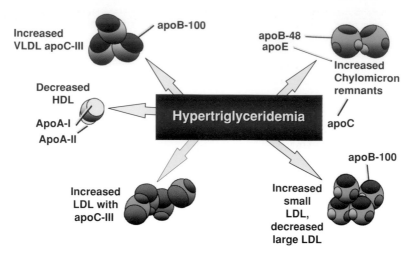

Figure 2.4 High TG – lipoprotein abnormalities. VLDL apoC-III: very low density lipoproteins that contain apolipoprotein, C-III apoB-100: apolipoprotein, B-100 apoB-48: apolipoprotein, B-48 apoE: apolipoprotein, EHDL: high density lipoproteins, ApoA-I: apolipoprotein,A-I ApoA-II: apolipoprotein, A-II LDL with apoC-III: low density lipoproteins that contain apolipoprotein, C-III ApoC: apolipoprotein C (C-I, C-II, or C-III), TG: triglyceride

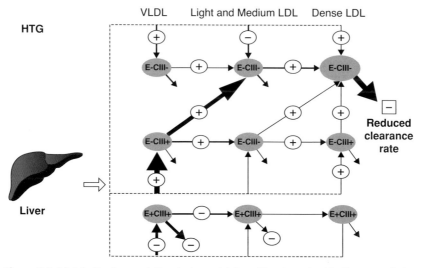

Figure 2.5 Metabolic dysregulation in hypertriglyceridemia and with dietary carbohydrate. In hypertriglyeridemia and with diets high in carbohydrate, liver secretion of VLDL shifts from apoE-containing to those with apoC-III, resulting in reduced VLDL clearance and increased convesion of VLDL to LDL. Accumulation of dense LDL is caused by increased flux from VLDL containing apoC-III, increased conversion from light and medium LDL to dense LDL, increased direct liver secretion of dense LDL with or without apoC-III, and reduced clearance of dense LDL. HTG = Hypertriglyceridemia; E-CIII−: Lipoproteins that do not contain apoE or apoC-III; E-CIII+: Lipoproteins that do not contain apoE but do contain apoC-III; E+CIII+: Lipoproteins that contain both apoE and apoC-III.

divergent insulin sensitivity, and widely different VLDL levels with a similar amount of insulin resistance [31]. Furthermore, the correlation between hyper-triglyceridemia and insulin resistance is not present in African Americans who have lower plasma TG levels and greater insulin resistance than whites [32].

A second metabolic hallmark of hypertriglyceridemia is delayed clearance of VLDL from the circulation [14,15]. ApoC-III is a strong candidate for this mechanism since it inhibits binding of apoE and apoB-100 to hepatic recep-tors and proteoglycan, and it is present in large amounts on triglyceride-rich VLDL [31]. However, in hypertriglyceridemia, clearance of all apoB lipopro-teins is diminished [15], both those with and without apoC-III, suggesting that additional mechanisms must be involved such as reduced activity of lipopro-tein lipase, hepatic lipase, or novel receptors such as GPIHBP1 (GPI-anchored HDL-binding protein 1) or proteoglycan [4]. Reduced apoE or the apoE to C-III ratio is associated with hypertriglyceridemia reflecting reduced ability of the lipoproteins to be taken up by the liver. Thus, both hyperproduction and inhib-ited clearance of VLDL are both likely involved in the most common form of hypertriglyceridemia.

Atherogenicity of TG-rich lipoproteins has been linked to their apoC-III con-tent. VLDL and LDL that have apoC-III stimulate a range of processes that are involved in atherosclerosis including activation of both monocytes and endothe-lial cells to produce adhesion molecules and proinflammatory transcription fac-tors that induce inflammatory mediators TNFa and IL1b [33,34]; activation of proinflammatory transcription factors NFkB, rhoA, and PKC [33,34]; activation of insulin resistance pathways in endothelial cells reducing their production of nitric oxide causing vascular dysfunction [35]; and increased oxidation and pro-teoglycan binding [36]. ApoC-III itself confers on VLDL these effects, although the lipids in VLDL may have additional proinflammatory effects on vascular cells.

Low-density lipoprotein, the primary lipoprotein for risk assesssment and treatment

LDL is the most prevalent atherogenic lipoprotein in the plasma of most peo-ple, reflecting the metabolic structure of the human lipoprotein system. LDL is measured clinically by its content of cholesterol with good rationale since cholesterol is its major molecular component, and cholesterol from LDL is the most prevalent lipid in atherosclerosis. LDL carries the majority of cholesterol even in populations that have very low LDL cholesterol concentrations, demon-strating that humans have an LDL-centric lipoprotein system even under ideal dietary conditions.

LDL exports cholesterol from the liver to peripheral tissues and organs. Since cells can make their own supply of cholesterol to use for membrane function-ing, there is only need for a very small amount of LDL in plasma. Healthy life protected against atherosclerosis can be sustained by plasma LDL cholesterol concentrations much lower than in most human populations (e.g., 20 to 40 mg/dL). This is demonstrated in several clinical settings: (i) by people who have defective synthesis of VLDL and LDL ("hypobetalipoproteinemia") [17]; (ii) by people who have very high levels of LDL receptors produced by a non-functional hepatic LDL receptor-degrading protein PCSK9 [37]; (iii) by the lower range of some Asian populations whose diets is very low in saturated fat and cholesterol [38]; and (iv) by strict vegetarians in the USA [39].

The biological rationale, if any, for the LDL-centric lipoprotein system of humans compared to the VLDL- or HDL-centric systems of many animals is unexplained. It may be that a low concentration of LDL is needed to deliver cholesterol to steroid-producing organs such as adrenal, gonads, and placenta, and to the fetus, perhaps especially during metabolically stressful conditions such as pregnancy when the need is much higher than usual. It is also difficult to understand the necessity for LDL when we have VLDL to transport cholesterol, except perhaps that the much shorter life of VLDL in circulation and its generally 5- to 10-fold lower concentration than LDL may produce too much fluctuation in circulating cholesterol. Long-lived LDL speculatively could have a role in maintaining an even supply of cholesterol to cells throughout the day. Some rodent species and other animals who do not ordinarily have atherosclerosis do not have much LDL, even if they are fed an atherogenic diet, and in them HDL and to a lesser extent VLDL are the main lipid transporters. Making the lipoprotein system of these animals closer to humans by overexpression of apoB-100 and inducing deficiency of LDL receptors together, or by one of these modifications plus an atherogenic diet, gives them atherosclerosis [40]. It could be that LDL is an unwelcome quirk of the physiology of humans [41]. A high LDL level reflects not only our inherent physiology but also a diet rich in saturated fat and cholesterol and the effects of aging that reduces LDL receptors, and the interaction between them.

A key metabolic feature of LDL is its long time in the circulation, 1.5 to 4 days. Its slow removal from the circulation is regulated by the number of LDL receptors, mainly on the liver. It is thought that the lengthy time in the circulation provides an LDL with many opportunities to enter the arterial wall, and a longer time in circulation is associated with higher LDL concentrations and more atherosclerosis.

LDL is often viewed as a terminal product of the metabolism of the TG-rich lipoproteins. In fact LDL is also secreted by the liver and mixes with the LDL that is formed from VLDL. The concentration of LDL is influenced by several metabolic paths as shown in Figure 2.6: (i) secretion rate of VLDL; (ii) conversion rate of VLDL to LDL; (iii) removal rate of VLDL before it becomes LDL; (iv) secretion rate of LDL; and (v) removal rate of LDL. There are several key metabolic processes that influence how much VLDL is converted into LDL and how much is removed from the circulation after partial lipolysis of its TG; these

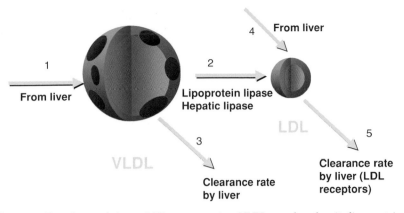

Figure 2.6 Regulators of plasma LDL concentration. VLDL: very low density lipoproteins, LDL: low density lipoproteins.

involve apoC-III, apoE and lipoprotein lipase and were described earlier. In general, in people with high TG, more of their LDL comes from VLDL, and in those with low TG, more of the LDL is directly secreted [15]. Classically, the removal rate of LDL has paramount importance to establish the LDL concentration, and it is regulated normally by the activity of LDL receptors, most prevalent in the liver [42]. Thus, competitive metabolic processes link and dissociate VLDL and LDL metabolism. This metabolic diversity is basis for the main lipoprotein phenotypes, hypertriglyceridemia (high VLDL), hypercholesterolemia (high LDL), and combined hyperlipidemia (high VLDL and LDL).

Clinical application: familial hypercholesterolemia

Familial hypercholesterolemia occurs in 1 in 500 individuals, who carry a defective allele in the LDL receptor gene that reduces the function of the receptors or prevents them from being synthesized [42]. A less common variant of familial hypercholesterolemia produces a truncated apoB that lacks the sequence that binds to the LDL receptor. Affected heterozygotes have LDL cholesterol concentrations that are well outside the normal distribution (e.g., 250–400 mg/dL), and the condition is apparent from early childhood. Heterozygous familial hypercholesterolemia requires lipid testing of all family members so that treatment can be started early in life to prevent atherosclerosis and CHD that occurs in young adulthood and middle age. Since one allele is normal, diet and drug treatments together are usually very effective in normalizing LDL by a combination of increasing LDL receptors and reducing the cholesterol burden from the diet. Homozygous familial hypercholesterolemia is still more severe and clinical CHD appears in childhood. Homozygotes are minimally responsive to diet and drug treatment and treatment requires LDL apheresis. Familial hypercholesterolemia may coexist with genes or behaviors that cause hypertriglyceridemia, resulting in combined hyperlipidemia. Familial hypercholesterolemia is not the same metabolically as the much more common "non-ideal" LDL cholesterol concentrations as defined by guidelines, which can be completely secondary to diet, or the combination of other undiscovered milder genetic variation in lipid genes.

Lipoprotein(a)

Lipoprotein(a) [Lp(a)] is an unusual apoB lipoprotein that may be viewed as an LDL that has a very large protein, apolipoprotein(a), complexed to its apoB [43,44]. Apo(a) has antithrombolytic and atherogenic properties and spends the longest time in circulation of all the apoB lipoproteins, about 4–5 days. Apo(a) has huge variation in its size resulting from size variation in a portion of the protein that has genetically determined repeating sequences. Furthermore, the smaller the Apo(a) size, the higher the Lp(a) concentration. Measurement of Lp(a) is complicated by its isoform variation that produces variability in affinity to some of the antibodies used in its measurement. Lp(a) concentration has a wide range without precedence from essentially zero to over 100 mg/dL; it is slightly higher in those with hypercholesterolemia but otherwise unrelated to concentrations of the other lipoproteins; is considered to be genetically determined; and responds minimally if at all to diet and drugs that are used to treat other lipid disorders. Lp(a), as an independent risk factor for CHD, is again unusual in that risk does not increase until after the upper half of the distribution, e.g., > 25 mg/dL, and the relative risk is modest even for levels > 150 mg/dL (relative risk 1.3) [45]. Furthermore, having a low-molecular-weight isoform of Apo(a), while moderately correlated with a high Lp(a) concentration, may have more relevance for risk than the concentration [46]. Thus, Lp(a) may be important just to a small portion of the population. Notwithstanding, I and colleagues who have lipid specialty practices have patients who have aggressive coronary atherosclerosis with no other risk factor except a very high Lp(a) concentration.

Clinical application: measuring the apoB lipoproteins

Low-density lipoprotein cholesterol
The primary lipid for risk assessment and treatment is LDL, quantified by its cholesterol concentration [2]. LDL-C is difficult to measure directly because its separation from VLDL requires exacting, time-consuming laboratory procedures and specialized equipment. The standard clinical measurement of LDL-C is an estimate determined from other lipid measurements. The calculation takes plasma total cholesterol and subtracts from it HDL cholesterol and VLDL cholesterol, yielding LDL cholesterol [2]. HDL cholesterol is measured easily since VLDL and LDL together can be removed from plasma by precipitation procedures, leaving only HDL in the supernatant. VLDL-C is then estimated by dividing the plasma total TG by 5. This calculation depends on the ratio of

plasma total TG to VLDL-C being approximately 5 universally. In most people, the resulting LDL-C estimate is quite robust since concentrations of VLDL-C are fairly low, less than 30 mg/dL. Thus mild errors in the estimate of VLDL-C will only mildly affect the LDL-C value. However, LDL-C may be seriously underestimated in hypertriglyceridemia and after eating since these conditions increase the plasma TG concentration more than VLDL-C, thereby increasing the true ratio of total TG to VLDL-C. Clinicians must be aware of the limitations of the standard LDL-C measurement.

Non-high-density lipoprotein cholesterol
The combination of VLDL cholesterol and LDL cholesterol, named "non-HDL cholesterol" [2], or perhaps better "atherogenic cholesterol," is a measurement that generally predicts CVD better than LDL-C, as would be anticipated by its including the two lipoprotein types that promote atherosclerosis and predict CVD [47]. Non-HDL cholesterol is a simple calculation of the difference between total and HDL cholesterol. Since even a large meal raises VLDL-C minimally, non-HDL cholesterol can be used in the non-fasting state, and it is valid in patients with hypertriglyceridemia. Treatment thresholds and targets for non-HDL-C are described in NCEP ATP-III [2], for use in patients with high TG, but they can be used just as well in any patient as the primary lipid target.

Apolipoprotein B
Apolipoprotein B level is the actual concentration of VLDL and LDL since each has one molecule of apoB. ApoB is an excellent predictor of CHD, generally superior to LDL-C and even to non-HDL-C [48–50]. One reason for the superiority of apoB is that, in hypertriglyceridemia, LDL contains less cholesterol than normal. ApoB counts each LDL the same whatever its cholesterol content. The rationale for measuring apoB is that the concentration of VLDL and LDL is more relevant to atherosclerosis than how much cholesterol they carry. Epidemiological studies that compared cholesterol with apoB usually support this concept [50]. ApoB is a straightforward immunochemical measurement in total plasma, requiring no computation from other measurements. ApoB is not affected acutely by diet and it can quantify risk in hypertriglyceridemia. The current limitation for apoB is the lack of a national standardization program for accuracy and consistency over time. However, this is surmountable as it was for the lipid risk factors, and apoB eventually could be used as a primary target.

There are several sophisticated methods that measure many types of VLDL, LDL, and HDL according to their size. Density gradient ultracentrifugation using a vertical rotor system directly measures the cholesterol concentration of the lipoprotein subtypes [51] from which estimates are made of lipoprotein concentrations. Nuclear magnetic resonance uses the lipid content of the lipoproteins to estimate concentration of the subtypes, and then applies a proprietary algorithm to compute the concentration of LDL, known as the LDL particle number

[52]. Clinicians must be aware that these measurements are only estimates of apoB or lipoprotein particle concentrations. Nuclear magnetic resonance measurements predicted CHD similarly but not superiorly to the standard lipid risk factors [53,54].

Low-density lipoprotein size and density
Like all lipoprotein classes, LDL exists in a range of sizes related to the core lipid content of TG and cholesterol ester. People with high plasma total TG tend to have smaller LDL (and larger VLDL) whereas those with hypercholesterolemia tend to have larger LDL (and smaller VLDL) [55,56]. Few people have "pure" large or small LDL, but differ in the size distribution. It has been hypothesized that small LDL is more atherogenic than large or medium size LDL [57]. However, the universality of LDL-C as a predictor of CHD across all population groups [2], and the similarity of effects of LDL-lowering treatments in them [58,59], argue for all types of LDL to be atherogenic. LDL-C predicts CHD in those who have low TG, who are not overweight, do not have type 2 diabetes, and in women, groups that have large size LDL; and LDL-C predicts CHD in the opposite type of patients, e.g., men and type 2 diabetics who tend to have small LDL. As LDL-C increases in the population, size of LDL tends to increase. Thus, the cholesterol theory of CHD is founded on the assumption that large cholesterol-rich LDL causes CHD. That patients with hypercholesterolemia have large LDL and high incidence of CHD is *prima facie* evidence for the atherogenicity of large LDL. Indeed, prospective studies demonstrate that large LDL predicts atherosclerosis and CHD [55,60,61]. Furthermore, statins reduce the concentration of all sizes of LDL, and their benefits to CHD are universal across population groups that have large or small LDL [58]. Finally, across a wide range of populations, neither LDL size nor the concentration of small dense LDL adds to CHD prediction in multiple variable analysis beyond the standard lipid risk factors [53–55]. A preponderance of small LDL may simply be a marker for atherogenic VLDL and its remnants.

High-density lipoprotein, the protective lipoprotein

HDL, the smallest lipoprotein, is uniquely established to transport cholesterol, mainly from peripheral tissues such as the arterial vasculature to the liver (Figure 2.7) [62,63]. Most of the plasma HDL has been secreted by the liver. The liver secretes HDL into plasma in its most primitive form, a combination of two molecules of an essential protein, apolipoprotein A-I, phospholipid, and a meager amount of unesterified cholesterol. A small percentage, perhaps 20%, is secreted by the intestine, and may be a cholesterol absorption mechanism in addition to that provided by chylomicrons [4]. Nascent HDL is shaped like a disk because its lacks hydrophobic lipids such as cholesterol ester and triglyceride that form the core of lipoproteins. HDL then goes into action in the circulation, stimulating the efflux of cholesterol from cells such as macrophages in the

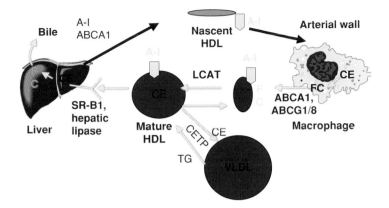

Figure 2.7 HDL metabolism and reverse cholesterol transport. ApoA-I, ApoA-I; ABCA, ABCA1; ABCG, ABCG1/4; CE, cholesterol ester; CEPT, cholesterol ester transport protein; FC, free cholesterol; LCAT, lecithin cholesterol acyl transferase; SR-B1, scavenger receptor B1; TG, triglyceride. The liver secretes ApoA-I combined with phospholipid. At the liver cell surface, cholesterol is added by the transporter ABCA1. The nascent discoidal HDL takes up cholesterol from macrophages and other peripheral cells by the action of ABCA1. LCAT esterifies the cholesterol which forms a core of cholesterol ester, changing the shape to a sphere. The small spherical HDL takes up additional cholesterol from peripheral cells by the action of ABCG1/4. HDL transfers its cholesterol ester to VLDL by the action of CEPT, transfers it to the liver by the action of SR-B1 and hepatic lipase, and becomes smaller. HDL then may re-enter the circulation to engage in another cycle of cholesterol uptake. This process is known as reverse cholesterol transport.

vascular wall (Figure 2.7). ApoA-I mobilizes cellular cholesterol by activating the hydrolysis of cholesterol ester stored in lipid-rich vesicles in macrophages. The unesterified cholesterol is transported to the cell surface and to HDL by a transport protein ABCA1. Once in the HDL, much of the cholesterol is re-esterified to cholesterol ester by the enzyme, lecithin cholesterol acyl transferase, coalesces in the hydrophobic interior of the HDL, creating a spherical form. Spherical HDL enlarges further by similar processes. At any time, HDL exists in plasma in many sizes ranging from a small disk, a small sphere, a plump sphere, and even an obese sphere the size of small LDL. The metabolic point of this process is to present excess cellular cholesterol to the liver for secretion into bile. Since humans cannot catabolize the cholesterol molecule, the body's cholesterol content can be reduced only by fecal excretion.

Cholesterol in HDL does not necessarily end up in bile. The liver may recycle it into making new VLDL and LDL. Circulating HDL may transfer its cholesterol ester to circulating VLDL, receiving a triglyceride molecule in return, by the action of cholesterol ester transfer protein (CETP). The clinical implications of this CETP-mediated process are arguably the strongest controversy in the lipid field [64,65]. Surely, a metabolic pathway that returns HDL cholesterol ester to the liver should be superior to one that transfers it to atherogenic apoB lipoproteins; and intuitively CETP is a logical target for pharmacological inhibition. The fundamental unanswered question is whether CETP is a necessary part of the reverse cholesterol pathway. That is, whether cholesterol transport out of HDL directly to the liver can be made to be a major route for cholesterol flux or whether HDL cholesterol normally goes first to apoB lipoproteins and with them to the liver. That CETP is active in humans is proven by people with genetic variants in the promotor of CETP gene that lowers its activity, producing higher HDL cholesterol and lower LDL cholesterol [66]; and by pharmacological inhibitors of CETP that do the same [64,65]. The first inhibitor of CETP was discontinued because it increased CVD, a toxic effect that may or may not have been related to CETP inhibition; and others are currently in clinical development.

High-density lipoprotein: function and dysfunction

The problem of understanding the implications of CETP inhibition may be generalized to any treatment that affects HDL concentration. Although many individual molecular mechanisms involving HDL cholesterol are known from basic science, it is unknown which are the major ones in humans and how they fit together into a metabolic pathway for reverse cholesterol transport. On the one hand, we can confidently state that the involvement of HDL in mobilizing cellular cholesterol and delivering it to the liver, a process called reverse cholesterol transport, is essential for normal cholesterol homeostasis and necessary to prevent the development of atherosclerosis. But on the other hand, we do not have a way to evaluate how diet and drug interventions affect the critical function of HDL in reverse cholesterol transport. Thus, we are left with the imperfect surrogate marker, HDL concentration.

Current views on HDL include the idea of dysfunctionality [67,68]. This can be framed as dysfunctional metabolism or dysfunctional HDL particles. An example of dysfunctional metabolism is the hypercatabolism of HDL as shown by a rapid rate of clearance of ApoA-I from the circulation, and reduced concentration of the mature large spherical HDL. Both are present in patients with low HDL concentrations who have hypertriglyceridemia, obesity, insulin resistance, or type 2 diabetes [69,70].

HDL has actions other than reverse cholesterol transport. HDL has anti-inflammatory actions related to its content of antioxidant enzymes such as paroxonase, and carries prooxidant enzymes such as phospholipases [67,68,71]. This raises the concept of "proinflammatory HDL," supported by experiments in cell culture associating it with coronary atherosclerosis, and a high plasma level of HDL-associated phospholipase. Apolipoprotein C-III exists in HDL and may reduce its protective action to inhibit adhesion of monocytes to endothelial cells [34]. ApoC-III in HDL is not a protective marker for CHD, unlike ApoA-I, its principal protein; in fact, HDL apoC-III is associated with increased CHD [72,73].

Clinical application: causes of low high-density lipoprotein cholesterol
Low HDL concentrations, measured either by its cholesterol or ApoA-I concentration, are associated with many of the same conditions that cause high TG, overweight, insulin resistance, type 2 diabetes, sedentary habits, and high carbohydrate diets. The association between low HDL and high TG is only moderate with correlation coefficients 0.6, as fitting to the complexity of metabolism of both TG-rich lipoproteins and HDL [72]. Metabolism of TG-rich lipoproteins is directly linked to HDL formation and enlargement. Lipid and protein components of chylomicrons and VLDL detach during lipolysis and form small HDL particles or attach to pre-existing HDL. Thus, impaired metabolism of TG-rich lipoproteins is associated with low HDL concentration.

Some agents affect HDL and TG in the same direction. Drinking alcoholic beverages and postmenopausal estrogen treatment raise HDL and TG. Testosterone lowers HDL and TG. Since we do not have a way as yet to evaluate the function of HDL in reverse cholesterol transport, we cannot be confident that these or any changes in HDL concentration affect atherosclerosis in the direction expected from the relation of HDL concentrations and CHD risk [59,65]. There is also no clear relation between genetic variants in enzymes or transporters in HDL metabolism that cause either very low or high HDL cholesterol concentrations and CHD [74].

Atherogenic dyslipidemia and residual risk for coronary heart disease

The LDL theory of CHD is firmly established from basic science, metabolism, genetics, epidemiology, and response to treatments. Appropriately, LDL remains the cornerstone of lipid treatment to reduce CHD [2]. CHD persists even with maximal LDL-lowering treatment by statins, albeit at a reduced rate [58]. High TG and low HDL-C are two of the causes of this "residual risk," and themselves are caused by overweight, diet, lack of exercise, and type 2 diabetes, increasing in prevalence worldwide [75]. They are the two lipid components of the metabolic syndrome (Table 2.1). Atherogenic dyslipidemia is a term that refers to the abnormal lipid metabolism in these conditions. The term is useful to distinguish it from high LDL that is under different metabolic and environmental control. Although there are many lipid abnormalities associated with high TG and low HDL-C (Figure 2.4, Table 2.1) discussed in this chapter, high TG and low HDL-C suffice to quantify the lipid risk in atherogenic dyslipidemia. For this reason, I advocate a simple definition for atherogenic dyslipidemia that includes only TG and HDL-C, and risk assessment and treatment based on

Table 2.1 Dyslipidemia associated with type 2 diabetes and the metabolic syndrome

Major independent CVD risk factors
- ↓ in HDL cholesterol level
- ↓ in apolipoprotein A-I
- ↑ in TG, and TG-rich lipoprotein
- ↑ in non-HDL cholesterol
- ↑ in apolipoprotein B

Other independent risk factors
- ↑ in postprandial TG
- ↑ in LDL particle numbers (measured by NMR)
- ↑ in apolipoprotein CIII

Other lipoprotein manifestations
- Small, dense LDL
- Small HDL (discoidal [prebeta-1] and small spherical [alpha-3])

NMR, nuclear magnetic resonance.

them and LDL-C, as described in national guidelines. An apolipoprotein-based system that uses apoB and ApoA-I is an alternative that needs comprehensive evaluation, for example, to determine if they capture fully the risk associated with TG-rich lipoproteins. The increasing worldwide prevalence of metabolic syndrome, type 2 diabetes, and its lifestyle causes is a disturbing development that gives important clinical meaning to the dysmetabolic processes of atherogenic dyslipidemia.

References

1. Ezzati J, Vander Hoorn S, Lopez AD, et al. Comparative quantification of mortality and burden of disease attributable to selected risk factors. In: Lopez AD, Mathers CD, Ezzati M, Jamison DT, Murray CJ (eds) *Global Burden of Disease and Risk Factors*. Oxford University Press, New York. 2006; pp. 241–68.
2. National Cholesterol Education Program (NCEP) Expert Panel on Detection, Evaluation, and Treatment of High Blood Cholesterol in Adults (Adult Treatment Panel III). Third Report of the National Cholesterol Education Program (NCEP) Expert Panel on Detection, Evaluation, and Treatment of High Blood Cholesterol in Adults (Adult Treatment Panel III). Final report. *Circulation* 2002;106:3143–421.
3. Iqbal J, Hussain MM. Intestinal lipid absorption. *Am J Physiol Endocrinol Metab* 2009;296:E1183–94.
4. Williams KJ. Molecular processes that handle – and mishandle – dietary lipids. *J Clin Invest* 2008:118:3247–59.
5. Campos H, Khoo C, Sacks FM. Diurnal and acute patterns of postprandial apolipoprotein B-48 in VLDL, IDL, and LDL from normolipidemic humans. *Atherosclerosis* 2005;181:345–51.

6. Zheng CY, Ikewaki K, Walsh BW, Sacks FM. Metabolism of apoB lipoproteins of intestinal and hepatic origin during constant feeding of small amounts of fat. *J Lipid Res* 2006;47:1171–9.

7. Parks EJ, Skokan LE, Timlin MT, Dingfelder CS. Dietary sugars stimulate fatty acid synthesis in adults. *J Nutr* 2008;138:1039–46.

8. Sarwar N, Danesh J, Eiriksdottir G, et al. Triglycerides and risk of coronary heart disease: 10,158 incident cases among 262,525 participants in 29 western prospective studies. *Circulation* 2007;115:450–8.

9. Bansal S, Buring JE, Rifai N, Mora S, Sacks FM, Ridker PM. Fasting compared with nonfasting triglycerides and risk of cardiovascular events in women. *JAMA* 2007;298:309–16.

10. Patsch J, Miesenböck G, Hopferwieser T, et al. Relation of triacylglycerol metabolism and coronary artery disease. *Arterioscler Thromb* 1992;12:1336–45.

11. Zilversmit DB. Atherogenic nature of triacylglycerols, postprandial lipidemia, and triacylglycerol-rich remnant lipoproteins. *Clin Chem* 1995;41:153–8.

12. Chen YD, Swami S, Skowronski R, Coulston AM, Reaven G. Effect of variations in dietary fat and carbohydrate intake on postprandial lipemia in patients with noninsulin dependent diabetes mellitus. *J Clin Endocrinol Metab* 1993;76:347–51.

13. Ginsberg HN, Fisher EA. The ever-expanding role of degradation in the regulation of apolipoprotein B metabolism. *J Lipid Res* 2009;50(Suppl):S162–6.

14. Ooi EM, Barrett PH, Chan DC, Watts GF. Apolipoprotein C-III: understanding an emerging cardiovascular risk factor. *Clin Sci* 2008;114:611–24.

15. Zheng C, Furtado J, Khoo C, Sacks FM. Apolipoprotein C-III and the metabolic basis for hypertriglyceridemia and the dense LDL phenotype. *Circulation* 2010;121: 1722–34.

16. Sundaram M, Zhong S, Khalil MB, et al. Expression of apolipoprotein C-III in McA-RH7777 cells enhances VLDL assembly and secretion under lipid-rich conditions. *J Lipid Res* 2010;51:150–61.

17. Tarugi P, Averna M, Di Leo E, et al. Molecular diagnosis of hypobetalipoproteinemia: an ENID review. *Atherosclerosis* 2007;195:e19–327.

18. Wang H, Eckel RH. Lipoprotein lipase: from gene to obesity. *Am J Physiol Endocrinol Metab* 2009;297:E271–88.

19. Bradley WA, Gotto AM Jr, Gianturco SH. Expression of LDL receptor binding determinants in very low density lipoproteins. *Ann N Y Acad Sci* 1985;454:239 47.

20. Rapp JH, Lespine A, Hamilton RL, et al. Triglyceride-rich lipoproteins isolated by selective-affinity anti-apolipoprotein B immunosorption from human atherosclerotic plaque. *Arterioscler Thromb Vasc Biol* 1994;14:1767–74.

21. Brunzell JD, Deeb SS. Familial lipoprotein lipase deficiency, apo C-II deficiency, and hepatic lipase deficiency. In: Scriver CR, Beaudet AL, Sly WS, Valle D (eds) *The Metabolic and Molecular Bases of Inherited Disease*. McGraw-Hill, New York. 2001; pp. 2789–816.

22. Rahalkar AR, Giffen F, Har B, et al. Novel LPL mutations associated with lipoprotein lipase deficiency: two case reports and a literature review. *Can J Physiol Pharmacol* 2009;87:151–60.

23. Zheng C, Murdoch SJ, Brunzell JD, Sacks FM. Lipoprotein lipase bound to apolipoprotein B lipoproteins accelerates clearance of postprandial lipoproteins in humans. *Arterioscler Thromb Vasc Biol* 2006;26:891–6.

24. de Silva HV, Lauer SJ, Wang J, et al. Overexpression of human apolipoprotein C-III in transgenic mice results in an accumulation of apolipoprotein B48 remnants that is corrected by excess apolipoprotein E. *J Biol Chem* 1994;269:2324–35.

25. Mahley RW, Weisgraber KH, Huang Y. Apolipoprotein E: structure determines function, from atherosclerosis to Alzheimer's disease to AIDS. *J Lipid Res* 2009;50(Suppl):S183–8.

26. Mendivil CO, Furtado J, Lel J, Sacks FM. Metabolism of very-low-density lipoprotein and low-density lipoprotein containing apolipoprotein C-III and not other small apolipoproteins. *Arterioscler Thromb Vasc Biol* 2010;30:239–45.

27. Wang CS, Hartsuck J, McConathy WJ. Structure and functional properties of lipoprotein lipase. *Biochim Biophys Acta* 1992;1123:1–17.

28. Ginsberg HN, Le NA, Goldberg IJ, et al. Apolipoprotein B metabolism in subjects with deficiency of apolipoproteins CIII and AI: evidence that apolipoprotein CIII inhibits catabolism of triglyceride-rich lipoproteins by lipoprotein lipase in vivo. *J Clin Invest* 1986;78:1287–95.

29. Kamagate A, Dong HH. FoxO1 integrates insulin signaling to VLDL production. *Cell Cycle* 2008;7:3162–70.

30. McLaughlin T, Abbasi F, Cheal K, Chu J, Lamendola C, Reaven GM. Use of metabolic markers to identify overweight individuals who are insulin resistant. *Ann Intern Med* 2003;139:802–9.

31. Lee SJ, Moye LA, Campos H, Williams GH. Sacks FM. Hypertriglyceridemia but not diabetes status is associated with VLDL containing apolipoprotein CIII in patients with coronary heart disease. *Atherosclerosis* 2003;167:293–302.

32. Sumner AE, Finley KB, Genovese DJ, Criqui MH, Boston RC. Fasting triglyceride and the triglyceride-HDL cholesterol ratio are not markers of insulin resistance in African Americans. *Arch Intern Med* 2005;165:1395–400.

33. Kawakami A, Aikawa M, Alcaide P, Luscinskas FW, Libby P, Sacks FM. Apolipoprotein CIII induces expression of vascular cell adhesion molecule-1 in vascular endothelial cells and increases adhesion of monocytic cells. *Circulation* 2006;114:681–7.

34. Kawakami A, Aikawa M, Libby P, Alcaide P, Luscinskas FW, Sacks FM. Apolipoprotein CIII in apolipoprotein B lipoproteins enhances the adhesion of human monocytic cells to endothelial cells. *Circulation* 2006;113:691–700.

35. Kawakami A, Osaka M, Tani M, et al. Apolipoprotein CIII links hyperlipidemia with vascular endothelial function. *Circulation* 2008;118:731–42.

36. Hiukka A, Stahlman M, Pettersson C, et al. ApoCIII-Enriched LDL in type 2 diabetes displays altered lipid composition, increased susceptibility for sphingomyelinase, and increased binding to biglycan. *Diabetes* 2009;58:2018–26.

37. Abifadel M, Rabès JP, Devillers M, et al. Mutations and polymorphisms in the proprotein convertase subtilisin kexin 9 (PCSK9) gene in cholesterol metabolism and disease. *Hum Mutat* 2009;30:520–9.

38. Keys A. *Seven Countries*. Harvard University Press. 1980.

39. Sacks FM, Castelli WP, Donner A, Kass EH. Plasma lipids and lipoproteins in vegetarians and controls. *New Engl J Med* 1975;292:1148–51.

40. Sanan DA, Newland DL, Tao R, et al. Low density lipoprotein receptor-negative mice expressing human apolipoprotein B-100 develop complex atherosclerotic lesions on a chow diet: no accentuation by apolipoprotein (a). *Proc Natl Acad Sci USA* 1998;95:4544–9.

41. Babin PJ, Gibbons GF. The evolution of plasma cholesterol: direct utility of a "spandrel" of hepatic lipid metabolism. *Prog Lipid Res* 2009;48:73–91.

42. Goldstein JL, Brown MS. The LDL receptor. *Arterioscler Thromb Vasc Biol* 2009;29:431–8.

43. Hobbs HH, White AL. Lipoprotein(a): intrigues and insights. *Curr Opin Lipidol* 1999;10:225–36.

44. Anuurad E, Boffa MB, Koschinsky ML, Berglund L. Lipoprotein(a): a unique risk factor for cardiovascular disease. *Clin Lab Med* 2006;26:751–72.

45. Emerging Risk Factors Collaboration, Erqou S, Kaptoge S, Perry PL, et al. Lipoprotein(a) concentration and the risk of coronary heart disease, stroke, and nonvascular mortality. *JAMA* 2009;302(4):412–23.

46. Rifai N, Ma J, Sacks FM, et al. Apolipoprotein(a) size and lipoprotein(a) concentration and future risk of angina pectoris with evidence of severe coronary atherosclerosis in men: the Physicians' Health Study. *Clin Chem* 2004;50:1364–71.

47. Miller M, Ginsberg HN, Schaefer EJ. Relative atherogenicity and predictive value of non-high-density lipoprotein cholesterol for coronary heart disease. *Am J Cardiol* 2008;101:1003–8.

48. Thompson A, Danesh J. Associations between apolipoprotein B, apolipoprotein AI, the apolipoprotein B/AI ratio and coronary heart disease: a literature-based meta-analysis of prospective studies. *J Intern Med* 2006;259(5):481–92.

49. Pischon T, Girman CJ, Sacks FM, Rifai N, Stampfer MJ, Rimm EB. Non-high-density lipoprotein cholesterol and apolipoprotein B in the prediction of coronary heart disease in men. *Circulation* 2005;112:3375–83.

50. Sniderman A, Williams K, Cobbaert C. ApoB versus non-HDL-C: what to do when they disagree. *Curr Atheroscler Rep* 2009;11:358–63.

51. Kulkarni KR, Garber DW, Marcovina SM, Segrest JP. Quantification of cholesterol in all lipoprotein classes by the VAP-II method. *J Lipid Res* 1994;35:159–68.

52. Jeyarajah EJ, Cromwell WC, Otvos JD. Lipoprotein particle analysis by nuclear magnetic resonance spectroscopy. *Clin Lab Med* 2006;26:847–70.

53. Mora S, Otvos JD, Rifai N, Rosenson RS, Buring JE, Ridker PM. Lipoprotein particle profiles by nuclear magnetic resonance compared with standard lipids and apolipoproteins in predicting incident cardiovascular disease in women. *Circulation* 2009;119:931–9.

54. Ip S, Lichtenstein AH, Chung M, Lau J, Balk EM. Systematic review: association of low-density lipoprotein subfractions with cardiovascular outcomes. *Ann Intern Med* 2009;150:474–84.

55. Sacks FM, Campos H. Low density lipoprotein and cardiovascular disease: a reappraisal. (Clinical Review 163). *J Clin Endocrinol Metab* 2003;88:4525–32.

56. Mora S. Advanced lipoprotein testing and subfractionation are not (yet) ready for routine clinical use. *Circulation* 2009;119:2396–404.

57. Musliner TA, Krauss RM. Lipoprotein subspecies and risk of coronary disease. *Clin Chem* 1988;34(8B):B78–83.

58. Cholesterol Treatment Trialists' (CTT) Collaborators. Efficacy and safety of cholesterol-lowering treatment: prospective meta-analysis of data from 90 056 participants in 14 randomised trials of statins. *Lancet* 2005;366:1267–78.

59. Briel M, Ferreira-Gonzalez I, You JJ, et al. Association between change in high density lipoprotein cholesterol and cardiovascular disease morbidity and mortality: systematic review and meta-regression analysis. *BMJ* 2009;338:b92.

60. Campos H, Moye LA, Glasser SP, Stampfer MJ, Sacks FM. Low density lipoprotein size, pravastatin treatment, and coronary events. *JAMA* 2001;286:1468–74.
61. Mora S, Szklo M, Otvos JD, et al. LDL particle subclasses, LDL particle size, and carotid atherosclerosis in the Multi-Ethnic Study of Atherosclerosis (MESA). *Atherosclerosis* 2007;192:211–17.
62. Tall AR. Cholesterol efflux pathways and other potential mechanisms involved in the athero-protective effect of high density lipoproteins. *J Intern Med* 2008;263:256–73.
63. deGoma EM, deGoma RL, Rader DJ. Beyond high-density lipoprotein cholesterol levels evaluating high-density lipoprotein function as influenced by novel therapeutic approaches. *J Am Coll Cardiol* 2008;51:2199–211.
64. Chapman MJ, Le Goff W, Guerin M, Kontush A. Cholesteryl ester transfer protein: at the heart of the action of lipid-modulating therapy with statins, fibrates, niacin, and cholesteryl ester transfer protein inhibitors. *Eur Heart J* 2010;31:149–64.
65. Joy T, Hegele RA. The end of the road for CETP inhibitors after torcetrapib? *Curr Opin Cardiol* 2009;24:364–71.
66. Boekholdt SM, Sacks FM, Jukema JW, et al. Cholesteryl ester transfer protein TaqIB variant, high-density lipoprotein cholesterol levels, cardiovascular risk, and efficacy of pravastatin treatment: individual patient meta-analysis of 13,677 subjects. *Circulation* 2005;111:278–87.
67. Barter PJ, Puranik R, Rye KA. New insights into the role of HDL as an anti-inflammatory agent in the prevention of cardiovascular disease. *Curr Cardiol Rep* 2007;9:493–8.
68. Navab M, Anantharamaiah GM, Reddy ST, Van Lenten BJ, Fogelman AM. HDL as a biomarker, potential therapeutic target, and therapy. *Diabetes* 2009;58:2711–17.
69. Brinton EA, Eisenberg S, Breslow JL. Human HDL cholesterol levels are determined by apoA-I fractional catabolic rate, which correlates inversely with estimates of HDL particle size. *Arterioscler Thromb* 1994;14:707–20.
70. Gylling H, Vega GL, Grundy SM. Physiologic mechanisms for reduced apolipoprotein A-I concentrations associated with low HDL cholesterol in patients with normal plasma lipids. *J Lipid Res* 1992;33:1527–39.
71. Nicholls SJ, Hazen SL. Myeloperoxidase, modified lipoproteins, and atherogenesis. *J Lipid Res* 2009;50:S346–51.
72. Sacks FM, Alaupovic P, Moye LA, et al. Very low density lipoproteins, apolipoproteins B, C-III, and E and risk of recurrent coronary events in the Cholesterol and Recurrent Events (CARE) Trial. *Circulation* 2000;102:1886–92.
73. Onat A, Hergenç G, Sansoy V, et al. Apolipoprotein C-III, a strong discriminant of coronary risk in men and a determinant of the metabolic syndrome in both genders. *Atherosclerosis* 2003;168:81–9.
74. Rader DJ. Lecithin: cholesterol acyltransferase and atherosclerosis: another high-density lipoprotein story that doesn't quite follow the script. *Circulation* 2009;120:549–52.
75. Fruchart JC, Sacks F, Hermans MP, et al. The Residual Risk Reduction Initiative: a call to action to reduce residual vascular risk in patients with dyslipidemia. *Am J Cardiol* 2008;102(10 Suppl):1–34K.

Chapter 3

Tobacco and risk for cardiovascular disease

C. Barr Taylor and Mickey Trockel

The 2004 Surgeon General's report, the first report on the overall health consequences of smoking since the initial report 40 years previously, concludes that smoking causes subclinical atherosclerosis, coronary heart disease (CHD), stroke, and abdominal aortic aneurysm [1]. Use of tobacco remains the most preventable cause of death. In 2005, an estimated 21% of adults in the USA were smoking or using other forms of tobacco. This means that an estimated 45 million US citizens continue to use tobacco. The report estimated that tobacco use causes 88 000 deaths from cardiovascular disease (CVD) in males and 55 000 deaths from CVD in females each year in the USA. In this chapter we review mechanisms about how tobacco use may increase risk for CVD, and also look at associations among smoking and metabolic risk factors. We conclude with a discussion of the implications of some of these findings for intervention.

Smoking and ischemic heart disease

The 2004 Surgeon General's report summarized new data, since the previous comparable report in 1990, supporting a causal association between smoking and myocardial infarction (MI). Across various racial and ethnic groups smoking has been identified as a strong risk factor for MI in women younger than 50 years of age [2,3], even though the incidence of MI is very low in this population. Risk for CHD in women increases with number of cigarettes smoked [4]. Some authors have found an apparently paradoxical benefit of smoking in in-hospital mortality [5], a difference not totally accounted for by baseline risk profile [6]. However, a recent meta-analysis found that the combined odds ratio (OR) in

Metabolic Risk for Cardiovascular Disease, 1st edition. Edited by R. H. Eckel.
© 2011 American Heart Association. By Blackwell Publishing Ltd.

former smokers compared with current smokers was 0.54 (95% CI, 0.46–0.62) [7]. A subsequent Cochrane Review demonstrated similar pooled results [8].

Many studies have demonstrated potential pathways and mechanisms for how cigarette smoking causes cardiovascular dysfunction and atherosclerosis. These are summarized in Figure 3.1.

Smoking, atherogenesis, and thrombosis

Atherosclerosis is the most common cause of clinically important CVD. Atherosclerosis is a complex process involving interactions of the blood (serum and blood cells) with the arterial walls and within the arterial wall itself. Smoking and the products of smoking in the bloodstream affect many of these physiological processes [9]. The effects of smoking on biological mechanisms leading to atherogenesis and thrombosis were reviewed in detail in the Surgeon General's report [1]. The main findings are summarized below.

Smoking and endothelial injury or endothelial dysfunction

Endothelial dysfunction is associated with an increased adhesion of circulating monocytes and T-lymphocytes to the endothelium as well as with their subsequent migration into the intimal layer of the arterial wall. These cells, in the presence of modified low-density lipoprotein (LDL) cholesterol (e.g., oxidized LDL cholesterol), become foam cells and accumulate in the intima, a key element in the early phases of atherogenesis. In recent years, more subtle functional changes in the endothelium have been associated with smoking [10]. Smoking may also promote other risk factors to increase endothelial dysfunction. For instance, smoking increases hypercholesterolemia [11].

Compared with non-smokers, smokers released smaller amounts of tissue plasminogen activator (TPA) when stimulated by substance P, which suggests tobacco use may contribute to thrombosis by increasing endothelial cell dysfunction [12,13].

Smoking and thrombosis/fibrinolysis

Smoking increases thrombosis, which in the context of atherosclerosis may be a main underlying factor causing acute MI and sudden death [14]. Smoking increases thrombosis in part through effects on endothelium but also by increasing platelet activation and platelet adhesion [15,16]. Smoking has an immediate deleterious effect by increasing platelet thrombus formation [17]. Evidence also strongly suggests that smoking has synergistic effects with other medications (e.g., oral contraceptives) to increase thrombosis [18,19]. In addition, smoking increases plasma fibrinogen, an independent cardiovascular risk factor [20].

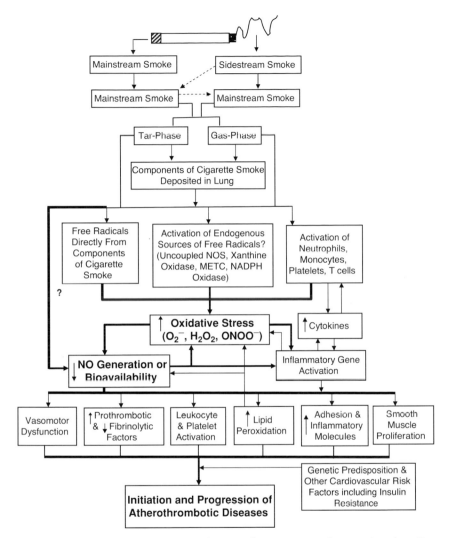

Figure 3.1 Potential pathways and mechanisms for cigarette smoking-mediated cardiovascular dysfunction. The bold boxes and arrows in the flow diagram represent the probable central mechanisms in the complex pathophysiology of cigarette-smoking-mediated atherothrombotic disease. H_2O_2 hydrogen peroxide; METC mitochondial electron transport chain; NADPH nicotinamide adenine dinucleotide phosphate reduced form; NO nitric oxide; NOS nitric oxide synthase; $ONOO^-$ peroxinitrite; O_2^- superoxide. (Reproduced from Ambrose and Barua, *J Am Coll Cardiol* 2004;43:1731–7, with permission from Elsevier.)

Smoking and inflammation

Inflammation plays a central role in atherosclerosis [21] and smoking induces a systemic inflammatory response [22,23]. For instance, smoking increases leukocyte counts, and higher counts are associated with increased CHD, stroke, and sudden death [20]. Smoking is also associated with an elevation of the C-reactive protein level [24] which has been associated with risks for CHD, stroke, and peripheral arterial disease.

Smoking, lipids, and lipid metabolism

Smoking is associated with higher concentrations of total, LDL and very low density lipoprotein (VLDL) cholesterol. The most consistent evidence indicates that smoking decreases levels of high-density lipoprotein (HDL) cholesterol in smokers compared with non-smokers [1]. Smoking may also seriously affect lipid metabolism and LDL modification, which has implications for metabolic syndrome. Smokers have higher levels of serum malondialdehyde [25], which may modify LDL cholesterol to promote uptake by macrophages and decrease cholesterol transport from cell membranes to plasma. Malondialdehyde may be a marker of oxidation, and evidence indicates that smoking may promote lipid peroxidation, which is hypothesized to be one key element in the causal pathway of atherogenesis [26]. In laboratory studies, cigarette smoke stimulated the generation of oxidized LDL cholesterol in human plasma [27].

Smoking and cardiovascular function

Even though there is no evidence that smoking is associated with chronic hypertension, there is evidence that smoking acutely increases peripheral vascular resistance and increases blood pressure [28,29]. In carefully controlled experiments in healthy humans, cigarette smoking increased blood pressure and sympathetic nervous system stimulation of both the blood vessels and the heart [30]. Acute and episodic increases in blood pressure, coupled with an increased heart rate, increase oxygen demands of the myocardium. However, in population studies, cigarette smokers tend to have, on average, lower blood pressures than do non-smokers [31].

Smoking, decreased oxygen supply, and increased blood rheology

Smoking has a negative impact on coronary blood flow by causing an immediate constriction of both proximal and distal coronary arteries as well as an increase in coronary vessel tone and hence resistance [32]. Smoking also compromises the oxygen supply to the myocardium by raising levels of carbon monoxide, which binds to the hemoglobin in erythrocytes to form carboxyhemoglobin, which has a diminished oxygen-carrying capacity.

As described in the Surgeon General's report [1], the net result of all of these mechanisms (reduced oxygen-carrying capacity of hemoglobin and compromised microcirculation from increased blood viscosity and leukocytes) is a reduction in the oxygen delivery capacity of blood both to the heart and to peripheral tissues. When oxygen demand is increased, resulting tissue hypoxemia may create a critical imbalance of oxygen need with diminished supply in a person with underlying coronary or peripheral atherosclerosis. Smoking is associated with significant myocardial perfusion abnormalities [33], thus explaining the increased risk for MI events, unstable angina, and sudden deaths observed in smokers with CHD [32].

Smoking and the metabolic syndrome

Smoking appears to increase metabolic risk. In a recent study of 1146 male subjects living in Taiwan [34], individuals who currently smoked had higher prevalence of metabolic syndrome than those who had never smoked and those who had quit smoking. The adjusted odds ratios for current smoking amount showed statistically significant dose-dependent associations with metabolic syndrome, high triglyceride level, and low HDL-C level. Current smokers with ≥ 20 pack-years had significantly increased risk of developing metabolic syndrome, high triglyceride level, and low HDL-C level. The higher risk of development of metabolic syndrome, high triglyceride level, and low HDL-C level was insignificant in former smokers.

Similar findings were reported from a Japanese population [35]. Compared with never smokers the odds ratio of developing metabolic syndrome (using the Japanese criteria) for current smokers was 1.20 [CI, 1.07–1.35) and for past smokers 1.21 (CI, 1.08–1.37). In current smokers, the odds ratio of metabolic syndrome increased with number of cigarettes smoked. After quitting, metabolic syndrome risk remained elevated for 10 to 20 years, depending on number of cigarettes smoked. These findings are consistent with previous studies suggesting metabolic syndrome is more frequent in current smokers than in those who have never smoked [36,37].

Increased risk for metabolic syndrome attributable to tobacco smoking may begin early in life. Recent analysis of NHANES III data indicates that among adolescents in the USA, metabolic syndrome prevalence is 1.2% among non-tobacco exposed, 5.4% among those exposed to environmental tobacco smoke, and 8.7% among active smokers [38]. Multiple regression analysis demonstrated increased risk of metabolic syndrome among adolescents exposed to environmental smoke (OR 4.7; CI, 1.7–12.9) and adolescents who were actively smoking (OR 6.1; CI, 2.8–13.4), controlling for socioeconomic status and other risk factors. The authors also demonstrated a dose–response relationship between serum cotinine levels and metabolic syndrome. Rates for metabolic syndrome by serum cotinine levels were 2.5%, 2.9%, and 6.7%, respectively, for the lowest, middle, and highest serum cotinine level terciles.

Smoking and metabolic syndrome risk factors

Insulin resistance is the key pathophysiological mechanism of metabolic syndrome. Smokers are at greater risk of developing insulin resistance [39,40] and subsequent diabetes than non-smokers [41–43]. Smoking increases a number of cardiac risk factors that increase with the metabolic syndrome. As mentioned above, smoking is associated with higher levels of LDL and lower levels of HDL-C. Smoking has also been associated with higher triglyceride levels [34,36].

Smoking cessation and weight gain

Smoking may have a positive impact on at least one metabolic syndrome risk factor: weight gain. Smoking cessation is associated with a statistically significant increase in bodyweight among quitters, although the estimates of post-cessation weight gain range considerably. Klesges et al. [44] found that estimates of weight gain associated with cessation range from 0.2 to 8.2 kg depending on the sample, study design, and follow-up period. Through their meta-analysis of these studies, the authors concluded that smokers gain an average of 2.9 kg after quitting. The reasons for this weight gain are not known and efforts to reduce weight gain have had minimal effect. Women smokers have greater concern with weight gain after cessation and those with high rates of concern are less likely to quit their habit [45]. Furthermore, women with body image dissatisfaction are more likely to resume smoking with post-cessation weight gain [46]. The overall public and personal health benefits of tobacco use cessation far outweigh the slightly increased risk from the increased weight.

Smoking, metabolic risk, and mental health issues

Several studies have found an association between depression and the metabolic syndrome. In an Israeli population of men and women who underwent a routine health check, metabolic syndrome was predicted by depressive symptoms, after controlling for age, education, smoking status, and other factors [47]. The separate predictive value of smoking was not given. Depression among women, but not men, was associated with a 1.94-fold risk of having the metabolic syndrome, and with an elevated risk of having two of its five components: elevated waist circumference (OR 2.23) and elevated glucose levels (OR 2.44). In addition, a positive trend was observed toward an association with the other three components: low high-density lipoprotein, hypertension, and elevated triglycerides. Among men depression was associated with elevated waist circumference only (OR 1.77).

This potential association is important because depression is a risk factor for smoking and for relapse on cessation in patients with CHD [48,49]. For instance, depression during hospitalization, as measured by a score on the Beck Depression Inventory of ≥ 16, was associated with a much greater relapse to smoking by 4 weeks compared to pre-MI smokers with lower Beck Depression Inventory score (incidence rate ratio 2.40; CI, 1.48–3.80) and 1-year follow-up (adjusted OR 3.77; 95% CI, 1.31–10.82). The authors found that the relationship was partly mediated by stronger nicotine withdrawal symptoms experienced by smokers with higher depressive symptoms [49]. Psychosocial interventions are effective post-MI in reducing depressive symptoms, and such therapies may obviate the need for antidepressants in patients with CVD [50,51]. In one of the few studies that examined the effects of a psychological intervention in depressed patients who smoked pre-MI and who were hospitalized for the event, the authors found that cognitive behavior therapy (CBT) did not significantly reduce post-MI smoking across all intervention patients with a history of smoking. However, CBT did reduce post-MI smoking among the subgroup of depressed patients with adequate perceived social support (OR 0.68; CI, 0.47–0.98) [52]. The focus of the intervention was on treating depression and social isolation and not on smoking cessation.

There may be subgroups of patients with mental health problems at particular risk for interactions among tobacco use, metabolic syndrome, and CVD. Recent evidence suggests that patients with schizophrenia, a group of patients with very high rates of tobacco use, have nicotinic cholinergic receptor abnormalities [53]. One theory is that schizophrenic patients need high nicotine concentrations to compensate for the decrease in effectiveness and/or number of nicotinic receptors. In a recent large study of antipsychotic medications for schizophrenia, the investigators found a higher rate of metabolic syndrome at baseline than in matched, non-schizophrenic populations [54]. The problem is further compounded by use of some antipsychotic medications that increase metabolic syndrome rates, leading to what has been described as an epidemic within an epidemic [55]. Taken together these studies suggest that some populations with mental disorders may be at particularly high risk for tobacco use and metabolic syndrome and the interactive consequences of these two risk factors. Relapse rates tend to be high in this population [56], suggesting that a sustained intervention effort is important.

Adverse life events, smoking, and the metabolic syndrome

A number of studies have begun to examine the possibility that there may be developmental factors that influence chronic disease risk, lifestyle, and mental health issues. For instance, Parker et al. [57] found that "childhood catch-up growth in men," considered a marker of suboptimal maternal nutrition, accounted for significant variation in a summary measure of metabolic syndrome during middle age. At the same time, smoking was independently associated with metabolic syndrome and most of the variation in metabolic syndrome was accounted for by factors measured in adulthood [57]. Adverse childhood experiences are associated with smoking in adolescence and adulthood [58] and significantly predict CVD in adults even after traditional risk factors, including smoking, are adjusted for [59].

Genetic factors

Recently, attempts have been made to examine genes and cigarette smoking. One hypothesis would be that there are common genetic links between tobacco use and other problems, like metabolic syndrome. There is consistent evidence from twin and adoption studies that genetic factors play a role in the etiology of cigarette smoking. Nevertheless, according to a recent review, there is as yet a lack of convincing evidence correlating genetic variants with specific smoking-related phenotypes [60].

Effectiveness of tobacco cessation in patients with cardiovascular disease

The general principles of tobacco use cessation have been discussed in a number of reports. The basic recommendations from the Treating Tobacco Use and Dependence guideline are listed in Table 3.1.

The long-standing recommendations [61] are that, at each visit, physicians should:

- *Ask* each patient about tobacco use – and document it in the medical record.
- *Advise* each smoker to quit. Make advice strong and positive: focus on benefits of quitting rather than harms of continued tobacco use; link the advice to the smoker's specific clinical condition or reason for visit.
- *Assess* each smoker's willingness to make a quit attempt. Is the tobacco user ready to set a 'quit date' in the next 30 days? If not, explore his barriers to taking action and help him to overcome them. If so, help him to formulate a plan based on smoker's experiences in quitting; your assessment of his likelihood of difficulty; and smoker's preferences about treatment.
- *Assist* each smoker to make a quit attempt. Offer medication and refer to counseling.
- *Arrange* follow-up – in your office, either with you or with an allied health professional, or through community services, accessed through http://gosmokefree.co.uk or www.smokefree.gov, or other websites.

Based on various reviews, the Surgeon General recommends five first-line agents (sustained-release bupropion, nicotine gum, inhaler, nasal spray, and patch) and, if the first are not effective, two second-line (clonidine and nortriptyline) for tobacco users in general. The 2008 Public Health Service guideline

Table 3.1 Treating tobacco use and dependence: findings and recommendations

Tobacco dependence is a chronic condition that often requires repeated intervention. Because effective tobacco dependence treatments are available, every patient who uses tobacco should be offered at least one of these treatments.

- Patients *willing* to try to quit tobacco use should be provided treatments identified as effective in this guideline.
- Patients *unwilling* to try to quit tobacco use should be provided a brief intervention designed to increase their motivation to quit.

It is essential that clinicians and healthcare delivery systems (including administrators, insurers, and purchasers) institutionalize the consistent identification, documentation, and treatment of every tobacco user seen in a healthcare setting.

Brief tobacco dependence treatment is effective, and every patient who uses tobacco should be offered at least brief treatment.

There is a strong dose–response relation between the intensity of tobacco dependence counseling and its effectiveness.

Treatments involving person-to-person contact (via individual, group, or proactive telephone counseling) are consistently effective, and their effectiveness increases with treatment intensity (e.g., minutes of contact).

Three types of counseling and behavioral therapies were found to be especially effective and should be used with all patients attempting tobacco cessation:

- Provision of practical counseling (problem-solving/skills training).
- Provision of social support as part of treatment (intra-treatment social support).
- Help in securing social support outside of treatment (extra-treatment social support).

Numerous effective pharmacotherapies for smoking cessation now exist. Except in the presence of contraindications, these should be used with all adult patients attempting to quit smoking.

Source: http://www.surgeongeneral.gov/tobacco/smokesum.htm, last accessed 3/30/08.

The AHRQ, CDC, and NCI have produced a quick reference guide for clinicians that covers the recommendations in detail: http://www.surgeongeneral.gov/tobacco/tobaqrg.htm, last accessed 3/30/08.

added varenicline to the list of first-line medications [61]. The safety of these medications needs to be considered when prescribing them for patients with cardiovascular disease [62]. A few reports of acute MI and stroke in patients taking nicotine replacement therapy (NRT) have been reported. Most of these events occurred in patients who also were smoking or who had an unknown smoking status while taking NRT [63]. Subsequent trials have evaluated the safety of NRT for patients with stable angina or a history of MI two or more weeks in the past [64–66]. These trials have not found a significant effect of NRT on the rate of cardiovascular events. However, no trial has assessed the safety of NRT in patients with more unstable or acute CVD [67]. Current clinical guidelines recommend against use of nicotine replacement for patients with unstable angina or an MI in the past two weeks because of a lack of data to support the safety of NRT use among this group of patients. Patients using nicotine replacement products need to be cautious not to use any other products (including cigarettes) containing nicotine.

One study found that the use of sustained-release bupropion in patients with CVD was safe and was associated with higher cessation rates. Continuous abstinence rates from weeks 4 to 26 and 4 to 52 were more than double for sustained-release bupropion compared with placebo (27 vs. 11%; 22 vs. 9%, $P < 0.001$) [68]. Nortriptyline is a tricyclic antidepressant. Drugs from this class should be used with extreme caution in patients with CVD.

Results from cessation trials using varenicline have been very encouraging [69]. This drug, when given alone, mimics the effects of nicotine on dopamine release in the nucleus accumbens – a part of the brain associated with reward and addiction – but attenuates this response to a subsequent nicotine challenge and reduces nicotine self-administration [70]. Clinical trials have found that varenicline is more effective than placebo [71] and may be more effective than bupropion and NRT [72].

An analysis by the US Food and Drug Administration (FDA) found that varenicline and bupropion might be associated with an increased risk of suicidal thoughts and behavior, including among patients with no psychiatric history (http://www.fda.gov/cder/dsn/2009_v2_no1/DSN_Vol2Num1.pdf). The label for varenicline has been updated to include a warning about serious psychiatric events and to advise patients who experience such events to stop taking the product immediately and contact a clinician. Bupropion already carries a black box warning related to increased risk of suicide.

Several new approaches to smoking cessation have been suggested [70,73]. Rimonabant, a cannabinoid CB1 receptor antagonist, was considered a promising new approach to cessation. Preclinically, this compound reduces nicotine self-administration, reduces dopamine turnover in the nucleus accumbens, and attenuates reinstatement of nicotine-seeking behavior. However, it was never approved in the USA and was withdrawn from markets in other nations where it had been approved because of greater than expected rates of psychiatric problems. Nicotine "vaccines" have been proposed as a way to raise antibodies in the blood that limit the amount of nicotine that penetrates into the brain, thereby reducing the psychopharmacological responses to the drug [70]. The vaccines also reduce dopamine turnover in the nucleus accumbens and reinstatement of nicotine-seeking behavior after nicotine readministration. The three vaccines have been well tolerated and show signs of good efficacy; however, the increase in antibody titer, evoked by the treatment, shows significant inter-individual variation and is generally short-lived.

Inpatient tobacco use cessation programs

Extensive work has been done on developing and evaluating interventions to provide smoking cessation interventions to inpatients. In a meta-analysis of smokers admitted to hospital because of CVD and provided an intervention with follow-up support, the odds of quitting smoking were significantly increased (OR 1.81; 95% CI, 1.54–2.15, 11 trials), but less intensive interventions did not produce convincing results [74]. One trial of intensive intervention, including counseling and pharmacotherapy for smokers admitted with CVD, assessed clinical and healthcare utilization endpoints, and found significant reductions in all-cause mortality and hospital readmission rates over a two-year follow-up period [75]. The authors conclude that a high-intensity behavioral intervention beginning during a hospital stay and including at least one month of supportive contact after discharge promotes smoking cessation. Interventions of lower intensity or shorter duration have not been shown to be effective in this setting. The authors also note that "there is insufficient direct evidence to conclude that adding NRT or bupropion to intensive counseling increases cessation rates over what is achieved by counseling alone, but the evidence of benefit for NRT has strengthened in this update and the point estimates are compatible with research in other settings showing that NRT and bupropion are effective" [74]. Smith and Burgess [76], in a study of 256 acute MI and coronary artery bypass graft patients, compared the effects of a minimal intervention consisting of physician and nurse advice and two pamphlets with an intensive intervention consisting of the minimal intervention plus 60 minutes of bedside counseling, take-home materials, and up to seven nurse-initiated post-discharge counseling calls for two months. One-year self-reported abstinence was 62% vs. 46% for the intensive vs. minimal intervention ($P < 0.01$), confirmed abstinence was 54% vs. 35%, respectively ($P < 0.01$). Continuous one-year abstinence was 57% vs. 39%, respectively ($P < 0.01$) and was significantly higher for CABG vs. acute MI patients ($P < 0.05$). The study suggests that even a more intensive intervention confers a better long-term outcome.

Recently the US Joint Commission on Accreditation of Healthcare Organizations (JCAHO) has created performance measures to help improve inpatient tobacco use cessation in patients with CVD. The measures stipulate that all patients admitted for an MI or congestive heart failure who were using tobacco in the year before admission should receive counseling about smoking cessation. The measures are based on the proportion of patients in each specific disease category who are provided intervention among the total number in each category who meet criteria. Performance on these measures is reported on the Joint Commission website (http://www.jointcommission.org/). As important as it is to identify patients with CVD who were using tobacco before admission and to offer intervention, a more meaningful approach would be to provide a performance measure based on post-hospitalization outcome.

Taylor et al. [77] have argued for at least a 25% six-months cessation rate target for any patient who used tobacco before admission. Six-months cessation rates for inpatients with CVD have been even higher [67] and a 50% six-months cessation rate target should be considered. Smith and Taylor [78] have provided a step-by-step guide for implementing an inpatient smoking cessation program.

Age, gender, ethnicity, and smoking

Current cigarette use prevalence among US high school students increased from 27.5% in 1991 to 36.4% in 1997, decreased to 21.9% in 2003, and remained stable from 2003 to 2007 [79]. Subgroup analysis from the same CDC report indicates these trends were similar across gender, grade level, and Hispanic vs. white subgroups. Smoking among black students increased from 12.6% in 1991 to 22.7% in 1997, then decreased to 11.6% by 2007. It is somewhat reassuring that rates have returned to levels seen two decades ago but an alarming number of adolescents continue to be exposed to this major risk for developing atherosclerosis.

Among US adults, 2007 CDC data demonstrate that prevalence of current cigarette smoking varies significantly across age, gender, and racial/ethnic subgroups [80]. Prevalence was lower among adults over age 65 (8.3%) compared to 18 to 24 (22.2%), 25 to 44 (22.6%), and 45 to 64 (21%) age groups. More men (22.3%) were currently smoking than women (17.4%). The prevalence rates of current cigarette smoking across racial/ethnic groups in increasing order were: Asians (9.6%), Hispanics (13.3%), blacks (19.8%), whites (21.4%), and Indians/Alaska Natives (36.4%).

Available evidence supports behavioral smoking cessation for adolescents but is insufficient to guide treatment decisions for pharmacotherapy interventions for youth who want to quit smoking [81]. Current literature suggests older adult smokers can quit at high rates, particularly following hospitalization for CVD, and nicotine replacement is safe and effective in this population [82].

Although progress has been made in smoking cessation research among women and African Americans, a dearth of evidence persists for evidence-based interventions among other minority groups [83]. The need for such evidence is underscored by a report demonstrating open-label trial abstinence rates among smokers receiving combined bupropion, nicotine replacement, and counseling were markedly different for whites (60%), African Americans (38%), and Hispanics (41%) [84]. A review of six studies looking at smoking cessation pharmacotherapy among non-white populations concluded that data from these studies support the use of bupropion and nicotine patch in non-white patients and cited a lack of congruent pharmacotherapy studies in Hispanic, American Indian/Alaskan Native, and other minority groups [85].

Summary

In spite of major gains in reducing tobacco use, it remains the most preventable cause of death in the USA. Tobacco use causes subclinical atherosclerosis, CHD, stroke, and abdominal aortic aneurysm. Tobacco use increases CVD risk through a variety of mediators including mechanisms that accelerate atherogenesis and thrombosis, impair endothelial function, increase inflammation, and decrease oxygen supply. Tobacco use also has a major effect on the metabolic syndrome. Tobacco smoke appears to increase the risk of developing metabolic syndrome directly and also to increase many metabolic syndrome risk factors. Complex interactions appear to occur among tobacco use, metabolic risk, and mental health problems. Patients with depression, schizophrenia, and alcohol dependence and abuse, and perhaps other mental health problems, merit very aggressive help with tobacco use cessation. Fortunately, a number of effective approaches are available to promote tobacco use cessation. The advent of the JCAHO measures has provided an impetus for implementation of inpatient tobacco use cessation programs as appropriate for patients admitted for an acute MI or for congestive heart failure. An important next step would be to ensure that all patients with CVD are provided tobacco use cessation programs and to base the effectiveness of these programs on outcome. A six-months 50% tobacco cessation rate is a good target for patients with CVD or metabolic syndrome identified in any healthcare setting. As a nation we have done well with reducing tobacco use but we must do better.

References

1. United States Department of Health and Human Services. *The Health Consequences of Smoking: A Report of the Surgeon General*. Atlanta, GA: US Department of Health and Human Services, Centers for Disease Control and Prevention, National Center for Chronic Disease Prevention and Health Promotion, Office on Smoking and Health. 2004.
2. Croft P, Hannaford PC. Risk factors for acute myocardial infarction in women: evidence from the Royal College of General Practitioners' oral contraception study. *BMJ* 1989;298:165–8.
3. Rosenberg L, Kaufman DW, Helmrich SP, Miller DR, Stolley PD, Shapiro S. Myocardial infarction and cigarette smoking in women younger than 50 years of age. *JAMA* 1985;253:2965–9.
4. Stampfer MJ, Hu FB, Manson JE, Rimm EB, Willett WC. Primary prevention of coronary heart disease in women through diet and lifestyle. *N Engl J Med* 2000;343: 16–22.
5. Barbash GI, White HD, Modan M, et al. Significance of smoking in patients receiving thrombolytic therapy for acute myocardial infarction: experience gleaned from the International Tissue Plasminogen Activator/Streptokinase Mortality Trial. *Circulation* 1993;87:53–8.

6. Gourlay SG, Rundle AC, Barron HV. Smoking and mortality following acute myocardial infarction: results from the National Registry of Myocardial Infarction 2 (NRMI 2). *Nicotine Tob Res* 2002;4(1):101–7.

7. Wilson K, Gibson N, Willan A, Cook D. Effect of smoking cessation on mortality after myocardial infarction: meta-analysis of cohort studies. *Arch Intern Med* 2000;160:939–44.

8. Critchley J, Capewell S. Smoking cessation for the secondary prevention of coronary heart disease. *Cochrane Database Syst Rev* 2004(1):CD003041.

9. Powell JJT, Worrell PP, MacSweeney SST, Franks PPJ, Greenhalgh RRM. Smoking as a risk factor for abdominal aortic aneurysm. *Ann N Y Acad Sci* 1996;800:246–8.

10. Celermajer DS, Sorensen KE, Georgakopoulos D, et al. Cigarette smoking is associated with dose-related and potentially reversible impairment of endothelium-dependent dilation in healthy young adults. *Circulation* 1993;88(5 Pt 1):2149–55.

11. Heitzer T, Yla-Herttuala S, Luoma J, et al. Cigarette smoking potentiates endothelial dysfunction of forearm resistance vessels in patients with hypercholesterolemia: role of oxidized LDL. *Circulation* 1996;93:1346–53.

12. Newby DE, McLeod AL, Uren NG, et al. Impaired coronary tissue plasminogen activator release is associated with coronary atherosclerosis and cigarette smoking: direct link between endothelial dysfunction and atherothrombosis. *Circulation* 2001;103:1936–41.

13. Newby DE, Wright RA, Labinjoh C, et al. Endothelial dysfunction, impaired endogenous fibrinolysis, and cigarette smoking: a mechanism for arterial thrombosis and myocardial infarction. *Circulation* 1999;99:1411–15.

14. Burke AP, Farb A, Malcom GT, Liang YH, Smialek J, Virmani R. Coronary risk factors and plaque morphology in men with coronary disease who died suddenly. *N Engl J Med* 1997;336:1276–82.

15. Lakier JB. Smoking and cardiovascular disease. *Am J Med* 1992;93(1A):8–12S.

16. Lassila R, Seyberth HW, Haapanen A, Schweer H, Koskenvuo M, Laustiola KE. Vasoactive and atherogenic effects of cigarette smoking: a study of monozygotic twins discordant for smoking. *BMJ* 1988;297:955–7.

17. Fusegawa Y, Goto S, Handa S, Kawada T, Ando Y. Platelet spontaneous aggregation in platelet-rich plasma is increased in habitual smokers. *Thromb Res* 1999;93:271–8.

18. Lidegaard O. Smoking and use of oral contraceptives: impact on thrombotic diseases. *Am J Obstet Gynecol* 1999;180(6 Pt 2):S357–63.

19. Roy S. Effects of smoking on prostacyclin formation and platelet aggregation in users of oral contraceptives. *Am J Obstet Gynecol* 1999;180(6 Pt 2):S364–8.

20. Danesh J, Collins R, Appleby P, Peto R. Association of fibrinogen, C-reactive protein, albumin, or leukocyte count with coronary heart disease: meta-analyses of prospective studies. *JAMA* 1998;279:1477–82.

21. Ross R. Atherosclerosis – an inflammatory disease. *N Engl J Med* 1999;340:115–26.

22. Bermudez EA, Rifai N, Buring JE, Manson JE, Ridker PM. Relation between markers of systemic vascular inflammation and smoking in women. *Am J Cardiol* 2002;89:1117–19.

23. Levitzky YS, Guo CY, Rong J, et al. Relation of smoking status to a panel of inflammatory markers: the Framingham offspring. *Atherosclerosis*. 2008;201:217–24.

24. Tracy RP, Psaty BM, Macy E, et al. Lifetime smoking exposure affects the association of C-reactive protein with cardiovascular disease risk factors and subclinical disease in healthy elderly subjects. *Arterioscler Thromb Vasc Biol* 1997;17:2167–76.

25. Samet JM. The 1990 Report of the Surgeon General: The Health Benefits of Smoking Cessation. *Am Rev Respir Dis* 1990;142:993–4.

26. Steinberg D, Parthasarathy S, Carew TE, Khoo JC, Witztum JL. Beyond cholesterol: modifications of low-density lipoprotein that increase its atherogenicity. *N Engl J Med* 1989;320:915–24.

27. Frei B, Forte TM, Ames BN, Cross CE. Gas phase oxidants of cigarette smoke induce lipid peroxidation and changes in lipoprotein properties in human blood plasma: protective effects of ascorbic acid. *Biochem J* 1991;277(Pt 1):133–8.

28. Cryer PE, Haymond MW, Santiago JV, Shah SD. Norepinephrine and epinephrine release and adrenergic mediation of smoking-associated hemodynamic and metabolic events. *N Engl J Med* 1976;295:573–7.

29. Koch A, Hoffmann K, Steck W, et al. Acute cardiovascular reactions after cigarette smoking. *Atherosclerosis* 1980;35:67–75.

30. Narkiewicz K, van de Borne PJ, Hausberg M, et al. Cigarette smoking increases sympathetic outflow in humans. *Circulation* 1998;98:528–34.

31. Friedman GD, Klatsky AL, Siegelaub AB. Alcohol, tobacco, and hypertension. *Hypertension* 1982;4(5 Pt 2):III143–50.

32. Quillen JE, Rossen JD, Oskarsson HJ, Minor RL, Jr., Lopez AG, Winniford MD. Acute effect of cigarette smoking on the coronary circulation: constriction of epicardial and resistance vessels. *J Am Coll Cardiol* 1993; 22642–7.

33. Deanfield JE, Shea MJ, Wilson RA, Horlock P, de Landsheere CM, Selwyn AP. Direct effects of smoking on the heart: silent ischemic disturbances of coronary flow. *Am J Cardiol* 1986;57:1005–9.

34. Chen CC, Li TC, Chang PC, et al. Association among cigarette smoking, metabolic syndrome, and its individual components: the metabolic syndrome study in Taiwan. *Metabolism* 2008;57:544–8.

35. Wada T, Urashima M, Fukumoto T. Risk of metabolic syndrome persists twenty years after the cessation of smoking. *Intern Med* 2007;46:1079–82.

36. Ishizaka N, Ishizaka Y, Toda E, Hashimoto II, Nagai R, Yamakado M. Association between cigarette smoking, metabolic syndrome, and carotid arteriosclerosis in Japanese individuals. *Atherosclerosis* 2005;181:381–8.

37. Nakanishi N, Takatorige T, Suzuki K. Cigarette smoking and the risk of the metabolic syndrome in middle-aged Japanese male office workers. *Ind Health* 2005;43:295–301.

38. Weitzman M, Cook S, Auinger P, et al. Tobacco smoke exposure is associated with the metabolic syndrome in adolescents. *Circulation* 2005;112:862–9.

39. Facchini FS, Hollenbeck CB, Jeppesen J, Chen YD, Reaven GM. Insulin resistance and cigarette smoking. *Lancet* 1992;339:1128–30.

40. Ronnemaa T, Ronnemaa EM, Puukka P, Pyorala K, Laakso M. Smoking is independently associated with high plasma insulin levels in nondiabetic men. *Diabetes Care* 1996;19:1229–32.

41. Foy CG, Bell RA, Farmer DF, Goff DC, Jr., Wagenknecht LE. Smoking and incidence of diabetes among US adults: findings from the Insulin Resistance Atherosclerosis Study. *Diabetes Care* 2005;28:2501–7.

42. Hu FB, Manson JE, Stampfer MJ, et al. Diet, lifestyle, and the risk of type 2 diabetes mellitus in women. *N Engl J Med* 2001;345:790–7.
43. Rimm EB, Chan J, Stampfer MJ, Colditz GA, Willett WC. Prospective study of cigarette smoking, alcohol use, and the risk of diabetes in men. *BMJ* 1995;310:555–9.
44. Klesges RC, Meyers AW, Klesges LM, La Vasque ME. Smoking, body weight, and their effects on smoking behavior: a comprehensive review of the literature. *Psychol Bull* 1989;106:204–30.
45. Pomerleau CS, Zucker AN, Stewart AJ. Characterizing concerns about post-cessation weight gain: results from a national survey of women smokers. *Nicotine Tob Res* 2001;3:51–60.
46. Dobmeyer AC, Peterson AL, Runyan CR, Hunter CM, Blackman LR. Body image and tobacco cessation: relationships with weight concerns and intention to resume tobacco use. *Body Image* 2005;2:187–92.
47. Toker S, Shirom A, Melamed S. Depression and the metabolic syndrome: gender-dependent associations. *Depress Anxiety* 2007;25:661–9.
48. Perez GH, Nicolau JC, Romano BW, Laranjeira R. Depression: a predictor of smoking relapse in a 6-month follow-up after hospitalization for acute coronary syndrome. *Eur J Cardiovasc Prev Rehabil* 2008;15:89–94.
49. Thorndike AN, Regan S, McKool K, et al. Depressive symptoms and smoking cessation after hospitalization for cardiovascular disease. *Arch Intern Med* 2008;168:186–91.
50. Barth J, Critchley J, Bengel J. Efficacy of psychosocial interventions for smoking cessation in patients with coronary heart disease: a systematic review and meta-analysis. *Ann Behav Med* 2006;32:10–20.
51. Barth J, Critchley J, Bengel J. Psychosocial interventions for smoking cessation in patients with coronary heart disease. *Cochrane Database Syst Rev* 2008(1):CD006886.
52. Trockel M, Burg M, Jaffe A, Barbour K, Taylor CB. Smoking behavior postmyocardial infarction among ENRICHD trial participants: cognitive behavior therapy intervention for depression and low perceived social support compared to care as usual. *Psychosom Med* 2008;70:875–82.
53. Levin ED, Rezvani AH. Nicotinic interactions with antipsychotic drugs, models of schizophrenia and impacts on cognitive function. *Biochem Pharmacol* 2007;74:1182–91.
54. McEvoy JP, Meyer JM, Goff DC, et al. Prevalence of the metabolic syndrome in patients with schizophrenia: baseline results from the Clinical Antipsychotic Trials of Intervention Effectiveness (CATIE) schizophrenia trial and comparison with national estimates from NHANES III. *Schizophr Res* 2005;80:19–32.
55. Fenton WS, Chavez MR. Medication-induced weight gain and dyslipidemia in patients with schizophrenia. *Am J Psychiatry* 2006;163:1697–704; quiz 858–9.
56. Evins AE, Cather C, Culhane MA, et al. A 12-week double-blind, placebo-controlled study of bupropion sr added to high-dose dual nicotine replacement therapy for smoking cessation or reduction in schizophrenia. *J Clin Psychopharmacol* 2007;27:380–6.
57. Parker L, Lamont DW, Unwin N, et al. A lifecourse study of risk for hyperinsulinaemia, dyslipidaemia and obesity (the central metabolic syndrome) at age 49–51 years. *Diabet Med* 2003;20:406–15.
58. Anda RF, Croft JB, Felitti VJ, et al. Adverse childhood experiences and smoking during adolescence and adulthood. *JAMA* 1999;282:1652–8.

59. Dong M, Giles WH, Felitti VJ, et al. Insights into causal pathways for ischemic heart disease: adverse childhood experiences study. *Circulation* 2004;110:1761–6.
60. Munafo MR, Johnstone EC. Genes and cigarette smoking. *Addiction* 2008;103:893–904.
61. Treating tobacco use and dependence: 2008 update US Public Health Service Clinical Practice Guideline executive summary. *Respir Care* 2008;53:1217–22.
62. Joseph AM, Fu SS. Smoking cessation for patients with cardiovascular disease: what is the best approach? *Am J Cardiovasc Drugs* 2003;3:339–49.
63. Benowitz NL, Gourlay SG. Cardiovascular toxicity of nicotine: implications for nicotine replacement therapy. *J Am Coll Cardiol* 1997;29:1422–31.
64. Nicotine replacement therapy for patients with coronary artery disease. Working Group for the Study of Transdermal Nicotine in Patients with Coronary artery disease. *Arch Intern Med* 1994;154:989–95.
65. Joseph AM, Antonuccio DO. Lack of efficacy of transdermal nicotine in smoking cessation. *N Engl J Med* 1999;341:1157–8.
66. Tzivoni D, Keren A, Meyler S, Khoury Z, Lerer T, Brunel P. Cardiovascular safety of transdermal nicotine patches in patients with coronary artery disease who try to quit smoking. *Cardiovasc Drugs Ther* 1998;12:239–44.
67. Thomson CC, Rigotti NA. Hospital- and clinic-based smoking cessation interventions for smokers with cardiovascular disease. *Prog Cardiovasc Dis* 2003;45:459–79.
68. Tonstad S, Farsang C, Klaene G, et al. Bupropion SR for smoking cessation in smokers with cardiovascular disease: a multicentre, randomised study. *Eur Heart J* 2003;24:946–55.
69. Cahill K, Stead LF, Lancaster T. Nicotine receptor partial agonists for smoking cessation. *Cochrane Database Syst Rev* 2007(1):CD006103.
70. Fagerstrom K, Balfour DJ. Neuropharmacology and potential efficacy of new treatments for tobacco dependence. *Exp Opin Investig Drugs* 2006;15:107–16.
71. Hays JT, Ebbert JO, Sood A. Efficacy and safety of varenicline for smoking cessation. *Am J Med* 2008;121(4 Suppl 1):S32–42.
72. Wu P, Wilson K, Dimoulas P, Mills EJ. Effectiveness of smoking cessation therapies: a systematic review and meta-analysis. *BMC Public Health* 2006;6:300.
73. Henningfield JE, Shiffman S, Ferguson SG, Gritz ER. Tobacco dependence and withdrawal: science base, challenges and opportunities for pharmacotherapy. *Pharmacol Ther* 2009;123:1–16.
74. Rigotti NA, Munafo MR, Stead LF. Interventions for smoking cessation in hospitalised patients. *Cochrane Database Syst Rev* 2007(3): CD001837.
75. Mohiuddin SM, Mooss AN, Hunter CB, Grollmes TL, Cloutier DA, Hilleman DE. Intensive smoking cessation intervention reduces mortality in high-risk smokers with cardiovascular disease. *Chest* 2007;131:446–52.
76. Smith PM, Burgess E. Smoking cessation initiated during hospital stay for patients with coronary artery disease: a randomized controlled trial. *CMAJ* 2009;180:1297–303.
77. Taylor CB, Miller NH, Cameron RP, Fagans EW, Das S. Dissemination of an effective inpatient tobacco use cessation program. *Nicotine Tob Res.* 2005;7:129–37.
78. Smith PM, Taylor CB. *Implementing an Inpatient Smoking Cessation Program.* Lawrence Erlbaum, New York. 2006.
79. Cigarette use among high school students – United States, 1991–2007. *MMWR Morb Mortal Wkly Rep* 2008;57:686–8.

80. Cigarette smoking among adults – United States, 2007. *MMWR Morb Mortal Wkly Rep* 2008;57:1221–6.

81. Curry SJ, Mermelstein RJ, Sporer AK. Therapy for specific problems: youth tobacco cessation. *Annu Rev Psychol* 2009;60:229–55.

82. Doolan DM, Froelicher ES. Smoking cessation interventions and older adults. *Prog Cardiovasc Nurs* 2008;23:119–27.

83. Doolan DM, Froelicher ES. Efficacy of smoking cessation intervention among special populations: review of the literature from 2000 to 2005. *Nurs Res* 2006;55(4 Suppl):S29–37.

84. Covey LS, Botello-Harbaum M, Glassman AH, et al. Smokers' response to combination bupropion, nicotine patch, and counseling treatment by race/ethnicity. *Ethn Dis* 2008;18:59–64.

85. Robles GI, Singh-Franco D, Ghin HL. A review of the efficacy of smoking-cessation pharmacotherapies in nonwhite populations. *Clin Ther* 2008;30:800–12.

Chapter 4

Nutrition and risk for cardiovascular disease

Alice H. Lichtenstein

There is a wide range of dietary approaches purported to decrease the risk of developing cardiovascular disease (CVD). Some were first identified early in the 20th century whereas others have been recognized more recently. Some have stood the test of time and others have not. None are without controversy, both past and present. We now understand that what appears to be inconsistent evidence to support a relationship between diet and CVD risk reduction is likely attributable to previously unrecognized confounders such as biological variability, co-linearity of diet variables, interaction among diet and biological factors, and differences in the strength of the relationship between clinical outcomes and biomarkers.

It is difficult, if not impossible, to directly assess the efficacy of dietary interventions on CVD risk because of the difficulty in modifying dietary intakes of large groups of individuals over long periods of time and the cost associated with such efforts. Hence, most dietary interventions with the intent of reducing CVD risk are evaluated on the basis of biomarkers.

Traditionally, plasma lipid, lipoprotein and apoprotein concentrations were used as biomarkers to evaluate diet interventions intended to reduce CVD risk. More recently, a wider range of biomarkers is used. Due to the amount of data available, for the most part, this chapter will be limited to a discussion of diet-lipoprotein relationships.

Level of dietary fat

Dietary fat serves as a major energy source for humans. One gram of fat contributes 9 kcal, a little more than twice that contributed by protein or carbohydrate (4 kcal per gram), and somewhat more than that contributed by alcohol

Metabolic Risk for Cardiovascular Disease, 1st edition. Edited by R. H. Eckel.
© 2011 American Heart Association. By Blackwell Publishing Ltd.

(7 kcal per gram). The two major issues to consider with regard to the amount of fat in the diet and CVD risk are bodyweight and plasma lipoprotein profiles.

Bodyweight

Long-term data on the effect of dietary fat amount (percent of energy) on bodyweight suggests that dramatic reductions in intake, approximately 10% of energy, results in only modest weight loss, 1.0 kg, over a 12-month period in normal weight subjects and 3 kg in overweight or obese subjects [1]. Some evidence suggests that the dietary fiber content may be a mitigating factor [2]. These data would suggest that substituting fruits, vegetables, and whole grains for fat instead of fat-free cookies, cakes, and snack foods, may have some value in promoting weight loss within the context of low-fat diets. In a longer-term study, the Women's Health Initiative, counseling postmenopausal women to reduce their dietary fat intake resulted in a modest decline in intake but was not accompanied by more favorable weight loss patterns when compared to women who did not receive the dietary counseling [3].

Five studies were included in a meta-analysis evaluating the effect of a high fat and protein/low carbohydrate diet relative to conventional or low-fat diets on bodyweight [4]. Six-month data suggested a potential advantage of the higher fat and protein/low carbohydrate diet compared to the conventional low-fat diets for bodyweight reduction. However, an advantage of one diet over the other was lost at the 12-month time point. A 2-year intervention trial has indicated that at the six-month time point a high-fat/low-carbohydrate diet results in more weight loss than "Mediterranean" or low-fat diets [5]. However, at the 2-year time point bodyweight loss was similar for the high-fat/low-carbohydrate and "Mediterranean" diets, and greater than for the low-fat diet. The retention rates were highest for the low-fat diet and lowest for the high-fat/low-carbohydrate diet. In the most recent study subjects were counseled and provided with intensive support to consume one of four diets: low-fat/average-protein, low-fat/high-protein, high-fat/average-protein and high-fat/high-protein for 2 years [6]. Regardless of diet composition, mean weight loss averaged about 6 kg and was similar among the diet groups. Maximal weight loss was achieved at about 6 months, maintained for an additional 6 months, and then about half was regained during the last 12 months. Satiety, hunger, satisfaction with the diet, and attendance at group sessions were similar for all diets. Attendance at group sessions was the strongest predictor of weight loss. Yet to be determined is whether bodyweight loss will be sustained and the impact of the weight loss or stabilization on CVD events.

Lipoprotein profiles

When considering the effect of level of dietary fat, usually expressed in terms of percent of energy, on plasma lipoprotein profiles and CVD risk, the focus is primarily on triglyceride and high-density lipoprotein (HDL) cholesterol concentrations or the total cholesterol to HDL cholesterol ratio. Relatively consistent evidence indicates that increasing the carbohydrate content of the diet at the expense of fat results in dyslipidemia [7–9].

The majority of the evidence suggests that carbohydrate-induced hypertriglyceridemia results from an increased rate of hepatic fatty acid synthesis [10,11] and subsequent production of hepatic triglyceride-rich particles, very-low-density lipoprotein (VLDL) [12–14]. In some cases delayed triglyceride clearance has also been observed [15]. The metabolic response to a low-fat diet can vary depending on experimental setting or characteristics of the study subjects. Within the context of a stable bodyweight, replacement of dietary fat with carbohydrate results in higher triglyceride and VLDL cholesterol concentrations, lower HDL cholesterol concentrations and a higher (less favorable) total cholesterol to HDL cholesterol ratio [16–21]. These effects are blunted when an individual is in negative energy balance, the carbohydrate source is rich in fiber, and perhaps when subjects are engaging in regular physical activity [7,19,20]. Sedentary individuals characterized by visceral adiposity are at particularly high risk for carbohydrate-induced hypertrygliceridemia [9]. It has yet to be determined whether elevated insulin concentrations or insulin resistance, per se, alters VLDL synthesis or clearance.

The more moderate the shifts in the fat to carbohydrate ratio of the diet, the more moderate the change in triglyceride and HDL cholesterol concentrations [22]. Moderate carbohydrate restriction and weight loss have been reported to provide equivalent but non-additive improvements in the atherogenic dyslipidemic pattern characterized by elevated triglyceride concentrations and total cholesterol/HDL cholesterol ratios [23]. Of note, after 2 years of consuming either a low-fat/average-protein, low-fat/high-protein, high-fat/average-protein or high-fat/high-protein diet, plasma lipid-related risk factors and fasting insulin concentrations were improved similarly by all the diets [6].

Low HDL cholesterol concentrations are an independent risk factor for CVD [24]. Low-fat diets are of particular concern in individuals with diabetes or metabolic syndrome, who tend to have low HDL cholesterol concentrations [7,25]. Nonetheless, there are no data with which to predict the effect of the dyslipidemia caused by low-fat diets on CVD event incidence. Current recommendations for the general population, and individuals with impaired insulin sensitivity, are to consume a diet moderate in fat, between 25% and 35% of energy [24,26].

Type of dietary fat and plasma lipoprotein concentrations

Studies performed in the mid 1960s demonstrated that changes in dietary fatty acid profiles altered plasma total cholesterol concentrations in most individuals

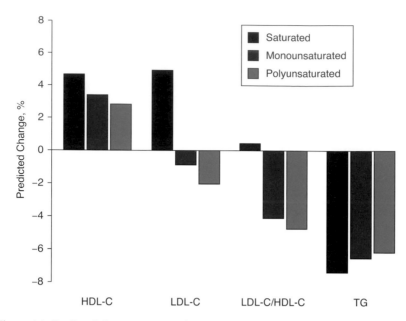

Figure 4.1 Predicted changes in serum lipids and lipoproteins on the basis of dietary fat type. Reproduced with permission from Hu FB, Willett WC. Optimal diets for prevention of coronary heart disease. *JAMA* 2002;288:2569–78. Copyright © (2002) American Medical Association. All rights reserved.

[27,28]. Many studies have since confirmed these early observations using a variety of different experimental designs [29]. When carbohydrate is displaced by saturated fatty acids, LDL cholesterol concentrations increase, whereas when carbohydrate is displaced by unsaturated fatty acids LDL cholesterol concentrations decrease, with the effect of polyunsaturated fatty acids greater than monounsaturated fatty acids [21,30] (Figure 4.1). When carbohydrate is displaced by saturated, monounsaturated or polyunsaturated fatty acids, HDL cholesterol concentrations are increased, with saturated fatty acids having the greatest effect and polyunsaturated fatty acids having the least effect. With respect to dietary fat on LDL cholesterol/HDL cholesterol ratios, there is little effect when carbohydrate is displaced by saturated fatty acids, whereas monounsaturated and polyunsaturated fatty acids decrease (more favorable) the ratio to a similar magnitude. Relative to carbohydrate, all types of dietary fat decrease triglyceride concentrations. Changes in LDL cholesterol concentrations induced by changes in the fatty acid profile of the diet are attributed to differences in the fractional catabolic rate of plasma LDL rather than production rate [31,32]. Differences in HDL cholesterol concentrations induced by changes in the fatty acid profile of the diet are attributed to differences in the production rates rather than fractional catabolic rate [33,34].

There is a certain level of heterogeneity reported for changes in plasma lipoprotein profiles in response to changes in dietary fatty acids. For the most part, this heterogeneity reported among studies is likely contributed to by study design differences such as the magnitude or type of dietary perturbation, length of study period, habituation to nutrient intakes prior to the start of the study period, background diet on which the dietary variable are superimposed in intervention studies, method of dietary assessment in observational studies, and differences among experimental subjects (e.g., age, sex, efficiency of cholesterol absorption, and initial blood lipid concentrations).

Dietary fatty acids – unique considerations

Saturated fatty acids

Early evidence demonstrated that foods relatively high in saturated fatty acids increase plasma total cholesterol concentrations and that not all saturated fatty acids had the same effect [27–29]. Saturated fatty acids with intermediate chain lengths – lauric (12:0), myristic (14:0), and palmitic (16:0) acids (Table 4.1) – increase plasma cholesterol concentrations whereas short-chain fatty acids (6:0 to 10:0) and stearic acid (18:0) result in little or no change in plasma cholesterol concentrations (Figure 4.2) [35]. The rapid conversion of stearic acid (18:0) to oleic acid (18:1) is the likely reason this saturated fatty acid has a relatively neutral effect on blood cholesterol concentrations [36]. The absorption of the short-chain saturated fatty acids directly into the portal vein is the likely reason these saturated fatty acids have a relatively neutral effect on blood cholesterol concentrations.

Foods high in saturated fatty acids, fats of animal origin (meat and dairy fat), contain a mixture of fatty acids. A linear relationship between saturated fatty acid intake and LDL cholesterol concentrations and saturated fat and cardiovascular disease risk has been reported [24,37]. Hence, current recommendations are to restrict saturated fat intake to less than 7% of energy intake [24,26].

Polyunsaturated fatty acids

A recent review by the American Heart Association concluded that "Aggregate data from randomized trials, case–control and cohort studies and long-term animal feeding experiments indicate that the consumption of at least 5% to 10% of energy from omega-6 polyunsaturated fatty acids reduces the risk of CHD relative to lower intakes. The data also suggest that higher intakes appear to be safe and may be even more beneficial (as part of a low-saturated-fat, low-cholesterol diet)" [38]. They further indicated that "To reduce omega-6 PUFA intakes from their current levels would be more likely to increase than to decrease risk for coronary heart disease." The current recommendation is to consume up to 10% of energy as polyunsaturated fatty acids [24,26].

Table 4.1 Dietary fatty acids

Code	Common name	Formula
Saturated		
12:0	lauric acid	$CH_3(CH_2)_{10}COOH$
14:0	myristic acid	$CH_3(CH_2)_{12}COOH$
16:0	palmitic acid	$CH_3(CH_2)_{14}COOH$
18:0	stearic acid	$CH_3(CH_2)_{16}COOH$
Monounsaturated		
16:1n-7 *cis*	palmitoleic acid	$CH_3(CH_2)_5CH=(c)CH(CH_2)_7COOH$
18:1n-9 *cis*	oleic acid	$CH_3(CH_2)_7CH=(c)CH(CH_2)_7COOH$
18:1n-9 *trans*	elaidic acid	$CH_3(CH_2)_7CH=(t)CH(CH_2)_7COOH$
Polyunsaturated		
18:2n-6,9 all *cis*	linoleic acid	$CH_3(CH_2)_4CH=(c)CHCH_2CH=(c)CH(CH_2)_7COOH$
18:3n-3,6,9 all *cis*	α-linolenic acid	$CH_3CH_2CH=(c)CHCH_2CH=(c)CHCH_2CH=(c)CH(CH_2)_7COOH$
18:3n-6,9,12 all *cis*	γ-linolenic acid	$CH_3(CH_2)_4CH=(c)CHCH_2CH=(c)CHCH_2CH=(c)CH(CH_2)_4COOH$
20:4n-6,9,12,15 all *cis*	arachidonic acid	$CH_3(CH_2)_4CH=(c)CHCH_2CH=(c)CHCH_2CH=(c)CHCH_2CH=(c)CH(CH_2)_3COOH$
20:5n-3,6,9,12,15 all *cis*	eicosapentaenoic acid	$CH_3(CH_2CH=(c)CH)_5(CH_2)_3COOH$
22:6n-3,6,9,12,15,18 all *cis*	docosahexaenoic acid	$CH_3(CH_2CH=(c)CH)_6(CH_2)_2COOH$

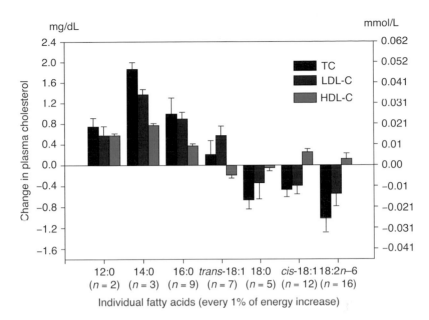

Figure 4.2 Changes (Δ) in total, LDL and HDL cholesterol concentrations of individual dietary fatty acids relative to oleic acid. TC = total cholesterol; LDL-C = low density lipoprotein-cholesterol; HDL-C = high density lipoprotein-cholesterol. (Reproduced from [35] with permission of *Am J Clin Nutr* (1997;65 (5 Suppl):1628–44S).)

Omega-3 polyunsaturated fatty acids

The three major dietary omega-3 polyunsaturated fatty acids (PUFAs) are alpha-linolenic acid (ALA, 18:3n-3), eicosapentaenoic acid (EPA, 20:5n-3), and docosahexaenoic acid (DHA,22:6n-3). The later two fatty acids are sometimes referred to as very-long-chain n-3 fatty acids. In the early 1980s it was reported that Greenland Inuits had a low prevalence of CHD compared with Scandinavian control subjects [39,40] and this was attributed to the high intake of marine foods by Inuits and the unique fatty acid profile of those foods.

Since that time a number of studies have reported an inverse association between dietary n-3 fatty acids, CVD and stroke risk [41]. Intervention data have demonstrated that EPA and DHA, but not ALA, benefit cardiovascular outcomes in primarily and secondary prevention studies [42]. The positive effects of EPA and DHA on cardiovascular outcomes, when provided at pharmacological levels (1–3 grams per day), is attributed to antiarrhythmic properties and effects on lowering plasma triglyceride concentrations, platelet reactivity, and blood pressure [43,44]. Of note, the relationship between arrhythmea and EPA and DHA has recently been questioned [45]. The major source of ALA in the diet is soybean and canola oils, whereas the major source of EPA and DHA is marine oils found in fish. The capacity of humans to convert ALA to EPA and

DHA is low [46,47]. For this reason the recommendation, with respect to CVD risk reduction, is to consume at least two fish meals per week [41]. For individuals with established disease the recommendation is to consume the equivalent of 1 gram of EPA+DHA per day. Due to their hypotriglyceridemic effect, 3 to 5 grams of EPA+DHA is recommended for individuals with chronically elevated triglyceride concentrations.

Trans *fatty acids*

The double bonds in fatty acids occur in the *cis* or *trans* configuration. The *cis* configuration is the most predominant form, representing the majority of double bonds in plant oils and animal fats. Dietary *trans* fatty acids occur naturally in meat and dairy products as a result of anaerobic bacterial fermentation in ruminant animals. *Trans* fatty acids are formed during hydrogenation of vegetable or fish oils. Traditionally, oils have been hydrogenated to increase viscosity (change a liquid oil into a semi-liquid or solid) and extend shelf life (decrease susceptibility to oxidation). The major dietary source of *trans* fatty acids worldwide is from hydrogenated fat, primarily in products made thereof, such as commercially fried foods and baked goods [48].

Since the 1990s attention has been focused on the effects of *trans* fatty acids on specific lipoprotein fractions [49,50]. Similar to saturated fatty acids, *trans* fatty acids increased LDL cholesterol concentrations. In contrast to saturated fatty acids, they do not raise HDL cholesterol concentrations. The changes result in a less favorable LDL cholesterol:HDL cholesterol ratio, with respect to CVD risk

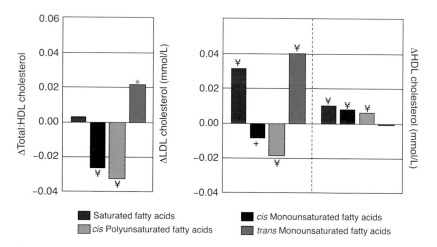

■ Saturated fatty acids
□ *cis* Polyunsaturated fatty acids
■ *cis* Monounsaturated fatty acids
■ *trans* Monounsaturated fatty acids

Figure 4.3 Predicted changes (Δ) in the ratio of serum total to HDL cholesterol and in LDL and HDL cholesterol concentrations when carbohydrates constituting 1% of energy are replaced isoenergetically with saturated, *cis* monounsaturated, *cis* polyunsaturated, or *trans* monounsaturated fatty acids. *$P < 0.05$; $^{+}P < 0.01$; $^{¥}P < 0.001$. (Reproduced from [21] with permission of *Am J Clin Nutr* (2003;77:1146–55).)

(Figure 4.3) [21,51]. A trend towards increased triglyceride concentrations is frequently reported. Some research has also suggested that *trans* fatty acids may increase lipoprotein (a) and high sensitivity C-reactive protein concentrations [48].

Dietary cholesterol and plasma lipoprotein concentrations

The observation that dietary cholesterol increased blood cholesterol concentrations and was associated with the development of CVD was originally made early in the early 20th century in rabbits [52]. In humans, a positive association has been repeatedly observed between dietary cholesterol and both plasma cholesterol concentrations and CVD risk [29,37,53].

The effect of dietary cholesterol on plasma lipoprotein concentrations is less than that of saturated and *trans* fatty acids and as such receives less emphasis with respect to dietary recommendations [24,26]. Of note, a relatively high degree of variability in response to dietary cholesterol among individuals has been reported [54].

With few exceptions, dietary cholesterol is present in foods of animal origin. Therefore, restricting saturated fat intake is likely to result in a decrease in dietary cholesterol intake.

Dietary carbohydrate

Fiber

Dietary soluble fiber, primarily β-glucan, has been reported to have a modest independent effect on decreasing blood total and LDL cholesterol concentrations. It has been estimated that 3 grams of soluble fiber (equivalent of three servings of oatmeal) reduce both total and LDL cholesterol concentrations by approximately 5 mg/dL [55]. When moderate carbohydrate diets are consumed, higher compared to lower fiber intakes are associated with lower LDL cholesterol, HDL cholesterol and triglycerides concentrations, similar total cholesterol/HDL cholesterol ratios, and lower postprandial plasma glucose concentrations [56,57].

Most evidence suggests that soluble fiber exerts its hypocholesterolemic effect by binding bile acids and cholesterol in the intestine, resulting in an increased fecal loss and altered colonic metabolism of bile acids [58]. The fermentation of fiber polysaccharides in the colon yields short-chain fatty acids. Some evidence suggests that these compounds may have hypocholesterolemic effects via alterations in hepatic metabolism. Interestingly, observational data has consistently associated dietary insoluble fiber from cereals, but not vegetable and fruits, with lower CVD risk and lower progression of atherosclerotic lesions [59,60]. Current recommendations for adults are for the consumption of 25–20 grams of dietary fiber daily.

Fructose

Observational data suggests that adults who consume higher amounts of sugar-sweetened beverages, frequently made from high-fructose corn syrup, are more likely to gain weight and be at increased risk for development of type 2 diabetes [61], and children who consume higher amounts of sugar-sweetened beverages are more likely to gain excess bodyweight [62]. Due to these relationships concern was raised about the potential relationship between fructose and high-fructose corn syrup and both bodyweight and CVD risk factors [63].

Recent intervention data have suggested that at least in the short term an increase in dietary fructose (~55% fructose/45% sucrose) either alone or as high-fructose corn syrup, relative to glucose or sucrose (50% fructose/50% sucrose), resulted in similar effects on insulin sensitivity or secretion, glucose kinetics, lipolysis, and glucose, insulin, C-peptide, triglycerides, HDL cholesterol and LDL cholesterol concentrations [64,65]. More recently, attention has been shifted from the type of carbohydrate to the form. It has been suggested that the purported relationship between fructose and bodyweight and CVD risk factors may be mediated via the physical form of the energy: liquid (beverage) versus solid (food) [66]. This is an active area of investigation at this time.

Protein

Type of protein

Target dietary recommendations for protein as a percent of energy have changed little over the years [24,26,67–70]. Dietary protein falls into two categories defined by origin: animal protein (primarily meat and dairy) and vegetable protein (primarily grains and legumes). For the most part, the former source of protein contributes the majority of dietary saturated and much of the monounsaturated fatty acids to the diet while the latter, with the exception of tropical oils (palm, palm kernel, and coconut), contributes the majority of the polyunsaturated and some of the monounsaturated fatty acids to the diet. The implications of fatty acids accompanying the sources of protein are discussed below.

Soy protein

The potential relationship between soy protein and the risk of developing CVD has a long history dating back to the 1940s [71]. Despite this relatively protracted lead time, attempts at more precisely defining this relationship were slow in coming and somewhat inconsistent [72]. Reinvigorated interest developed about the relationship between soy protein and lipoprotein concentrations in the mid 1990s [73]. At that time it was unclear whether the effect of soy on lipoprotein concentrations was attributable to the soy protein, per se, or other soybean derived factor(s) such as isoflavones. The most recent data suggests either a null or small LDL cholesterol-lowering effect of relativity large amounts of soy protein (25 to 50 grams) [74–76]. Soy-derived isoflavones do not appear to have an independent effect on lipoprotein concentrations [77–80]. Nevertheless, consumption of soy protein-rich foods may indirectly reduce CVD risk if they displace from the diet animal and full-fat dairy products that contain saturated fat and cholesterol.

Dietary supplements

Phytosterols

Plant sterols (phytosterols or stanols) are a group of alcoholic derivatives of cyclopentanoperhydrophenanthrene. They are structurally similar to cholesterol, differing only in the aliphatic side chain. The most common forms are sitosterol, campesterol, and stigmasterol. Plant sterols occur naturally in plants; their function is analogous to cholesterol in humans. In the gut, plant sterols have a higher affinity for micelles than cholesterol. The net result is displacement of cholesterol from micelles, both dietary and bile derived. This causes a decrease in the efficiency of cholesterol absorption by about 50% [81–84]. The resulting reduction in plasma cholesterol concentrations has been associated with an increase in the expression of LDL receptors on peripheral cells [81].

Two forms of plant sterols have been used to lower LDL cholesterol concentrations, plant sterols in their natural state and a saturated form of plant sterols, termed plant stanols. In addition, some plant sterol/stanol preparations used to lower LDL cholesterol concentrations are esterified to a fatty acid. As a group, these forms of plant stanols/sterols or stanol/sterol esters lower LDL cholesterol concentrations, on average, by 10% [81,82,85]. Maximal effects are observed at about 2 grams per day. By comparison the mean intake of naturally occurring plant sterols in the diet ranges from 150 mg to 350 mg per day and of plant stanols 15 mg to 50 mg per day. Intakes of plant sterols/stanols above 2 grams per day provide little additional benefit [82,86]. With respect to LDL cholesterol lowering, the efficacy of the different forms of plant sterols/stanols is similar.

Habitual consumption of plant sterols results in a small increase in plasma concentrations, greater than that of plant stanols. This has led to some concern about the potential adverse effects of increased plant sterol concentrations on CVD outcomes [85,87]. The data, in both mice models and humans, are inconsistent [88,89]. This issue is of particular concern because statin therapy increases the rate of plant sterol absorption [87].

Plant stanol/sterols are currently available in a wide variety of foods, drinks, and soft gel capsules. The choice of vehicle should be determined by availability and by other considerations, including caloric content. To sustain LDL cholesterol reductions from these products, individuals need to consume them daily, just as they would use lipid-lowering medication.

Policicosanols

Policosanols are a mixture of higher primary aliphatic alcohols originally isolated from sugarcane wax, wheatgerm, rice, beeswax, and other plants [90–92]. Early work suggested that plicosanols were highly efficacious as a cholesterol-lowering agent, decreasing LDL cholesterol concentrations up to 31% and increasing HDL cholesterol concentrations up to 29% (dose up to 20 mg/day) [92–94]. The vast majority of studies demonstrating the efficacy of policosanols on plasma lipoprotein profiles were conducted using a preparation of policosanols isolated from sugarcane wax [94]. More recent work conducted under controlled conditions in individuals with hypercholesterolemia [91,95–97] and heterozygous familial hypercholesterolemia [98,99] have consistently failed to support these earlier findings. At this time the evidence does not support the use of policosanols, regardless of source, to treat elevated LDL cholesterol concentrations or to optimize lipoprotein profiles.

Antioxidant nutrients

In the mid-1990s there was considerable interest in the potential benefit of antioxidant nutrients and CVD risk reduction [100–103]. Since that time a series of randomized controlled intervention trials have failed to demonstrate a benefit of vitamin E or other antioxidant vitamin supplementation on CVD risk [104, 105]. The most recent work focusing on vitamins C and E confirm these earlier trials [106]. At this time the data do not support a recommendation to use antioxidant vitamins for the prevention or management of CVD.

References

1. Roberts SB, Pi-Sunyer FX, Dreher M, et al. Physiology of fat replacement and fat reduction: effects of dietary fat and fat substitutes on energy regulation. *Nutr Rev* 1998;56(5 Pt 2):S29–41; discussion S9.
2. Yao M, Roberts SB. Dietary energy density and weight regulation. *Nutr Rev* 2001;59(8 Pt 1):247–58.
3. Howard BV, Van Horn L, Hsia J, et al. Low-fat dietary pattern and risk of cardiovascular disease: the Women's Health Initiative Randomized Controlled Dietary Modification Trial. *JAMA* 2006;295:655–66.
4. Nordmann AJ, Nordmann A, Briel M, et al. Effects of low-carbohydrate vs low-fat diets on weight loss and cardiovascular risk factors: a meta-analysis of randomized controlled trials. *Arch Intern Med* 2006;166:285–93.
5. Shai I, Schwarzfuchs D, Henkin Y, et al. Weight loss with a low-carbohydrate, mediterranean, or low-fat diet. *N Engl J Med* 2008;359:229–41.
6. Sacks FM, Bray GA, Carey VJ, et al. Comparison of weight-loss diets with different compositions of fat, protein, and carbohydrates. *N Engl J Med* 2009;360:859–73.
7. Hellerstein MK. Carbohydrate-induced hypertriglyceridemia: modifying factors and implications for cardiovascular risk. *Curr Opin Lipidol* 2002;13:33–40.

8. Parks EJ. Changes in fat synthesis influenced by dietary macronutrient concent. *Proc Nutr Soc* 2002;61:281–6.

9. Fried SK, Rao SP. Sugars, hypertriglyceridemia, and cardiovascular disease. *Am J Clin Nutr* 2003;78:873–80S.

10. Hudgins LC, Seidman CE, Diakun J, Hirsch J. Human fatty acid synthesis is reduced after the substitution of dietary starch for sugar. *Am J Clin Nutr* 1998;67:631–9.

11. Raben A, Holst JJ, Madsen J, Astrup A. Diurnal metabolic profiles after 14 d of an ad libitum high-starch, high-sucrose, or high-fat diet in normal-weight never-obese and postobese women. *Am J Clin Nutr* 2001;73:177–89.

12. Nestel PJ, Hirsch EZ. Triglyceride turnover after diets rich in carbohydrate or animal fat. *Australas Ann Med* 1965;14:265–9.

13. Nestel PJ, Carroll KF, Havenstein N. Plasma triglyceride response to carbohydrates, fats and caloric intake. *Metab Clin Exp* 1970;19:1–18.

14. Mittendorfer B, Sidossis LS. Mechanism for the increase in plasma triacylglycerol concentrations after consumption of short-term, high-carbohydrate diets. *Am J Clin Nutr* 2001;73:892–9.

15. Parks EJ, Krauss RM, Christiansen MP, Neese RA, Hellerstein MK. Effects of a low-fat, high-carbohydrate diet on VLDL-triglyceride assembly, production, and clearance. *J Clin Invest* 1999;104:1087–96.

16. Mancini M, Mattock M, Rabaya E, Chait A, Lewis B. Studies of the mechanisms of carbohydrate-induced lipaemia in normal man. *Atherosclerosis* 1973;17:445–54.

17. Grundy SM, Nix D, Whelan MF, Franklin L. Comparison of three cholesterol-lowering diets in normolipidemic men. *JAMA* 1986;256:2351–5.

18. Garg A, Grundy SM, Koffler M. Effect of high carbohydrate intake on hyperglycemia, islet function, and plasma lipoproteins in NIDDM. *Diabetes Care* 1992;15:1572–80.

19. Lichtenstein AH, Ausman LM, Carrasco W, Jenner JL, Ordovas JM, Schaefer EJ. Short-term consumption of a low-fat diet beneficially affects plasma lipid concentrations only when accompanied by weight loss: hypercholesterolemia, low-fat diet, and plasma lipids. *Arterioscler Thromb* 1994;14:1751–60.

20. Kasim-Karakas SE, Almario RU, Mueller WM, Peerson J. Changes in plasma lipoproteins during low-fat, high-carbohydrate diets: effects of energy intake. *Am J Clin Nutr* 2000;71:1439–47.

21. Mensink RP, Zock PL, Kester AD, Katan MB. Effects of dietary fatty acids and carbohydrates on the ratio of serum total to HDL cholesterol and on serum lipids and apolipoproteins: a meta-analysis of 60 controlled trials. *Am J Clin Nutr* 2003;77:1146–55.

22. Ginsberg HN, Kris-Etherton P, Dennis B, et al. Effects of reducing dietary saturated fatty acids on plasma lipids and lipoproteins in healthy subjects: the DELTA Study, protocol 1. *Arterioscler Thromb Vasc Biol* 1998;18:441–9.

23. Krauss RM, Blanche PJ, Rawlings RS, Fernstrom HS, Williams PT. Separate effects of reduced carbohydrate intake and weight loss on atherogenic dyslipidemia. *Am J Clin Nutr* 2006;83:1025–31; quiz 205.

24. Expert Panel on Detection Evaluation and Treatment of High Blood Cholesterol in Adults. Executive Summary of The Third Report of The National Cholesterol Education Program (NCEP) Expert Panel on Detection, Evaluation, And Treatment of High Blood Cholesterol In Adults (Adult Treatment Panel III). *JAMA* 2001;285:2486–97.

25. Bantle JP, Wylie-Rosett J, Albright AL, et al. Nutrition recommendations and interventions for diabetes: a position statement of the American Diabetes Association. *Diabetes Care* 2008;31(Suppl 1):S61–78.

26. Lichtenstein AH, Appel LJ, Brands M, et al. Diet and lifestyle recommendations revision 2006: a scientific statement from the American Heart Association Nutrition Committee. *Circulation* 2006;114:82–96.

27. Hegsted DM, McGandy RB, Myers ML, Stare FJ. Quantitative effects of dietary fat on serum cholesterol in man. *Am J Clin Nutr* 1965;17:281–95.

28. Keys A, Anderson JT, Grande F. Serum cholesterol response to change in the diet. *Metab Clin Exp* 1965;14:747–58.

29. Clarke R, Frost C, Collins R, Appleby P, Peto R. Dietary lipids and blood cholesterol: quantitative meta-analysis of metabolic ward studies. *BMJ* 1997;314:112–17.

30. Hu FB, Willett WC. Optimal diets for prevention of coronary heart disease. *JAMA* 2002;288:2569–78.

31. Shepherd J, Packard CJ, Grundy SM, Yeshurun D, Gotto AM, Jr., Taunton OD. Effects of saturated and polyunsaturated fat diets on the chemical composition and metabolism of low density lipoproteins in man. *J Lipid Res* 1980;21:91–9.

32. Matthan NR, Welty FK, Barrett PH, et al. Dietary hydrogenated fat increases high-density lipoprotein apoA-I catabolism and decreases low-density lipoprotein apoB-100 catabolism in hypercholesterolemic women. *Arterioscler Thromb Vasc Biol* 2004;24:1092–7.

33. Velez-Carrasco W, Lichtenstein AH, Li Z, et al. Apolipoprotein A-I and A-II kinetic parameters as assessed by endogenous labeling with [(2)H(3)]leucine in middle-aged and elderly men and women. *Arterioscler Thromb Vasc Biol* 2000;20:801–6.

34. Marsh JB, Welty FK, Schaefer EJ. Stable isotope turnover of apolipoproteins of high-density lipoproteins in humans. *Curr Opin Lipidol* 2000;11:261–6.

35. Kris-Etherton PM, Yu S. Individual fatty acid effects on plasma lipids and lipoproteins: human studies. *Am J Clin Nutr* 1997;65(5 Suppl):1628–44S.

36. Bonanome A, Grundy SM. Effect of dietary stearic acid on plasma cholesterol and lipoprotein levels. *N Engl J Med* 1988;318:1244–8.

37. Institute of Medicine. *Dietary Reference Intakes: energy, carbohydrate, fiber, fat, fatty acids, cholesterol, protein and amino acids*. National Academy of Sciences, Washington, DC. 2005.

38. Harris WS, Mozaffarian D, Rimm EB, et al. Omega-6 fatty acids and risk for cardiovascular disease: a science advisory from the American Heart Association Nutrition Subcommittee of the Council on Nutrition, Physical Activity, and Metabolism; Council on Cardiovascular Nursing; and Council on Epidemiology and Prevention. *Circulation* 2009;119:902–7.

39. Kromann N, Green A. Epidemiological studies in the Upernavik district, Greenland: incidence of some chronic diseases 1950–1974. *Acta Medica Scand* 1980;208:401–6.

40. Dyerberg J, Bang HO. A hypothesis on the development of acute myocardial infarction in Greenlanders. *Scand J Clin Lab Invest Suppl* 1982;161:7–13.

41. Kris-Etherton PM, Harris WS, Appel LJ, American Heart Association. Nutrition C. Fish consumption, fish oil, omega-3 fatty acids, and cardiovascular disease. *Circulation* 2002;106:2747–57.

42. Wang C, Harris WS, Chung M, et al. n-3 Fatty acids from fish or fish-oil supplements, but not alpha-linolenic acid, benefit cardiovascular disease outcomes in

primary- and secondary-prevention studies: a systematic review. *Am J Clin Nutr* 2006;84(1):5–17.

43. De Caterina R, Zampolli A. Omega-3 fatty acids, atherogenesis, and endothelial activation. *J Cardiovasc Med* 2007;8Suppl 1:S11–14.

44. Harris WS, Miller M, Tighe AP, Davidson MH, Schaefer EJ. Omega-3 fatty acids and coronary heart disease risk: clinical and mechanistic perspectives. *Atherosclerosis* 2008;197:12–24.

45. Brouwer IA, Raitt MH, Dullemeijer C, et al. Effect of fish oil on ventricular tachyarrhythmia in three studies in patients with implantable cardioverter defibrillators. *Eur Heart J* 2009;30(7):820–6.

46. Burdge G. Alpha-linolenic acid metabolism in men and women: nutritional and biological implications. *Curr Opin Clin Nutr Metab Care* 2004;7:137–44.

47. Burdge GC, Calder PC. Conversion of alpha-linolenic acid to longer-chain polyunsaturated fatty acids in human adults. *Reprod Nutr Devel* 2005;45:581–97.

48. Mozaffarian D, Katan MB, Ascherio A, Stampfer MJ, Willett WC. Trans fatty acids and cardiovascular disease. *N Engl J Med* 2006;354:1601–13.

49. Mensink RP, Katan MB. Effect of dietary trans fatty acids on high-density and low-density lipoprotein cholesterol levels in healthy subjects. *N Engl J Med* 1990;323:439–45.

50. Lichtenstein AH, Ausman LA, Jalbert SM, Schaefer EJ. Comparison of different forms of hydrogenated fats on serum lipid levels in moderately hypercholesterolemic female and male subjects. *N Engl J Med* 1999;340:1933–40.

51. Ascherio A, Katan MB, Zock PL, Stampfer MJ, Willett WC. Trans fatty acids and coronary heart disease. *N Engl J Med* 1999;340:1994–8.

52. Finking G, Hanke H. Nikolaj Nikolajewitsch Anitschkow (1885–1964) established the cholesterol-fed rabbit as a model for atherosclerosis research. *Atherosclerosis* 1997;135:1–7.

53. Stamler J, Shekelle R. Dietary cholesterol and human coronary heart disease: the epidemiologic evidence. *Arch Pathol Lab Med* 1988;112:1032–40.

54. Katan MB, Beynen AC. Characteristics of human hypo- and hyperresponders to dietary cholesterol. *Am J Epidemiol* 1987;125:387–99.

55. Brown L, Rosner B, Willett WW, Sacks FM. Cholesterol-lowering effects of dietary fiber: a meta-analysis. *Am J Clin Nutr* 1999;69:30–42.

56. Anderson JW, Randles KM, Kendall CW, Jenkins DJ. Carbohydrate and fiber recommendations for individuals with diabetes: a quantitative assessment and meta-analysis of the evidence. *J Am Coll Nutr* 2004;23:5–17.

57. Queenan KM, Stewart ML, Smith KN, Thomas W, Fulcher RG, Slavin JL. Concentrated oat beta-glucan, a fermentable fiber, lowers serum cholesterol in hypercholesterolemic adults in a randomized controlled trial. *Nutr J* 2007;6:6.

58. Lipsky H, Gloger M, Frishman WH. Dietary fiber for reducing blood cholesterol. *J Clin Pharmacol* 1990;30:699–703.

59. Erkkila AT, Herrington DM, Mozaffarian D, Lichtenstein AH. Cereal fiber and whole-grain intake are associated with reduced progression of coronary-artery atherosclerosis in postmenopausal women with coronary artery disease. *Am Heart J* 2005;150(1):94–101.

60. Steffen LM, Jacobs DR, Jr., Stevens J, Shahar E, Carithers T, Folsom AR. Associations of whole-grain, refined-grain, and fruit and vegetable consumption with risks of

all-cause mortality and incident coronary artery disease and ischemic stroke: the Atherosclerosis Risk in Communities (ARIC) Study. *Am J Clin Nutr* 2003;78:383–90.

61. Schulze MB, Manson JE, Ludwig DS, et al. Sugar-sweetened beverages, weight gain, and incidence of type 2 diabetes in young and middle-aged women. *JAMA* 2004;292:927–34.

62. Ludwig DS, Peterson KE, Gortmaker SL. Relation between consumption of sugar-sweetened drinks and childhood obesity: a prospective, observational analysis. *Lancet* 2001;357:505–8.

63. Bray GA, Nielsen SJ, Popkin BM. Consumption of high-fructose corn syrup in beverages may play a role in the epidemic of obesity. *Am J Clin Nutr* 2004;79:537–43.

64. Stanhope KL, Griffen SC, Bair BR, Swarbrick MM, Keim NL, Havel PJ. Twenty-four-hour endocrine and metabolic profiles following consumption of high-fructose corn syrup-, sucrose-, fructose-, and glucose-sweetened beverages with meals. *Am J Clin Nutr* 2008;87:1194–203.

65. Sunehag AL, Toffolo G, Campioni M, Bier DM, Haymond MW. Short-term high dietary fructose intake had no effects on insulin sensitivity and secretion or glucose and lipid metabolism in healthy, obese adolescents. *J Pediatr Endocrinol Metab* 2008;21:225–35.

66. Wolf A, Bray GA, Popkin BM. A short history of beverages and how our body treats them. *Obes Rev* 2008;9:151–64.

67. Expert Panel on Detection, Evaluation, and Treatment of High Blood Cholesterol in Adults. Report of the National Cholesterol Education Program Expert Panel on Detection, Evaluation, and Treatment of High Blood Cholesterol in Adults. *Arch Intern Med* 1988;148:36–69.

68. Expert Panel on Detection, Evaluation, and Treatment of High Blood Cholesterol in Adults. Summary of the second report of the National Cholesterol Education Program (NCEP) Expert Panel on Detection, Evaluation, and Treatment of High Blood Cholesterol in Adults (Adult Treatment Panel II). *JAMA* 1993;269:3015–23.

69. Krauss RM, Deckelbaum RJ, Ernst N, et al. Dietary guidelines for healthy American adults. A statement for health professionals from the Nutrition Committee, American Heart Association. *Circulation* 1996;94:1795–800.

70. Krauss RM, Eckel RH, Howard B, et al. AHA Dietary Guidelines: revision 2000: a statement for healthcare professionals from the Nutrition Committee of the American Heart Association. *Circulation* 2000;102:2284–99.

71. Carroll KK, Kurowska EM. Soy consumption and cholesterol reduction: review of animal and human studies. *J Nutr* 1995;125(3 Suppl):594–7S.

72. Vega-Lopez S, Lichtenstein AH. Dietary protein type and cardiovascular disease risk factors. *Prev Cardiol* 2005;8:31–40.

73. Anderson JW, Johnstone BM, Cook-Newell ME. Meta-analysis of the effects of soy protein intake on serum lipids. *N Engl J Med* 1995;333:276–82.

74. Kreijkamp-Kaspers S, Kok L, Grobbee DE, et al. Effect of soy protein containing isoflavones on cognitive function, bone mineral density, and plasma lipids in postmenopausal women: a randomized controlled trial. *JAMA* 2004;292:65–74.

75. Sacks FM, Lichtenstein AH, Van Horn L, et al. Soy Protein, Isoflavones, and Cardiovascular Health: An American Heart Association Science Advisory for Professionals From the Nutrition Committee. *Circulation* 2006;113:1034–44.

76. Dewell A, Hollenbeck PLW, Hollenbeck CB. Clinical Review: A critical evaluation of the role of soy protein and isoflavone supplementation in the control of plasma cholesterol concentrations. *J Endocrinol Metab* 2006;91:772–80.

77. Balk E, Chung M, Chew P, et al. *Effects of Soy on Health Outcomes. Evidence Report/Technology Assessment No. 126.* (Prepared by Tufts-New England Medical Center Evidence-based Practice Center under Contract No. 290–02–0022.) AHRQ Publication No. 05-E024–2. Rockville, MD: Agency for Healthcare Research and Quality. 2005.

78. Lichtenstein AH, Jalbert SM, Adlercreutz H, et al. Lipoprotein response to diets high in soy or animal protein with and without isoflavones in moderately hypercholesterolemic subjects. *Arterioscler Thromb Vasc Biol* 2002;22:1852–8.

79. Dewell A, Hollenbeck PL, Hollenbeck CB. Clinical review: a critical evaluation of the role of soy protein and isoflavone supplementation in the control of plasma cholesterol concentrations. *J Clin Endocrinol Metab* 2006;91:772–80.

80. Demonty I, Lamarche B, Jones PJ. Role of isoflavones in the hypocholesterolemic effect of soy. *Nutr Rev* 2003;61(6 Pt 1):189–203.

81. Plat J, Mensink RP. Effects of plant stanol esters on LDL receptor protein expression and on LDL receptor and HMG-CoA reductase mRNA expression in mononuclear blood cells of healthy men and women. *FASEB J* 2002;16:258–60.

82. Katan MB, Grundy SM, Jones P, et al. Efficacy and safety of plant stanols and sterols in the management of blood cholesterol levels. *Mayo Clin Proc* 2003;78:965–78.

83. Ostlund RE, Jr. Phytosterols and cholesterol metabolism. *Curr Opin Lipidol* 2004;15:37–41.

84. de Jong A, Plat J, Mensink RP. Metabolic effects of plant sterols and stanols. *J Nutr Biochem* 2003;14:362–9.

85. Gylling H, Miettinen TA. The effect of plant stanol- and sterol-enriched foods on lipid metabolism, serum lipids and coronary heart disease. *Ann Clin Biochem* 2005;42 (Pt 4):254–63.

86. Law M. Plant sterol and stanol margarines and health. *BMJ* 2000;320:861–4.

87. Patch CS, Tapsell LC, Williams PG, Gordon M. Plant sterols as dietary adjuvants in the reduction of cardiovascular risk: theory and evidence. *Vasc Health Risk Manag* 2006;2:157–62.

88. Wilund KR, Yu L, Xu F, et al. No association between plasma levels of plant sterols and atherosclerosis in mice and men. *Arterioscler Thromb Vasc Biol* 2004;24: 2326–32.

89. Weingartner O, Lutjohann D, Ji S, et al. Vascular effects of diet supplementation with plant sterols. *J Am Coll Cardiol* 2008;51:1553–61.

90. Reiner Z, Tedeschi-Reiner E. Rice policosanol does not have any effects on blood coagulation factors in hypercholesterolemic patients. *Coll Antropol* 2007;31:1061–4.

91. Lin Y, Rudrum M, van der Wielen RP, et al. Wheat germ policosanol failed to lower plasma cholesterol in subjects with normal to mildly elevated cholesterol concentrations. *Metab Clin Exp* 2004;53:1309–14.

92. Varady KA, Wang Y, Jones PJ. Role of policosanols in the prevention and treatment of cardiovascular disease. *Nutr Rev* 2003;61:376–83.

93. Gouni-Berthold I, Berthold HK. Policosanol: clinical pharmacology and therapeutic significance of a new lipid-lowering agent. *Am Heart J* 2002;143:356–65.

94. Chen JT, Wesley R, Shamburek RD, Pucino F, Csako G. Meta-analysis of natural therapies for hyperlipidemia: plant sterols and stanols versus policosanol. *Pharmacotherapy* 2005;25:171–83.

95. Cubeddu LX, Cubeddu RJ, Heimowitz T, Restrepo B, Lamas GA, Weinberg GB. Comparative lipid-lowering effects of policosanol and atorvastatin: a randomized, parallel, double-blind, placebo-controlled trial. *Am Heart J* 2006;152:982.e1–5.

96. Kassis AN, Jones PJ. Lack of cholesterol-lowering efficacy of Cuban sugar cane policosanols in hypercholesterolemic persons. *Am J Clin Nutr* 2006;84:1003–8.

97. Dulin MF, Hatcher LF, Sasser HC, Barringer TA. Policosanol is ineffective in the treatment of hypercholesterolemia: a randomized controlled trial. *Am J Clin Nutr* 2006;84:1543–8.

98. Greyling A, De Witt C, Oosthuizen W, Jerling JC. Effects of a policosanol supplement on serum lipid concentrations in hypercholesterolaemic and heterozygous familial hypercholesterolaemic subjects. *Br J Nutr* 2006;95:968–75.

99. Berthold HK, Unverdorben S, Degenhardt R, Bulitta M, Gouni-Berthold I. Effect of policosanol on lipid levels among patients with hypercholesterolemia or combined hyperlipidemia: a randomized controlled trial. *JAMA* 2006;295:2262–9.

100. Stampfer MJ, Hennekens CH, Manson JE, Colditz GA, Rosner B, Willett WC. Vitamin E consumption and the risk of coronary disease in women. *N Engl J Med* 1993;328:1444–9.

101. Rimm EB, Stampfer MJ, Ascherio A, Giovannucci E, Colditz GA, Willett WC. Vitamin E consumption and the risk of coronary heart disease in men. *N Engl J Med* 1993;328:1450–6.

102. Pietinen P, Ascherio A, Korhonen P, et al. Intake of fatty acids and risk of coronary heart disease in a cohort of Finnish men. The Alpha-Tocopherol, Beta-Carotene Cancer Prevention Study. *Am J Epidemiol* 1997;145:876–87.

103. Gaziano JM, Manson JE, Branch LG, Colditz GA, Willett WC, Buring JE. A prospective study of consumption of carotenoids in fruits and vegetables and decreased cardiovascular mortality in the elderly. *Ann Epidemiol* 1995;5:255–60.

104. Gibbons RJ, Abrams J, Chatterjee K, et al. ACC/AHA 2002 guideline update for the management of patients with chronic stable angina – summary article: a report of the American College of Cardiology/American Heart Association Task Force on Practice Guidelines (Committee on the Management of Patients With Chronic Stable Angina). *Circulation* 2003;107:149–58.

105. Lichtenstein AH. Nutrient supplements and cardiovascular disease – a heartbreaking story. *J Lipid Res* 2009;50(Suppl):S429–33.

106. Sesso HD, Buring JE, Christen WG, et al. Vitamins E and C in the prevention of cardiovascular disease in men: the Physicians' Health Study II randomised controlled trial. *JAMA* 2008;300:2123–33.

Chapter 5

Physical activity and cardiovascular health

William E. Kraus and William L. Haskell

Introduction

Cardiovascular diseases account for the majority of premature morbidity and mortality in the developed world. The influence of physical activity and the prevention and treatment of cardiovascular disease is therefore of great importance. In addressing the effects of physical activity on cardiovascular health one must address not only the influence on the development of symptomatic disease (for example, heart attack and stroke) but also the influence on metabolic risk factors that are known to be contributory to the development of symptomatic disease and are often indicative of subclinical asymptomatic vascular pathology. Most of the modifiable risk factors for cardiovascular diseases are metabolic in nature and are, in turn, modifiable by changes in physical activity. These metabolic risk factors include hypertension, atherogenic dyslipidemia, the axis of insulin resistance to metabolic syndrome to frank diabetes mellitus, and obesity. In turn, both physical inactivity and poor cardiorespiratory fitness are major risk markers for cardiovascular diseases.

In general, the science about the relation between physical activity and cardiovascular outcomes addresses physical activity performed in the context of dedicated sessions of exercise. The assumption is that the specified exercise activity is performed in addition to and on top of normal physical activity performed as a part of activities of daily living. The information is primarily confined to dynamic aerobic (endurance) exercise, as the long-term cardiovascular prevention benefits of resistance and flexibility exercises are relatively little studied to date [1]. An exception to this occurs when measures of total activity or occupational activity are used as exposure variables in prospective

Metabolic Risk for Cardiovascular Disease, 1st edition. Edited by R. H. Eckel.
© 2011 American Heart Association. By Blackwell Publishing Ltd.

cohort or case–control studies. The literature to date is well summarized in the *Physical Activity Guidelines Advisory Committee Report* delivered in June 2008 [2] which resulted in the *Physical Activity Guidelines for Americans* released by the US Department of Health and Human Services in October of the same year [3].

Special considerations

The relation between dynamic aerobic exercise and cardiovascular health outcomes, including cardiorespiratory fitness, is complex and can be thought of as a series of point estimates within a three-dimensional matrix of continuous variables: exercise exposure, disease activity, and magnitude of the response. The major limitation to exercise exposure recommendations for cardiovascular health outcomes is that any recommendation poorly conveys the concept that the location of any point estimate along each of these three axes is along a continuum of exposure and response, and should not be viewed as an absolute threshold below which no benefits accrue and above which benefits always accrue.

Continuum of exercise exposure

It is well accepted that aerobic exercise exposures can be characterized by an interaction between bout intensity, frequency, duration, and longevity of the program [4,5]. The product of these characteristics can be thought of as volume and can be represented by the total energy expenditure (EE) of the exercise exposure. Exercise volume is referred to as the major determinant of the exercise recommendation in some recent statements [6], thus allowing for the mixing of exercise bouts of varying intensity, frequency, and duration to achieve the volume goal. Volume can be expressed as kcal/kg/week, MET-hr, or MET-min per week, or as a representative distance of walking or running for a man or woman of given body mass. Recommendations are thought to be adopted for an individual's lifetime; thus the time course over which the benefits are achieved is usually not of much concern. However, it is clear that most benefits resulting from changes in physical activity and exercise patterns accrue over days, weeks, months, and even years of exposure, and that the study and understanding of such time lines are of scientific and clinical interest and should be investigated further.

Most of the data from experimental studies regarding dose response address the issue of varying intensities of exercise and do not control for bout duration, frequency, or volume of the exercise exposure. In most observational studies the major variable used as an exposure is activity amount (e.g., minutes, MET-min/day, distance/wk) with the other exposure frequently being activity intensity. As is apparent from the relation of exercise volume to the other variables, one cannot fix volume and also simultaneously study either intensity, frequency, or duration effects while controlling the other two. For example, there exist relatively few interventional experimental studies that study exercise intensity while controlling for energy expenditure and there are even fewer that study frequency or duration effects while controlling for energy expenditure. This makes the construction of precise exercise dose for any given response problematic.

Continuum of disease state

Cardiovascular disease is a continuum from asymptomatic fatty vascular streaks, to severe symptomatic coronary heart disease, to fatal myocardial necrosis and death. The same is true for cerebrovascular disease and stroke. It is the goal of this chapter to focus primarily on primary cardiovascular disease prevention. As part of that process, we have explored some treatment effects on cardiovascular risk factors (atherogenic dyslipidemia and hypertension), the favorable modulation of which, by pharmacological or lifestyle therapy, has been shown to be related to reductions in cardiovascular risk as well. The modulation of these risk markers may be the mechanism through which physical activity acts to reduce cardiovascular clinical events, as well.

Continuum of the exercise responses

The response of biological parameters to dynamic aerobic exercise, and likely to resistance training as well, is a continuum from undetectable changes to highly significant, robust and clinical important ones, likely highly dependent on the exercise exposure variables previously discussed. Consequently, it is likely that there is not a given minimal intensity, frequency, duration, or volume of exercise that results in a favorable response for any given outcome. Similarly, there is unlikely to be a level of any of these exercise variables for *optimal* outcome. Furthermore, increases in exercise exposure do have tangible adverse outcomes that are primarily musculoskeletal and cardiovascular. Thus, potential increases in favorable outcomes of increasing exercise exposure must be balanced by the potential for increases in unfavorable outcomes.

Physical activity and cardiovascular morbidity and mortality

In *Physical Activity and Health: A Report of the Surgeon General* (released in 1996) [7] it was concluded that "The epidemiologic literature supports an inverse association and a dose–response gradient between physical activity level or cardiorespiratory fitness and both cardiovascular disease (CVD) in general and coronary heart disease (CHD) in particular. A smaller body of research supports similar findings for hypertension. The biological mechanisms for these effects are plausible and supported by a wealth of clinical and observational studies. It is unclear whether physical activity provides a protective role against stroke." Since 1996 there has been a large volume of research directed at better defining the relation between physical activity and various CVD clinical outcomes, the mechanisms by which the cardiovascular benefits of physical activity are likely mediated and the characteristics of the dose of activity (type, intensity, frequency, session duration, and amount) associated with lower CVD clinical event rates.

The results of recently published studies continue to support a strong inverse relation between the amount of habitual physical activity performed and CHD and CVD morbidity or mortality. For both men and women at middle age or older, remaining sedentary is a major independent risk factor, with persons reporting moderate amounts of activity having a 20% lower risk and those reporting activity of higher amounts or intensity having approximately a 30% lower risk than least active persons. These may be underestimates of the risk reductions because multivariate models in many studies include adjustments for hypertension, dyslipidemia, and glucose tolerance, conditions that may represent biological intermediates in the causal pathway. While still limited, data indicate habitual physical activity benefits the cardiovascular health of people of various race and ethnicities.

Coronary heart disease

The results of studies investigating the relation between habitual physical activity and CHD morbidity and/or mortality published since 1996 quite consistently show lower event rates in more physically active men and women than for their least active counterparts. Most notable has been the large increase in the number of studies that have included data on women, with 11 studies reporting data on women and two more with data on men and women combined. In studies of women reporting CHD clinical events more than 200 000 subjects between 20 and 85 years of age were included. For prospective cohort studies the median relative risk of having a CHD clinical event for women reporting participation in moderate intensity or amount of physical activity compared to women reporting no or only light intensity activity was 0.78 while the relative risk for women performing vigorous or high amounts of activity as compared to women reporting no or light activity was 0.62. These relative risks are quite similar to those resulting from a meta-analysis of many of the same studies that were published between 1996 and 2003 [8]. The conclusion from this meta-analysis for CHD was that physical activity was associated with a lower risk of CHD (as well as CVD and stroke) in a dose–response fashion with pooled relative risks for both moderate amounts and high amounts being significant when compared to no or light activity. In the three case–control studies reported for women, the median relative risk for moderate versus no or light activity was 0.62 and for vigorous intensity or high amounts of activity versus no or light activity it was 0.44.

Of studies reporting on CHD in men, 16 were prospective cohort studies and four case–control studies. Approximately 124 000 men, ranging in age between 15 and 96 years at baseline, were included as subjects. Most studies reported on leisure-time physical activity (LTPA) with a few studies including occupational activity, commuting, and sports participation. Among the prospective cohort studies the median relative risk for moderate intensity or amount of activity versus no or light activity was 0.81 and for vigorous intensity or high amounts versus light or no activity it was 0.68. For the four case–control studies the median relative risk for moderate versus no or light activity was 0.65 and for vigorous intensity or high amounts versus no or light activity it was 0.53. These values are of a similar magnitude to those reported in a systematic review of studies published between 1953 and 2000 [9] and in a meta-analysis published in 2000 that included data from studies published before and after the Report of the Surgeon General [10]. The lower CHD event rate for more active men was reported for both non-fatal and fatal CHD with no systematic difference in CHD incidence versus CHD mortality.

Two prospective cohort studies and four case–control studies were published where the results for CHD events for men and women were combined. In the prospective cohort studies the median relative risk for moderate intensity or amount versus no or light activity was 0.74 and 0.63 for high intensity or amount versus no or light activity. In the case–control studies the relative risk for moderate activity versus no or light activity was 0.61 and for high amounts or intensity versus no or light activity it was 0.48.

Cardiovascular disease

In 11 prospective cohort studies published since 1996 that included data on the relation between habitual physical activity and CVD in women, the median relative risk for those reporting moderate intensity or amount versus no or light activity was 0.80 and for vigorous versus no or light activity it was 0.72. In the one case–control study reporting on CVD in women the relative risk for moderate intensity versus no or light activity was 0.89 and for high versus no or light activity was 0.71. Here again, the amount and quality of data evaluating the relation between physical activity and CVD clinical events in women has substantially increased since 1996 with at least 350 000 women included in the reported studies. Overall, the CVD data reported on men are very similar to those for women: in 10 prospective cohort studies the median relative risk for CVD events for moderate versus no or light activity was 0.78 and for high intensity or amount versus no or light activity it was 0.70. In the one case–control study the relative risk for moderate versus light activity was 0.65 and 0.67 for high versus no or light activity. While data are not provided in the reports, it is very likely that a majority of the CVD events included in these studies were the result of coronary heart disease.

Dose–response relations

The inverse association between CVD clinical events and habitual physical activity exists across a wide range of types, amounts, and intensities of activity. People at highest risk are those who are least active and spend much of their day sitting. When compared to very sedentary persons, men and women who perform small amounts of moderate-intensity activity, such as 60 minutes per week of walking at a brisk pace, exhibit fewer CVD clinical events. People who perform more activity and/or at a faster pace are at an even lower risk with much of the benefit derived when men and women are performing ≥ 150 minutes per week of moderate-intensity physical activity (3 to less than 6 MET, where 1 metabolic equivalent, or MET, represents the energy expenditure rate at rest for any given individual). Greater amounts of activity appear to provide greater benefit but the shape of the dose–response relation has not been well defined. Vigorous activity (greater than 6 MET) when performed for a similar duration as moderate-intensity activity results in greater energy expenditure and is associated with lower CVD event rates. Much of the recent data are based on LTPA but performing physical activity during an occupation, around the home or while commuting all appear to provide benefit.

Cerebrovascular disease and stroke

More physically active men and women generally have a lower risk of stroke incidence or mortality than the least active, with more active persons demonstrating a 25 to 30% lower risk for all strokes. A favorable relation exists between physical activity level separately for ischemic and hemorrhagic stroke but the data on these stroke subtypes are still quite limited. The benefits appear to be derived from a variety of activity types including activity during leisure time, occupation, and walking. Overall, the relation between activity and stroke is not influenced by sex or age, but very little data exist for race and ethnicity other than for non-Hispanic whites.

Cardiovascular disease metabolic risk factors

Hypertension

Both aerobic and progressive resistance exercise yield important reductions in systolic and diastolic BP in adult humans, although the evidence for aerobic exercise is more convincing. Traditional aerobic training programs of 40 minutes of moderate-to-high intensity exercise training 3 to 5 times per week and that involve more than 800 MET-min (13 kcal/kg/week equivalent to 12 miles) of aerobic exercise per week appear to have reproducible effects on blood pressure reduction.

Ten meta-analyses dealing with the effects of aerobic exercise on resting BP in adults have been published since 1996 [11–20]. Six of these meta-analyses were comprehensive [11,14–18] while four others focused on either women [12], older adults [20], overweight and obese subjects [13], or walking as the only intervention [19]. The most recent and inclusive meta-analysis that included data partitioned according to hypertensive, pre-hypertensive, and normotensive adults included a total of 72 studies, 105 exercise groups, and 3936 men and women with a between study age range of 21 to 83 years (median 47 years) [17]. Across all categories, mean reductions in resting BP ranged from 2 to 5 mmHg (2% to 4%) for resting systolic BP and 2 to 3 mmHg (2% to 3%) for resting diastolic BP. Reductions were greater in hypertensive subjects (systolic BP, –6.9 mmHg; diastolic BP, –4.9 mmHg), than in pre-hypertensive (systolic BP, –3.1 mmHg; diastolic BP, –1.7 mmHg) and normotensive (systolic BP, –2.4 mmHg; diastolic BP, –1.6 mmHg) subjects. Changes were equivalent to relative reductions of approximately 5% for both resting systolic and diastolic BP in hypertensive subjects, 1% (systolic BP) and 2% (diastolic BP) in pre-hypertensive subjects, and 2% for both resting systolic and diastolic BP in normotensive subjects. Significant reductions of 3.3 mmHg (2%) and 3.5 mmHg (4%) were also observed for daytime ambulatory systolic and diastolic BP with no significant change in night-time BP. Changes in ambulatory BP are especially noteworthy since the assessment of such may better predict target end-organ damage [21]. Changes in both resting and ambulatory BP were independent of changes in bodyweight [17]. Similar changes in resting BP were also found for other more inclusive meta-analyses [11,14–18] as well as meta-analyses that focused on women [12], older adults [20], overweight and obese subjects [13], and walking [19].

Resistance exercise for blood pressure

Three meta-analyses [18,22,23] have been conducted on the effects of progressive resistance exercise on resting systolic and diastolic BP since the release of the Surgeon General's report on physical activity and health in 1996 [7]. However, since two of these included the same data [18,23], the discussion is limited to the one that contained more complete data on progressive resistance training [23]. This meta-analysis included nine randomized controlled trials and 12 exercise groups comprising 341 men and women, aged 20 to 72 years (median 69 years). The vast majority of subjects were not hypertensive (baseline resting systolic/diastolic BP values, 131.6/80.9 mmHg) [23]. With the one static (isometric) training study deleted from the analysis, a statistically significant reduction of 3.1 mmHg was found for resting diastolic BP with a trend for a reduction in systolic BP of 3.1 mmHg. Similar and statistically significant reductions of 2% and 4% were also found for resting systolic and diastolic BP in an earlier meta-analysis that excluded static training studies [22].

Atherogenic dyslipidemia

For the purposes herein, atherogenic dyslipidemia is defined as the presence of abnormally low serum concentrations of high-density lipoprotein (HDL) cholesterol, elevated concentrations of high triglycerides (TG) and small, dense low-density lipoprotein (LDL) cholesterol. The response of serum lipoproteins to changes in habitual physical activity have been well studied [24,25]. In general, both HDL cholesterol and serum TG reproducibly and favorably respond to changes in habitual physical activity, with increases in HDL cholesterol and decreases in serum TG, mostly related to the volume of exercise training and responding with threshold volumes in the range of 7 to 15 miles per week of regular exercise (equating to 700 to 1200 kcal of energy expenditure per week). There is some evidence that women are less responsive than men to change in habitual exercise, perhaps due to the observation that those with the largest baseline abnormalities (lower HDL and higher TG) gain the greatest benefit and men on average have lower HDL and higher TG than do women. However, when weekly volume or energy expenditure is controlled for men and women, the gender-related differences seems to be mitigated. There is some inconsistent evidence that LDL cholesterol may respond favorably to exercise training under some conditions; when it does, it is at the same volume thresholds as observed for HDL and TG. Finally, more recent studies have observed that fractionated serum lipoproteins respond favorably to aerobic exercise training in a dose–response fashion that is related to the weekly volume of exercise [26,27].

There is a large volume of information about the exercise responsiveness of serum lipoproteins and dose–response effects, much of which was accumulated prior to the Surgeon General's Report in 1996. For this review of the literature regarding the relationship between habitual exercise and serum lipoproteins, we have relied mostly upon meta-analyses and reviews assembled since 1996. The relevant information is well summarized in two relatively recent reviews from Durstine et al. [24] and Leon & Sanchez [25]. Most of the information prior to 1996 is based upon responses in total cholesterol and fractionated lipids – HDL cholesterol, LDL cholesterol, and TG. Recently there has been some new information on the response of lipoprotein subfractions to exercise training [26,27].

As illustrated in a recent meta-analysis of exercise-induced effects on HDL cholesterol [28], the volume of exercise exposure is the primary determinant of exercise-induced modulations of HDL at an EE threshold of 10 to 20 kcal/kg per week.

Women seem to be more resistant to modulation of TG through exercise interventions than are men, although this is not a consistent finding. In some studies, TG appears to be responsive to lower volumes of exercise training than is HDL, mimicking the responses in insulin action to which TG levels are closely tied [27]. However, the sum of the literature seems to indicate that triglycerides are consistently, reproducibly and robustly responsive to exercise training of volumes that are comparable to those that induce changes in HDL

(10 to 20 kcal/kg per week) and that lower-intensity exercise results in more sustained changes in TG once the training stimulus is removed [27].

LDL cholesterol is generally found not to be responsive to exercise training interventions. When LDL is modulated with lowering of serum concentrations, it requires approximately 12 kcal/kg/wk of exercise to favorably influence LDL. Recently, studies of the modulation of fractionated lipoproteins with exercise training have shown that HDL, TG, and LDL size and number are favorably modulated in a dose–response fashion to exercise training related to training volume and that 14 kcal/kg of exercise per week was required for an effect different from that of a sedentary control group [27]. More work is needed to understand the magnitude, consistency, and mechanism of these effects.

As noted previously, little is known about the effects of resistance training, alone or in combination with aerobic exercise training, on serum lipoprotein variables, although several studies in progress are poised to address this issue.

Vascular health

Habitual aerobic exercise appears to induce favorable responses in measures of vascular health. Exercise training initially increases brachial artery flow-mediated dilation (BAFMD – a measure of endothelial vascular health) with later normalization of BAFMD as vessels become structurally larger. Habitual aerobic exercise appears to slow the progression of age-related central arterial stiffening in healthy subjects. Increased levels of habitual physical activity are associated with slowed progression of carotid intimal medial thickening in cross-sectional and prospective cohort studies. No significant dose–response data are available for any of these measures.

Brachial artery flow-mediated dilation

Dysfunction of endothelial cells is an early event in the process of atherosclerosis [29], and is associated with risk factors for cardiovascular disease [30–32]. These relations have led to the use of endothelium-mediated vascular responsiveness as a surrogate biomarker of vascular health. BAFMD is a non-invasive measure of endothelial function, has been shown to correlate with measures of coronary artery function [33,34], and independently predict cardiovascular events in patients with established disease [35–40]. Due to the non-invasive nature and relative ease of use of BAFMD it has become increasingly utilized as a research tool to monitor the efficacy of interventions on vascular health.

Carotid intimal-medial thickening

Most studies on this outcome are prospective or case–control observational studies. There are relatively few studies which examine the effects of exercise training on carotid intimal-medial thickening (CIMT) or progression. From seven available cross-sectional studies, four report lower CIMT in subjects with higher physical activity levels [41,42] or higher peak VO_2 [43,44]. The remaining three studies found no difference between active and sedentary groups [45–47]. The discrepancies between these study results could be related to differences in age and health of participants, methods of activity measurement and reporting, concomitant lifestyle changes, length of measurement, and differences in the techniques used to quantify CIMT.

The results from interventional studies make it even more difficult to draw definitive conclusions. From nine available studies [47–55], only three appear to have reported the effects of exercise training isolated from other concurrent treatments [47,50,52] and all of these showed no effect [55]. Unfortunately two of these studies were underpowered to detect CIMT progression and the third was a pharmaceutical trial where exercise served as a control and no changes were observed after four years [53].

A lack of adequately powered exercise interventional studies is understandable if one considers the small size of the pooled annual rates of changes in CIMT progression that occur among control groups from randomized placebo-controlled trials. For studies using multiple IMT measures from several interrogation angles and carotid segments, the mean maximum progression rate was 0.0176 mm/y with a median SD of 0.05 [56]. Given that sample size calculations rely heavily on rates of change, precision of the measurement, and projected effectiveness of the intervention, the subject numbers required and length of exercise training assessment period would have to be much longer than is traditional in such studies. For example for a 30% treatment effect, average change in mean maximum CIMT of 0.0352 ± 0.05 mm over 2 years, and using a two-tailed alpha, one would need 468 subjects in each arm of the trial to have 90% power.

Arterial stiffness

Central arterial stiffening occurs with aging [57] but is often both a consequence and mechanism of atherosclerotic vasculopathy. The investigation of arterial stiffness has increased in recent years due to the development of non-invasive assessment techniques [58–60]. However, there appears to be a lack of consensus regarding the most accurate and reliable method to measure arterial stiffness, complicating the determination of the efficacy of exercise training responses. The most frequently reported assessment methodologies are pulse wave velocity, pulse wave analysis, and distensibility/compliance (Δ diameter/Δ pressure).

Using these outcome measures, habitual aerobic exercise appears to slow the progression of age-related central arterial stiffening in healthy subjects as reported in several cross-sectional studies [57,61–63]. Furthermore, four training intervention studies report significant improvements in measures of central stiffness across gender and age ranges [61–64]. Interestingly, the benefits in central elastic arteries were not replicated in peripheral muscular arteries [62,65], suggesting that training-specific responses or different mechanisms are active in different arterial beds.

The effects of resistance training on central arterial stiffness are conflicting. Two cross-sectional studies report a decrease in central but not peripheral arterial compliance in comparison to sedentary controls [63,66]. In contrast, from four available case–controlled interventional studies, two report increases in measures of central arterial stiffness [67,68] and two report no significant effect [69,70]. These differences appear to be intensity-related with higher training intensities eliciting higher central stiffness values. Clearly, larger-scale prospective studies are warranted to clarify these discrepancies and to further elucidate the possible mechanisms involved in the observed changes.

Physical activity and cardiorespiratory fitness

Cardiorespiratory fitness is a sensitive and useful measure of changes in physical activity. It demonstrates dose–response relations between exercise volume and the various components of exercise exposure (intensity, frequency, duration, and longevity). It appears that one can acquire exercise exposure in bouts as small as 10 minutes each, while holding volume constant, although this is still somewhat controversial. Changes in fitness during exercise interventions correspond with changes in cardiovascular risk, but do not always correspond with changes in cardiovascular risk factors.

Cardiorespiratory fitness, as measured by a number of relatively simple and inexpensive clinical maneuvers, provides strong and independent prognostic information about overall morbidity and mortality. This relationship extends to men, women, and adolescents. It is valid in apparently healthy individuals; in patients with a broad range of maladies, including several types of cancer and cardiovascular disease; and in at-risk individuals with diabetes mellitus, metabolic syndrome, and hypertension [7,71,72]. Fitness is also a marker for functional capacity and ability to perform activities of daily living, especially in older individuals. Finally, it is used as an outcome measure of adherence and physical activity exposure in interventional studies. For example, men who improve their fitness (as assessed by exercise duration) improve their cardiovascular risk. In one report, there was an 8% lower long-term cardiovascular risk for every minute increase in exercise capacity [73]. Due to the correlation between fitness and health status, the responsiveness to changes in physical activity and its usefulness as a marker of physical activity levels, cardiorespiratory fitness is an important health outcome measure in and of itself and is often quoted as an outcome in health-related physical activity studies. That said, favorable changes in fitness do not always correspond to change in health outcomes in response to exercise recommendations [74].

Aerobic exercise training and heart failure

The recently completed HF-ACTION study produced useful information about the role of physical activity and exercise in the prevention of morbidity and mortality, as well as improvement in quality of life in patients with functional class II to IV congestive heart failure [75]. The population size of 2331 was randomized in a 1:1 fashion to supervised versus home-based exercise training for a period of from one to four years of follow-up where the exercise training group received supervised exercise for six months and were then transitioned to home-based exercise. The primary outcome of all-cause hospitalization and all-cause mortality showed a trend for significance and when the groups were adjusted for predictive outcome variables the analysis showed a significant benefit for exercise training [76]. This was also true for the cardiovascular hospitalization and mortality, heart failure hospitalization and cardiovascular mortality, as well as quality-of-life endpoints [77].

Physical Activity Guidelines for Americans

The release of the *Physical Activity Guidelines for Americans* by the Department of Health and Human Services in October 2008 [3] incorporated the findings of a thorough review of the literature relating physical inactivity, physical activity, and dedicated exercise to health outcomes ranging from body mass and body composition, to physical function, to metabolic diseases, to cardiovascular disease and cancer in youth, adults, and older Americans [2]. The findings and recommendations (Tables 5.1 and 5.2) address observations regarding aerobic, resistance and flexibility exercise, although the number of randomized clinical studies in populations of sufficient size to draw reasoned conclusions is limited for resistance and flexibility exercise. This should be an area of focus for future research.

Physical activity assessment and counseling in the clinic setting

The role of the physician in behavior change cannot be underestimated and this is as true for physical activity counseling as it is for nutrition, weight loss, and smoking cessation counseling [78,79]. The details of this issue are complex and are discussed in detail in seminal articles in the field. However, the physician can start by assessing physical activity in the clinical setting, by making it a "vital sign" that can be recorded and followed in parallel to others such as blood pressure and pulse, body mass and waist circumference, and others. Asking about and assessing physical activity with all patients, making it in essence a vital sign in every clinic visit, provides evidence to the patient that the clinician believes both that physical activity level is as important as other vital signs to the assessment of health status and that the patient should also. Until recently a readily administered physical activity assessment tool was not available. With the development of the Stanford Brief Physical Activity Score

Table 5.1 Classification of total weekly amounts of aerobic physical activity into four categories

Levels of physical activity	Range of moderate-intensity minutes a week	Summary of overal health benefits	Comment
Inactive	No activity beyond baseline	None	Being inactive is unhealthy
Low	Activity beyond baseline but fewer than 150 minutes per week	Some	Low levels of activity are clearly preferable to an inactive liefstyle
Medium	150 minutes to 300 minutes per week	Substantial	Activity at the high end of this range has additional and more extensive health benefits than activity at the low end
High	More than 300 minutes per week	Additional	Current science does not allow researchers to identify an upper limit of activity above which there are no additional health benefits

Source: *Physical Activity Guidelines for Americans*, US Dept of Health and Human Services, 2008; http://www.health.gov/paguidelines/ [3].

Table 5.2 Summary of the physical activity guidelines for Americans – adults

Minimum levels of physical activity for adults
Aerobic activity
- 150 minutes (30 minutes on 5 days per week) of moderate intensity aerobic activity
- 75 minutes (15 minutes on 5 days per week) of vigorous intensity exercise
- Any equivalent combination (for example 30 minutes of moderate intensity exercise on 2 days and 15 minutes of vigorous activity on 3 days)

Muscle strengthening activity
- Muscle strengthening activities involving all major musclr groups on 2 or more days per week

For additional benefits
- 300 minutes per week of moderate intensity activity
- 150 minutes of vigorous intensity exercise
- Any equivalent combination

Source: Physical Activity Guidelines Advisory Committee [2].

[80], a two-question self-assessment tool that can be administered in the waiting room, this barrier has been removed. The tool has been validated in working and retired populations, and also against the much longer and burdensome 7-Day Physical Activity Recall that is a standard in the research field [81]. It is reliable and accurate, allowing longitudinal assessment to be available for any given individual and the simple score can be recorded along with waist circumference, body mass index, and other more traditional markers of health status (e.g., temperature, pulse, and heart rate) as part of a normal vital sign profile.

Summary

The weight of evidence points toward a favorable relation between increases in habitual dynamic aerobic exercise and cardiovascular health outcomes, including coronary heart disease morbidity and mortality, stroke, control of blood pressure, atherogenic dyslipidemia, vascular function measures, and cardiorespiratory fitness. In many of these outcomes, including cardiovascular morbidity and mortality, there appears to be a more favorable response with increasing intensity of exercise bouts, although exercise volume is poorly controlled in some studies and may be the important mediating exercise parameter. Also, the more powerful relation between exercise intensity and outcomes does not hold for all outcomes in experimental studies, especially when weekly volume or energy expenditure is held constant [82]. In many if not most cardiovascular outcomes, favorable responses are notable and reproducible when the volume of physical activity exceeds 13 kcal/kg per week of energy expenditure. A combination of endurance exercise bouts with different intensities, durations, and frequencies per day and week can achieve this level of exercise, which is equivalent to 12 miles per week of walking or jogging at any intensity. As energy expenditure at a given perceived intensity is highly dependent upon baseline fitness level, gender, and type of activity, a volume target can be individualized with adjustment of bout intensity, duration, and frequency both initially and as greater fitness levels are achieved. Given that more volume is likely to result in greater benefits but also higher injury and cardiovascular risk, the ultimate volume goal should be approached upon the initiation of a program gradually, especially in initially sedentary individuals. As noted previously, little is known about the effects of resistance training, alone or in combination with aerobic exercise training, on cardiovascular risk parameters, although several studies in progress are poised to address this issue. Physicians in practice should assess physical activity levels at every visit, using tools readily accessible to the physician and patient and use this information to counsel about physical activity levels in daily life.

References

1. Williams MA, Haskell WL, Ades PA, et al. Resistance exercise in individuals with and without cardiovascular disease: 2007 update: a scientific statement from the American Heart Association Council on Clinical Cardiology and Council on Nutrition, Physical Activity, and Metabolism. *Circulation* 2007;116:572–84.

2. Physical Activity Guidelines Advisory Committee. *Physical Activity Guidelines Advisory Committee Report*. US Department of Health and Human Services: Washington DC. 2008.

3. *Physical Activity Guidelines for Americans*. US Department of Health and Human Services, 2008; http://www.health.gov/paguidelines/

4. Swain DP, Franklin BA. VO(2) reserve and the minimal intensity for improving cardiorespiratory fitness. *Med Sci Sports Exerc* 2002;34:152–7.

5. Wenger HA, Bell GJ. The interactions of intensity, frequency and duration of exercise training in altering cardiorespiratory fitness. *Sports Med* 1986;3:346–56.

6. Haskell WL, Lee IM, Pate RR, et al. Physical activity and public health: updated recommendation for adults from the American College of Sports Medicine and the American Heart Association. *Circulation* 2007;116:1081–93.

7. US Department of Health and Human Services. *Physical Activity and Health: A Report of the Surgeon General*. Atlanta, GA: US Department of Health and Human Services, Centers for Disease Control and Prevention, National Center for Chronic Disease Prevention and Health Promotion. 1996.

8. Oguma Y, Shinoda-Tagawa T. Physical activity decreases cardiovascular disease risk in women: review and meta-analysis. *Am J Prev Med* 2004;26:407–18.

9. Kohl HW, 3rd. Physical activity and cardiovascular disease: evidence for a dose response. *Med Sci Sports Exerc* 2001;33:S472–83; discussion S93–4.

10. Thompson PD, Buchner D, Pina IL, et al. Exercise and physical activity in the prevention and treatment of atherosclerotic cardiovascular disease: a statement from the Council on Clinical Cardiology (Subcommittee on Exercise, Rehabilitation, and Prevention) and the Council on Nutrition, Physical Activity, and Metabolism (Subcommittee on Physical Activity). *Circulation* 2003;107:3109 16.

11. Halbert JA, Silagy CA, Finucane P, Withers RT, Hamdorf PA, Andrews GR. The effectiveness of exercise training in lowering blood pressure: a meta-analysis of randomised controlled trials of 4 weeks or longer. *J Hum Hypertens* 1997;11:641–9.

12. Kelley GA. Aerobic exercise and resting blood pressure among women: a meta-analysis. *Prev Med* 1999;28:264–75.

13. Fagard RH. Physical activity in the prevention and treatment of hypertension in the obese. *Med Sci Sports Exerc* 1999;31:S624–30.

14. Fagard RH. Exercise characteristics and the blood pressure response to dynamic physical training. *Med Sci Sports Exerc* 2001;33:S484–92.

15. Kelley GA, Kelley KS, Tran ZV. Aerobic exercise and resting blood pressure: a meta-analytic review of randomized controlled trials. *Prev Cardiol* 2001;4:73–80.

16. Whelton SP, Chin A, Xin X, He J. Effect of aerobic exercise on blood pressure: a meta-analysis of randomized, controlled trials. *Ann Intern Med* 2002;136:493–503.

17. Cornelissen VA, Fagard RH. Effects of endurance training on blood pressure, blood pressure-regulating mechanisms, and cardiovascular risk factors. *Hypertension* 2005;46:667–75.

18. Fagard RH, Cornelissen VA. Effect of exercise on blood pressure control in hypertensive patients. *Eur J Cardiovasc Prev Rehabil* 2007;14:12–17.

19. Murphy MH, Nevill AM, Murtagh EM, Holder RL. The effect of walking on fitness, fatness and resting blood pressure: a meta-analysis of randomised, controlled trials. *Prev Med* 2007;44:377–85.

20. Kelley GA, Kelley KS. Aerobic exercise and resting blood pressure in older adults: a meta-analytic review of randomized controlled trials. *J Gerontol Med Sci* 2001;56A:M298–303.

21. Chobanian AV, Bakris GL, Black HR, et al. The Seventh Report of the Joint National Committee on Prevention, Detection, Evaluation, and Treatment of High Blood Pressure: The JNC 7 Report. *JAMA* 2003;289:2560–71.

22. Kelley GA, Kelley KS. Progressive resistance exercise and resting blood pressure: a meta-analysis of randomized controlled trials. *Hypertension* 2000;35:838–43.

23. Cornelissen VA, Fagard RH. Effect of resistance training on resting blood pressure: a meta-analysis of randomized controlled trials. *J Hypertens* 2005;23:251–9.

24. Durstine JL, Grandjean PW, Davis PG, Ferguson MA, Alderson NL, DuBose KD. Blood lipid and lipoprotein adaptations to exercise: a quantitative analysis. *Sports Med* 2001;31:1033–62.

25. Leon AS, Sanchez OA. Response of blood lipids to exercise training alone or combined with dietary intervention. *Med Sci Sports Exerc* 2001;33:S502–15; discussion S28–9.

26. Kraus WE, Houmard JA, Duscha BD, et al. Effects of the amount and intensity of exercise on plasma lipoproteins. *N Engl J Med* 2002;347:1483–92.

27. Slentz CA, Houmard JA, Johnson JL, et al. Inactivity, exercise training and detraining, and plasma lipoproteins. STRRIDE: a randomized, controlled study of exercise intensity and amount. *J Appl Physiol* 2007;103:432–42.

28. Kodama, S., Tanaka S, Saito K, et al. Effect of aerobic exercise training on serum levels of high-density lipoprotein cholesterol: a meta-analysis. *Arch Intern Med* 167:999–1008.

29. Verma S, Buchanan MR, Anderson TR. Endothelial function testing as a biomarker of vascular disease. *Circulation* 2003;108:2054–9.

30. Celermajer DS, Sorensen KE, Georgakopoulos D, et al. Cigarette smoking is associated with dose-related and potentially reversable impairment of endothelium dependent dilation in healthy young adults. *Circulation* 1993;88:2149–55.

31. Celermajer DS, Sorensen KE, Spiegelhalter DJ, Georgapoulos D, Robinson J, Deanfield JE. Aging is associated with endothelial dysfunction in healthy men years before the age-related decline in women. *J Am Coll Cardiol* 1994;24:471–6.

32. Taddei S, Virdis A, Mattei P, et al. Aging and endothelial function in normotensive subjects and patients with essential hypertension. *Circulation* 1995;91:1981–7.

33. Anderson TJ, Uehata A, Gerhard MD, et al. Close relation of endothelial function in the human coronary and peripheral circulations. *J Am Coll Cardiol* 1995;26:1235–41.

34. Takase B, Uehata A, Akima T, et al. Endothelium-dependent flow-mediated vasodilation in coronary and brachial arteries in suspected coronary artery disease. *Am J Cardiol* 1998;82:1535–9.

35. Neunteufl T, Katzenschlager R, Hassan A, et al. Systemic endothelial dysfunction is related to the extent and severity of coronary artery disease. *Atherosclerosis* 1997;129:111–18.

36. Neunteufl T, Heher S, Katzenschlager R, et al. Late prognostic value of flow-mediated dilation in the brachial artery of patients with chest pain. *Am J Cardiol* 2000;86:207–10.

37. Kaku B, Mizuno S, Ohsato K, et al. The correlation between coronary stenosis index and flow-mediated dilation of the brachial artery. *Jap Circ J* 1998;62:425–30.

38. Perticone F, Ceravolo R, Pujia A, et al. Prognostic significance of endothelial dysfunction in hypertensive patients. *Circulation* 2001;104:191–6.

39. Gokce N, Holbrook M, Hunter LM, et al. Acute effects of vasoactive drug treatment on brachial artery reactivity. *J Am Coll Cardiol* 2002;40:761–5.

40. Brevetti G, Silvestro A, Schiano V, Chiariello M. Endothelial dysfunction and cardiovascular risk protection in periperal arterial disease: additive value of flow-mediated dilation to ankle-brachial pressure index. *Circulation* 2003;108:2093–8.

41. Folsom AR, Eckfeldt JH, Weitzman S, et al. Relation of carotid artery wall thickness to diabetes mellitus, fasting glucose and insulin, body size, and physical activity. Atherosclerosis Risk in Communities (ARIC) Study Investigators. *Stroke* 1994;25:66–73.

42. Watarai T, Yamasaki Y, Ikeda M, et al. Insulin resistance contributes to carotid arterial wall thickness in patients with non-insulin-dependent-diabetes mellitus. *Endocr J* 1999;96:629–38.

43. Rauramaa R, Rankinen T, Tuomainen P, Vaisanen S, Mercuri M. Inverse relationship between cardiorespiratory fitness and carotid atherosclerosis. *Atherosclerosis* 1995;112:213–21.

44. Hagg U, Wandt B, Bergstrom G, Volkmann R, Gan L-M. Physical exercise capacity is associated with coronary and peripheral vascular function in healthy young adults. *Am J Physiol Heart Circ Physiol* 2005;289:H1627–34.

45. American College of Sports Medicine, American Heart Association. Recommendations for cardiovascular screening, staffing, and emergency policies at health/fitness facillities. *Med Sci Sports Exerc* 1998;30:1009–18.

46. Schmidt-Trucksass A, Grathwohl D, Frey I, et al. Relation of leisure-time physical activity to structural and functional arterial properties of the common carotid artery in male subjects. *Atherosclerosis* 1999;145:107–14.

47. Tanaka H, Seals DR, Monahan KD, Clevenger CM, DeSouza CA, Dinenno FA. Regular aerobic exercise and the age-related increase in carotid artery intima-media thickness in healthy men. *J Appl Physiol* 2002;92:1458–64.

48. Markus RA, Mack WJ, Azen SP, Hodis HN. Influence of lifestyle modification on atherosclerotic progression determined by ultrasonographic change in the common carotid intima-media thickness. *Am J Clin Nutr* 1997;65:1000–4.

49. Okada K, Maeda N, Tatsukawa M, Shimizu C, Sawayama Y, Hayashi J. The influence of lifestyle modification on carotid artery intima-media thickness in a suburban Japanese population. *Atherosclerosis* 2004;173:327–35.

50. Rauramaa R, Halonen P, Vaisanen SB, et al. Effects of aerobic physical exercise on inflammation and atherosclerosis in men: the DNASCO study: a six-year randomized, controlled trial. *Ann Intern Med* 2004;140:1007–14.

51. Wildman RP, Schott LL, Brockwell S, Kuller LH, Sutton-Tyrrell K. A dietary and exercise intervention slows menopause-associated progression of subclinical atherosclerosis as measured by intima-media thickness of the carotid arteries. *J Am Coll Cardiol* 2004;44:579–85.

52. Anderssen SA, Hjelstuen AK, Hjermann I, Bjerkan K, Holme I. Fluvastatin and lifestyle modification for reduction of carotid intima-media thickness and left ventricular mass progression in drug-treated hypertensives. *Atherosclerosis* 2005;178:387–97.

53. Chan SY, Mancini GBJ, Burns S, et al. Dietary measures and exercise training contribute to improvement of endothelial function and atherosclerosis even in patients given intensive pharmacologic therapy. *J Cardiopulm Rehab* 2006;26: 288–93.

54. Meyer AA, Kundt G, Lenschow U, Schuff-Werner P, Kienast W. Improvement of early vascular changes and cardiovascular risk factors in obese children after a six-month exercise program. *J Amer Coll Cardiol* 2006;48:1865–70.

55. Kadoglou NPE, Iliadis F, Liapis CD. Exercise and carotid atherosclerosis. *Eur J Vasc Endovasc Surg* 2008;35:264–72.

56. Bots ML, Evans GW, Riley WA, Grobbee DE. Carotid intima-media thickness measurements in intervention studies: design options, progression rates, and sample size considerations: a point of view. *Stroke* 2003;34:2985–94.

57. Vaitkevicius PV, Fleg JL, Engel JH, et al. Effects of age and aerobic capacity on arterial stiffness in healthy adults. *Circulation* 1993;88:1456–62.

58. O'Rourke MF, Staessen JA, Vlachopoulos C, Duprez D, Plante GeE. Clinical applications of arterial stiffness; definitions and reference values. *Am J Hypertens* 2002;15:426–44.

59. Van Bortel LM, Duprez D, Starmans-Kool MJ, et al. Clinical applications of arterial stiffness, Task Force III: recommendations for user procedures. *Am J Hypertens* 2002;15:445–52.

60. Pannier BM, Avolio AP, Hoeks A, Mancia G, Takazawa K. Methods and devices for measuring arterial compliance in humans. *Am J Hypertens* 2002;15:743–53.

61. Tanaka H, DeSouza CA, Seals DR. Absence of age-related increase in central arterial stiffness in physically active women. *Arterioscler Thromb Vasc Biol* 1998;18:127–32.

62. Tanaka H, Dinenno FA, Monahan KD, Clevenger CM, DeSouza CA, Seals DR. Aging, habitual exercise, and dynamic arterial compliance. *Circulation* 2000;102: 1270–5.

63. Miyachi M, Donato AJ, Yamamoto K, et al. Greater age-related reductions in central arterial compliance in resistance-trained men. *Hypertension* 2003;41:130–5.

64. Ikegami H, Satake M, Kurokawa T, Tan N, Sugiura T, Yamazaki Y. Effects of physical training on body composition, respiro-circulatory functions, blood constituents, and physical abilities. Part 1: men aged 30 years. *J Phys Fitness Japan* 1983;32:302–9.

65. Moreau KL, Donato AJ, Seals DR, DeSouza CA, Tanaka H. Regular exercise, hormone replacement therapy and the age-related decline in carotid arterial compliance in healthy women. *Cardiovasc Res* 2003;57:861–8.

66. Bertovic DA, Waddell TK, Gatzka CD, Cameron JD, Dart AM, Kingwell BA. Muscular strength training is associated with low arterial compliance and high pulse pressure. *Hypertension* 1999;33:1385–91.

67. Miyachi M, Kawano H, Sugawara J, et al. Unfavorable effects of resistance training on central arterial compliance: a randomized intervention atudy. *Circulation* 2004;110:2858–63.

68. Cortez-Cooper MY, DeVan AE, Anton MM, et al. Effects of high intensity resistance training on arterial stiffness and wave reflection in women. *Am J Hypertens* 2005;18:930–4.

69. Casey DP, Beck DT, Braith RW. Progressive resistance training without volume increases does not alter arterial stiffness and aortic wave reflection. *Exper Biol Med* 2007;232:1228–35.

70. Casey DP, Pierce GL, Howe KS, Mering MC, Braith RW. Effect of resistance training on arterial wave reflection and brachial artery reactivity in normotensive postmenopausal women. *Eur J Appl Physiol* 2007;100:403–8.

71. Blair SN, Kohl HW, 3rd, Paffenbarger RS, Jr., Clark DG, Cooper KH, Gibbons LW. Physical fitness and all-cause mortality: a prospective study of healthy men and women. *JAMA* 1989;262:2395–401.

72. Lee S, Kuk JL, Katzmarzyk PT, Blair SN, Church TS, Ross R. Cardiorespiratory fitness attenuates metabolic risk independent of abdominal subcutaneous and visceral fat in men. *Diabetes Care* 2005;28:895–901.

73. Blair SN, Kampert JB, Kohl HW, 3rd, et al. Influences of cardiorespiratory fitness and other precursors on cardiovascular disease and all-cause mortality in men and women. *JAMA* 1996;276:205–10.

74. Johnson JL, Slentz CA, Houmard JA, et al. Exercise training amount and intensity effects on metabolic syndrome (from Studies of a Targeted Risk Reduction Intervention through Defined Exercise). *Am J Cardiol* 2007;100:1759–66.

75. Whellan DJ, O'Connor CM, Lee KL, et al. Heart failure and a controlled trial investigating outcomes of exercise training (HF-ACTION): design and rationale. *Am Heart J* 2007;153:201–11.

76. O'Connor CM, Whellan DJ, Lee KL, et al. Efficacy and safety of exercise training in patients with chronic heart failure: HF-ACTION randomized controlled trial. *JAMA* 2009;301:1439–50.

77. Flynn KE, Pina IL, Whellan DJ, et al. Effects of exercise training on health status in patients with chronic heart failure: HF-ACTION randomized controlled trial. *JAMA* 2009;301:1451–9.

78. Pearson TA, Kopin LA. Compliance of providers to guidelines. In: Burke LE, Ockene IS (eds) *Compliance in Healthcare Research*. Armonk, NY: Futura Publishing Co. 2001; pp. 285–97.

79. Pearson TA, McBride PE, Miller NH, S.C. S. 27th Bethesda Conference: matching the intensity of risk factor management with the hazard for coronary disease events. Task Force 8: Organization of Preventive Cardiology Service. *J Am Coll Cardiol* 1996: 1039–47.

80. Taylor-Piliae RE, Norton LC, Haskell WL, et al. Validation of a new brief physical activity survey among men and women aged 60–69 years. *Am J Epidemiol* 2006;164:598–606.

81. Taylor-Piliae RE, Haskell WL, Iribarren C, et al. Clinical utility of the Stanford brief activity survey in men and women with early-onset coronary artery disease. *J Cardiopulm Rehabil Prev* 2007;27:227–32.

82. Swain DP, Franklin BA. Comparison of cardioprotective benefits of vigorous versus moderate intensity aerobic exercise. *Am J Cardiol* 2006;97:141–7.

Chapter 6

The obesity epidemic and cardiovascular risk

Paul Poirier

Introduction

Studies have permitted the identification of major risk factors for cardiovascular disease (CVD). Some of them are non-modifiable and include age, sex, and genetic susceptibility to CVD but many reflect our lifestyle habits such as smoking, blood pressure, plasma lipid/lipoprotein and glucose levels, diabetes, deleterious diet, lack of physical activity/exercise, overweight and obesity, and psychosocial factors [1]. Obesity has reached epidemic proportions in the USA as well as much of the industrialized world, and is increasing in prevalence in the developing world [2,3]. In the most widely used classification of body mass, bodyweight is expressed in terms of body mass index (BMI) [2]. In adults, obesity is defined as a BMI $\geq 30 \text{ kg/m}^2$, which is further subdivided into classes (Table 6.1) [3,4]. In youths between 2 and 18 years of age, obesity is defined as a BMI of 95th percentile or BMI of $\geq 30 \text{ kg/m}^2$, whichever is lower. For children under 2 years of age, BMI normative values are not available [3].

The most rapidly growing segment of the obese adult population comprises the severely obese individuals [5]. Between 1986 and 2000, individuals with a BMI > 30, 40, and 50 kg/m^2 are reported to have doubled, quadrupled, and quintupled, respectively, in the USA [6]. Data indicate that extreme obesity in children is increasing in prevalence, and these children are at high risk for multiple CVD risk factors. A proposed definition of severe childhood obesity is 99th percentile BMI, which correspond to a BMI of ~ 30 to 32 kg/m^2 for youths 10 to 12 years of age and 34 kg/m^2 for youths 14 to 16 years of age [3].

Thus, the improvement in risk factor recognition and management that developed through the years in modern cardiology may be counteracted by the

Metabolic Risk for Cardiovascular Disease, 1st edition. Edited by R. H. Eckel.
© 2011 American Heart Association. By Blackwell Publishing Ltd.

Table 6.1 Classification of body weight according to body mass index in adults and in children

Adults	
Underweight:	BMI $< 18.5 \, \text{kg}/\text{m}^2$
Normal or acceptable weight:	BMI 18.5–$24.9 \, \text{kg}/\text{m}^2$
Overweight:	BMI 25–$29.9 \, \text{kg}/\text{m}^2$
Obese:	BMI $\geq 30 \, \text{kg}/\text{m}^2$
Class 1:	BMI 30–$34.9 \, \text{kg}/\text{m}^2$
Class 2:	BMI 35.0–$39.9 \, \text{kg}/\text{m}^2$
Class 3:	BMI $\geq 40 \, \text{kg}/\text{m}^2$ (severe, extreme or morbid obesity)
Class 4:	BMI $\geq 50 \, \text{kg}/\text{m}^2$
Class 5:	BMI $\geq 60 \, \text{kg}/\text{m}^2$
Children (youths between 2 to 18 years of age)	
Overweight:	BMI of 85th to 94th percentile
Obese:	BMI of 95th percentile or BMI of $\geq 30 \, \text{kg}/\text{m}^2$, whichever is lower
Severe obesity:	99th percentile BMI
~ 30 to $32 \, \text{kg}/\text{m}^2$ for youths 10–12 years of age	
$34 \, \text{kg}/\text{m}^2$ for youths 14–16 years of age	

Source: [3,4]

rising incidence of obesity since it was suggested that the life-shortening effect of obesity could increase as the obese who are now at younger ages carry their elevated risk of death into middle and older ages [7]. However, obesity is a remarkably heterogeneous condition, where the distribution of the adipose tissue is of importance in determining the presence or absence of metabolic dysfunctions [8]. Obesity as defined by the BMI is undoubtedly associated with an increased rate of comorbidities and cardiovascular mortality [9,10] and obese individuals considered "at risk" are mostly characterized by features associated with the metabolic syndrome [8,9]; however, the existence of this entity as a syndrome has been challenged [11].

Definition of obesity

Obesity was depicted in 1998 by the American Heart Association as a major modifiable risk factor for CVD [12]. CVD risks have been also documented in obese children [3,13]. In children, high BMI predicts future adiposity, as well as future morbidity and death [3]. The estimate for years of life lost due to obesity differs among races and gender [14]. The epidemic of obesity is occurring on genetic backgrounds that have not changed, but it is nonetheless clear that genetics plays an important role in the development of obesity [15]. From the time of the early twin and adoption studies published in 1986, large groups of individuals have been evaluated for genetic defects related to the development of obesity [16,17]. These can be divided into two groups: the rare genes that produce significant obesity and a group of more common genes that underlie the propensity to develop obesity – the so-called "susceptibility" genes. Indeed, within a permissive environment, the more common genetic factors involved in obesity regulate the distribution of body fat, the metabolic rate and its response to exercise and diet, and the control of feeding and food preferences [18,19].

It appears that obesity as defined solely by BMI cannot always discriminate between the individuals at higher risk of developing CVD. Actually, non-obese overweight patients with excess visceral adiposity, thus at higher risk, may not be detected on the basis of BMI alone [20]. For these reasons, measurement of waist circumference (WC) and a set of metabolic markers has been proposed to detect individuals with the metabolic syndrome, and higher risk of developing CVD [9,21]. The metabolic syndrome is mostly encountered in individuals with increased adiposity or obesity and is characterized by a clustering of cardiovascular risk factors including central adiposity, insulin resistance, elevated blood pressure, dyslipidemia, and a proinflammatory-prothrombotic state. At present, two definitions are commonly employed to define the metabolic syndrome (Table 6.2).

Waist circumference or waist-to-hip ratio (WHR) has been used as a proxy measure for body fat distribution when investigating the health risk associated with obesity. Abdominal obesity has been reported as a risk factor for CVD worldwide and is likely to better refine clinical assessment of obesity risk [1, 20,22]. Although some uncertainty about the metabolic syndrome exists [11], it remains useful in identifying CVD risk that extends beyond LDL cholesterol [8,21,23]. Waist circumference measurements are not recommended routinely in children since reference values for children that identify risk over and above the risk from BMI category are not available [3]. Nevertheless, clinicians may add WC to the tools they use to assess risk. If they do, clinicians should use a high, age-specific, percentile cut-off point, such as 90th or 95th percentile, to evaluate risk [13].

Cardiovascular disease

Neurological disorders: stroke
Stroke is one of the leading causes of long-term disability and morbidity. Numerous studies have reported an association between BMI and WHR and stroke

Table 6.2 Definitions of the metabolic syndrome

ATPIII 2001 and ATPIII 2005	International Diabetes Federation 2005
	Central obesity (population specific): waist circumference ≥ 94 cm (M), ≥ 80 cm (F)
≥ 3 of the following:	Plus ≥ 2 of the following:
Central obesity: waist circumference > 102 cm (M), > 88 cm (F)	
Dyslipidemia: triglycerides ≥ 1.7 mmol/L or medication HDL cholesterol: < 1.0 mmol/L (M), < 1.1 mmol/L (F)	*Dyslipidemia:* triglycerides ≥ 1.7 mmol/L HDL cholesterol < 0.9 mmol/L (M), < 1.1 mmol/L (W)
Hypertension: $\geq 135/85$ mmHg or medication	*Hypertension:* $\geq 130/85$ mmHg or medication
Fasting plasma glucose: ≥ 6.1 mmol/L (2001) ≥ 5.6 mmol/L (2005)	*Fasting plasma glucose:* ≥ 5.6 mmol/L

BMI, body mass index; M, male; F, female.
Source: Alberti et al. [24].

[2]. Indeed, obesity is listed as a potential modifiable risk factor for stroke in men independently of cholesterol, systemic hypertension, and diabetes [25]. When BMI was examined as a continuous variable, each one-unit increase in BMI was associated with a multiple adjusted increase of 6% in the risk of total and ischemic stroke and 6% for hemorrhagic stroke in men [25]. In a large cohort of Finnish participants, it was reported that BMI predicted total and ischemic stroke risk among men and women [26]. Although there were no significant interactions between sex and WC or WHR on stroke risk, WC or WHR predicted total and ischemic stroke risk in men but not in women [26]. Of clinical relevance, the metabolic syndrome defined by the most used criteria predicted stroke in elderly Finnish subjects and if obesity, especially central obesity, was included in the definition of the metabolic syndrome, then the metabolic syndrome predicted stroke [27]. Several studies have examined the association between BMI and the risk of hemorrhagic stroke, and the results are inconsistent. Most studies have found an increased risk of hemorrhagic stroke among lean persons.

BMI in patients with stroke has been inversely related to total post-stroke mortality during a 5-year follow-up period. Overweight and obese stroke patients depicted a lower mortality rate than normal-weight and underweight patients

[28] and post-stroke mortality was inversely related to BMI in patients with hemorrhagic stroke or with ischemic stroke. Age may be an important determinant of this "obesity paradox" (see below). In fact, mortality risk in elderly people aged over 65 years showed that BMI in the overweight range was not associated with increased mortality, and moderate obesity was only associated with a moderately increased mortality risk, while studies on elderly patients over 70 years of age show an inverse association between BMI and mortality [29,30]. In contrast, high BMI was strongly associated with increased stroke mortality only among younger men (~ 54 years) who were overweight or obese in a Chinese population [31]. In this population, BMI was strongly related to blood pressure throughout the whole range of BMI levels studied. Similarly, blood pressure was strongly related to stroke mortality, with no evidence of any threshold within the range of baseline systolic blood pressure measurements studied (i.e., ~ 100 to 180 mmHg). However, despite these two trends, BMI was strongly associated with stroke mortality only for individuals with BMI $> 25 \, \text{kg/m}^2$. This emphasized the fundamental importance of blood pressure and age where a substantial excess risk of stroke death among those who are overweight or obese may be largely accounted for by a higher blood pressure [31].

Neurological disorders: dementia

High bodyweight is associated with an increased risk of Alzheimer disease, dementia, and neurodegenerative changes in old age independent of sociodemographic characteristics and common comorbidities [32,33]. In fact, midlife (40–45 years) status of increased BMI in the overweight and obese range was associated with higher risk, up to 36 years later, for both Alzheimer disease and vascular dementia in men and women [34]. More recently, it was observed that central obesity, defined as sagittal abdominal diameter, increases the risk for dementia independent of demographics, diabetes, cardiovascular comorbidities, and BMI [35]. Although diabetes and cardiovascular comorbidities including systemic hypertension and stroke are on the causal pathway between excess adiposity and risk for Alzheimer disease and vascular dementia, adjustment for these conditions did not attenuate the impact of overweight on Alzheimer disease and vascular dementia, suggesting that additional mechanisms exist. Adiposity is also one component of the metabolic syndrome, which has also been shown to cause cognitive decline, particularly in those with high levels of inflammation [36]. In addition, obesity in elderly women was shown to be associated with greater cerebral atrophy [37] and white matter hyperintensity [38].

Adipocytes secrete a large number of bioactive compounds including growth hormones and complement factors (Figure 6.1), some of which cross the blood–brain barrier and play a role in learning and memory [39–41]. It was found that leptin may contribute to amyloid beta deposition [42], and a large population study reported that leptin is associated with cognitive decline, even after

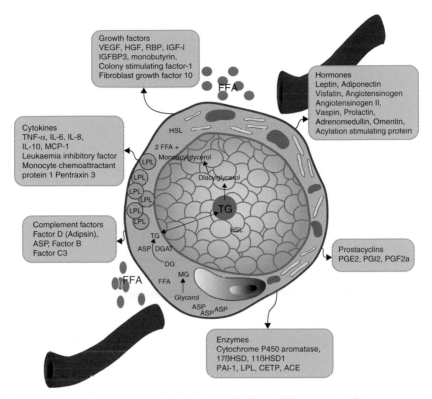

Figure 6.1 TNF; tumor necrosis factor, IL: interleukin, MCP; monocyte-chemoattractant protein, ASP; acylation stimulating protein, PAI; plasminogen activator inhibitor-1, LPL; lipoprotein lipase, CETP; cholesteryl ester transfer protein, ACE; angiotensin converting enzyme.

adjusting for BMI [43]. One limitation in the literature evaluating Alzheimer disease and obesity is that apolipoprotein E4 status, the major genetic risk factor for late-onset Alzheimer disease, is not available. Also, it is well-known that the subclinical phase and initial onset of dementia affects appetite and causes weight loss, skewing the temporal association between weight and dementia. Actually, weight loss precedes onset of dementia in elderly adults. Nonetheless, assessment of obesity before old age may be a more accurate representation of adiposity as the ratio of lean to fat mass changes with aging, resulting in a decreased BMI (sarcopenic obesity).

Coronary artery disease

Atherosclerosis begins in childhood (5–10 years) and is demonstrated predominantly as fatty streaks [44,45]. Postmortem examination of arteries from individuals 15 to 34 years of age [Determinants of Atherosclerosis in Youth (PDAY) study] who died from accidental injuries, homicides or suicides revealed that the extent of fatty streaks and even advanced lesions (fibrous plaques and plaques with calcification or ulceration) in the right coronary artery and abdominal aorta were associated with obesity and size of the abdominal panniculus [46]. In adults, it has been shown that: (i) maximal density of macrophages/mm^2 in atherosclerotic lesions is associated with visceral obesity [47]; (ii) reduced coronary flow reserve is related to body fat distribution and insulin resistance [48]; (iii) the metabolic syndrome is associated with lipid-rich plaque [49]; (iv) coronary artery calcium and abdominal aortic calcium are associated with visceral adipose tissue [50]; and (v) prospective evidence shows that abdominal obesity is associated with accelerated progression of carotid atherosclerosis in men independently of overall obesity and other risk factors [51].

Pathophysiology

Aside from the metabolic disturbances associated with the metabolic syndrome, other factors may play a role in the development of early atherosclerosis in obesity. In contrast to BMI-defined obesity, the components of the insulin resistance syndrome have been reported following coronary artery bypass graft to be associated with angiographic progression of atherosclerosis in non-grafted coronary arteries [52]. Pericardial fat may also play a role. The amount of pericardial fat assessed by echocardiography or magnetic resonance imaging correlates with the amount of visceral adiposity [50,53]. Among individuals free of clinical CVD, pericardial fat is correlated with multiple measures of adiposity and cardiovascular risk factors and correlations remained significant after adjustment for BMI and WC [50]. However, associations with pericardial fat were attenuated when considered simultaneously with visceral adipose tissue with regard to metabolic risk, suggesting that pericardial fat may be an overall marker of visceral fat accumulation [50]. Interestingly, pericardial fat was associated with coronary artery calcium and abdominal aortic calcium even after metabolic risk factors and visceral adipose tissue were accounted for [50]. Epicardial fat may be considered the visceral cardiac fat depot which commonly increases in subjects with increased abdominal obesity [54]. Under physiologically adapted circumstances, epicardial fat might function as a buffer in order to protect the cardiac muscle against exposure to excessively high circulating levels of fatty acids and probably to be used as a local energy source for myocardium when needed or to defend the myocardium against hypothermia and trauma [55]. In contrast, under pathological conditions, such as visceral obesity, increased epicardial fat deposit may be involved in the generation of cardiotoxic molecules leading to metabolic dysfunction [56]. From its close proximity to the coronary arteries, it has been proposed that epicardial fat might locally mediate the development of coronary artery disease [57]. In a human pathological study, it was observed that part of the left anterior descending artery with an intramyocardial course

was without any intimal atherosclerotic lesion, in contrast to the epicardial segment of the same artery in which atherosclerosis was documented [58]. Further,
in 203 patients who underwent cardiac catheterization, epicardial fat thickness
was correlated with the severity of angiographic disease [59]. Accordingly, in an
animal model using hypercholesterolemic rabbits, epicardial coronary arteries,
surrounded by adipose tissue, develop atherosclerosis whereas intramyocardial
segments of the same arteries remain unaffected [60]. Although speculative, local production of cytokines by epicardial fat could modulate underneath blood
vessel biology through paracrine signaling or through the vasa vasorum. Compared to subcutaneous fat, epicardial adipocyte produces more interleukin-1β,
interleukin-6, tumor necrosis factor alpha (TNF-α), CD45, and less adiponectin
[61]. Hence, the proinflammatory environment of adipose tissue and its close
proximity to epicardial coronary arteries could promote a proatherosclerotic
environment (Figure 6.1). Mononuclear cells could reach the subintimal space
through the adventitia as well as through the endothelium. Therefore, perivascular fat might contribute directly to perivascular inflammation and smooth
muscle cell proliferation [62]. Thus, epicardial fat may be considered the visceral fat depot of the heart.

Coronary artery disease revascularization procedure in obesity

Characteristics of obese patients in the catheterization laboratory are younger
age, more comorbidities, and with more single-vessel disease at baseline [?].
When percutaneous transluminal coronary angioplasty (PTCA) is indicated,
abnormal glucose tolerance and/or the metabolic syndrome may be important
for long-term prognosis [63,64]. Although presence of the metabolic syndrome
was not associated with restenosis in one study [65], abdominal obesity was
not directly measured and the authors defined obesity as a BMI $> 28.8\,\mathrm{kg/m^2}$
[65]. On the other hand, there was a trend toward more frequent target lesion
revascularization after coronary stenting in patients with obesity class II/III,
but this trend was strongly influenced by the presence of diabetes and systemic
hypertension [66]. Despite a widespread misperception, obesity has not been
reported to be associated with increased mortality or postoperative cerebrovascular accidents following CABG in numerous studies [67,68], yet an increased
incidence of sternal and superficial wound infection, saphenous vein harvest
site infection, and atrial dysrhythmias was observed [69–71]. This is also true
for the geriatric population (> 75 years) [72]. Further, severe obesity is not associated with increased mortality, but with an increased length of hospital stay,
a greater likelihood of renal failure, prolonged assisted ventilation, and longer
postoperative stay following cardiac surgery [71,73,74]. On the other hand, the
metabolic syndrome was reported to be a strong and independent risk factor for morbidity and mortality following CABG [75] as well as an increased
risk of developing postoperative complications such as atrial fibrillation and

renal failure [76]. More recently, the metabolic syndrome has also been documented as a risk factor for the development of aortic valve sclerosis and stenosis [77]. Patients with the metabolic syndrome had a faster progression of aortic stenosis and experienced more events, defined as aortic valve replacement or death [78], and experienced a two-fold risk (compared with patients without the syndrome) of developing dysfunction of an implanted aortic bioprosthesis [79].

Congestive heart failure

Cardiomyopathy is applied when cardiac structural (left ventricular dilatation) and hemodynamic (increased left ventricular wall stress) adaptations result in congestive heart failure [2]. With the recent interest in lipid partitioning, and the role of lipid byproducts as potential cytotoxic compounds, scientists have shown renewed interest in the fatty heart (obesity cardiomyopathy) and its pathophysiological relevance [2,80,81]. In humans, using magnetic resonance imaging and spectroscopic techniques, investigators have shown that intracellular accumulation of lipids is positively associated with BMI and inversely related to systolic function [82], and dynamic changes in triglyceride content and myocardial left ventricular diastolic function have been documented [83]. Alterations in cardiac fatty acid metabolism may play a causal role in the development of obesity-related cardiomyopathies [80,81]. The physiological mechanisms linking obesity with cardiac disease are poorly characterized but may involve adipokine signaling, altered insulin signaling, and changes in circulating glucose and lipids. In fact, the development of heart failure in the obese population may involve different pathophysiological mechanisms than in non-obese heart failure patients. Aside from the presence of diabetes and systemic and pulmonary hypertension, the presentation of heart failure in obese people is associated with a cluster of obesity-related pathogenic factors (i.e., elevated circulating free fatty acids and glucose, suppressed adiponectin levels, elevated insulin and leptin levels, to name a few) that are not generally found in non-obese heart failure patients.

Electrocardiogram and arrhythmias

There are several changes in the ECG associated with increasing obesity (Table 6.3). A prolonged QT interval is observed in a relatively high percentage of obese subjects and the association between abnormal QT_c and BMI is most evident in the severely obese [2]. Metabolic variables may be of importance to explain increased QT_c interval in obesity [84]. Obesity has been shown to be an independent risk factor for atrial fibrillation with an adjusted 50% risk increase for developing atrial fibrillation [2], and higher radiation dose during atrial fibrillation ablation procedures has been reported [85]. All of the metabolic syndrome components except elevated triglycerides have been reported to be

Table 6.3 ECG changes that may occur in obese individuals

Clinically significant
↑ Heart rate
↑ QRS interval
↑ QT$_c$ interval
False positive criteria for inferior myocardial infarction
Less clinically significant
↑ PR interval
↑ or ↓ QRS voltage
↑ QT dispersion
↑ SAECG (late potentials)
ST-T abnormalities
ST depression
Left axis deviation
Flattening of the T wave (inferolateral leads)
Left atrial abnormalities

associated to the development of atrial fibrillation, but elevated blood pressure and obesity contributed the most to the increased risk of new-onset atrial fibrillation [86]. Obesity can cause mechanical atrial stretch and dilatation resulting in a structural substrate predisposing to atrial fibrillation. The increased incidence of stroke in patients with obesity can be partially explained by its association with asymptomatic or undiagnosed atrial fibrillation.

The obesity paradox

Despite the fact that obesity has been shown to be an independent risk factor for CVD, many studies have reported that obese patients with established CVD have a better prognosis than do patients with ideal bodyweight; the so-called "obesity paradox." This paradox has been best described for patients with advanced systolic heart failure [2] and in overweight and mildly obese groups where a meta-analysis reported a better outcomes for cardiovascular events and total mortality [87] as well as in a large prospective population of patients (~ 22 500) with hypertension and coronary artery disease [88]. The improved survival of obese individuals is paradoxical principally because of the assumption that excessive weight is always and invariably injurious. As a matter of fact, among patients with congestive heart failure, subjects with higher BMI are at decreased risk for death and hospitalization compared with patients with a "healthy" BMI [2]. Further, obesity was associated, in a prospective cohort study, with lower all-cause and cardiovascular mortality after unstable angina/non-ST-segment elevation myocardial infarction treated with early revascularization [89].

The obesity paradox may reflect the lack of discriminatory power of BMI to adequately reflect body fat distribution [20,87,90]. Since BMI measures total body mass, i.e. both fat and lean mass, it may better represent the protective effect of lean body mass on mortality. This negative confounding may have been under-appreciated in prior studies that did not adjust for measures of abdominal obesity. It is possible that the favorable prognosis implications associated with mildly elevated BMI might actually reflect intrinsic limitations of BMI to differentiate adipose tissue from lean mass. The lack of specificity of BMI could dilute the adverse effects of excess fat with the beneficial effects of preserved or increased lean mass [91].

As an example, in patients with known CVD or following acute myocardial infarction, overall obesity as assessed by BMI has not been associated with myocardial infarction, cardiovascular mortality, and total mortality when abdominal obesity (WHR, WC) was integrated into the analysis [22,92,93]. In the Nurses Health Study, WHR and WC were independently strongly associated with increased risk of coronary artery disease among women with a BMI of $25\,kg/m^2$ or less [94] and in the Paris prospective study, sagittal diameter (i.e., abdominal obesity) was the only significant predictor of cardiac death [95]. In the Trandolapril Cardiac Evaluation (TRACE) registry, the mortality rate was increased 23% in men who were abdominally obese [93]. In postmenopausal women with established coronary artery disease from the Heart and Estrogen/progestin Replacement Study, it was reported that both BMI and WC were associated with mortality, but WC may be more important than BMI [96]. Indeed, for every category of BMI, mortality rates were higher for women whose WC was > 88 cm compared with those with a smaller WC. In contrast, for every category of WC, women of normal BMI had higher mortality than those who were overweight or obese [96]. Thus, higher levels of baseline WC were associated with a 22% increased risk of mortality after adjusting for BMI and traditional risk factors. In addition, after adjustment for WC, higher levels of baseline BMI were associated with a 20% decreased risk of mortality. Only women whose WC was < 88 cm had a decreased risk of mortality with increasing BMI [96]. Another issue to consider is that normal-weight patients may have a significantly higher percentage of high-risk coronary anatomy compared with obese patients [97]. This highlights the difficulty in precisely assessing potential increased CVD risk using BMI as an overall adiposity index in patients with known CVD.

Another limitation in most studies reporting an obesity paradox in patients with CVD is that non-intentional weight loss, which would be associated with a poor prognosis, is not assessed as BMI is measured only at the beginning of the study. Patients who have decompensated heart failure may lose weight because of extensive caloric demands associated with the increased work of breathing, and patients with show poor nutrient absorption by the edematous bowel may be at higher risk of recurrent CVD events. Adiposity in certain stressful pathological settings might on balance be salutary. Adipose tissue has been shown to produce soluble TNF receptor that is thought to neutralize the deleterious effects of TNFα on the myocardium, which may explain a protective effect of obesity in patients with heart failure [98]. Lastly, in hemodialysis patients, the obesity-survival paradox may be in part a reflection of better performance of activities of daily living. Studies in hemodialysis patients reported that patients with high body mass and normal lean body mass showed a decreased hazard ratio for death than individuals with high BMI and low lean body mass who did worse [99,100].

Despite the high correlation between WC and BMI, the combination of both indices may be very relevant in clinical practice because WC for a given BMI is a strong predictor of all-cause mortality. Studies reporting negative results between all-cause mortality and WC did not mutually adjust WC and BMI, a possible explanation for the inconsistent results [101,102]. Another example is that the excess health risk associated with a higher BMI declines with increasing age. An explanation for the lack of a positive association between BMI and mortality at older ages is that, in older persons, higher BMI is a poor measure of body fat and may simply represent a measure of increased physical activity with preserved lean mass. Sarcopenic obesity, which is defined as excess fat with loss of lean body mass, is a highly prevalent problem in the older individual. In fact, the ideal BMI may be higher in older adults than in middle-aged adults. It was recently reported in ~ 4000 persons aged ≥ 75 years that WHR rather than WC predicted mortality in non-smoking men and women, mainly because of the association with cardiovascular deaths [103]. In the Health Professionals Study, in men aged 65 years, WC and WHR were significantly related to CVD mortality [101]. It was found in the Cardiovascular Health Study in over 5000 patients aged ≥ 65 years with a mean BMI of 26.3 kg/m^2 (42% overweight) that higher BMI values indicated a lower mortality risk once the risk attributable to WC was accounted for, whereas WC values indicate a higher mortality risk once the risk attributable to BMI was accounted for [104]. Death rates were highest in individuals with a high WC within the overweight and obese BMI categories. Finally, in a large case–control study, WHR was found to be more strongly associated than was BMI with myocardial infarction, whereas the association with BMI was weak and intermediate for WC in older patients [105]. In order to discriminate low-risk vs. high-risk subjects, WHR may possibly be more useful. Further studies are needed to clarify the concept of the obesity paradox in patients with known CVD.

Assessment of adiposity in clinical practice

The introduction of WC as a simple risk measure in public health settings has already begun, but the simplification is under debate. Thresholds for WC to identify individuals with excess cardiovascular risk have been suggested but the choice of WC thresholds should be based on outcomes of importance, such as all-cause mortality or myocardial infarction. It seems from the data available that there is no basis for choosing thresholds because the mortality rate ratio increased steadily with WC. Nevertheless, there may be differences between different ethnic groups [105]. From a clinical viewpoint, both indices should probably be assessed and may be useful to better define "at risk" obesity [23,106]. It was observed in the IDEA (International Day for the Evaluation of Abdominal obesity), including 157 211 patients, that both WC and BMI were independently associated with the presence of CVD in both men and women [107]. Nevertheless, with all the knowledge available in the literature regarding obesity and CVD, assessment and management of obesity following diagnosis of acute coronary syndrome is simply inadequate [108].

Management

The aging of the population coupled with the explosive rise in metabolic risk factors will contribute to increasing prevalence of CVD over time. Numerous cardiovascular abnormalities may be encountered in obese subjects (Table 6.4) it

Table 6.4 Functional and structural changes that may occur in obese individuals

LV diastolic dysfunction
Left ventricular hypertrophy
Eccentric, concentric
Right ventricular hypertrophy
Altered left ventricular systolic function
Altered right ventricular systolic function
Pulmonary hypertension
Autonomic dysfunction
Arrhythmia, sudden death
Adipositas cordis (cardiomyopathy of obesity)

is not written properly in the PDF files that I have but this version seems correct. Health service usage and medical costs associated with obesity and related diseases have and will increase dramatically [109]. Abdominal obesity as assessed by WC (independently of ethnicity, gender, smoking status, and age) is associated with increased total healthcare expenditures, especially with the costs of inpatient care [110]. Efforts need to be taken to curb the underlying causes of increasing risk factors, such as pervasive overweight/obesity, physical inactivity, and growing similar trends among children. The general goals of weight loss and management are, at a minimum, (i) to prevent further weight gain, (ii) reduce bodyweight, and (iii) to maintain a lower bodyweight indefinitely. Current therapies available for weight management that cause weight loss by inducing a negative energy balance include dietary intervention, physical activity, pharmacotherapy, and bariatric surgery. Behavior modification to enhance dietary and activity compliance is an important component of all of these treatments. It is important to recognize that obese individuals may be limited in terms of exercise capacity [111] and it is imperative to inform patients about the results to be expected, to avoid unrealistic weight loss expectations. Identifying potential barriers to long-term weight loss is an important step in formulating an effective treatment intervention, especially after bariatric surgery in severely obese individuals. The key to long-term weight loss and maintenance is calorie reduction, coupled with an adjunctive exercise program and increased lifestyle activity.

Bodyweight normalization should not be the primary target, but rather some weight loss which can lead to substantial improvements in risk factors [112] and on the cardiovascular system (Table 6.5). The American Heart Association has addressed and reviewed a variety of weight loss approaches for the management and treatment of obesity [113]. Combining diet and an exercise program results in a greater weight loss with a sustained effect and prevents weight regain. In overweight/obese patients psychologically ready for weight loss, this approach should be emphasized and sustained for at least 6 months before considering pharmacotherapy. Although some drug classes may be beneficial from a risk factor standpoint, they may be deleterious from a bodyweight or a cardiac structure and/or function perspective [114]. The opposite may also be true since the pleiotropic effect of anti-obesity drugs may impact favorably on atherosclerotic processes and myocardial metabolism. This should always be kept in mind by clinicians [114].

In general, reducing food intake is most important for weight loss whereas a substantial amount of physical activity is important for weight maintenance. Reducing weight and, possibly more important, WC will result in beneficial impact on the metabolic profile and consequently on the overall CVD risk. There are numerous cardiovascular system benefits of weight reduction (Table 6.5) and a clinical trial involving patient with diabetes, called Look AHEAD, is testing whether weight loss by non-surgical means can reduce mortality [115]. Regarding this issue, it should be noted that, in recent years, emphasis has

Table 6.5 Benefits for the cardiovascular system from weight reduction

↓ blood volume
↓ stroke volume
↓ cardiac output
↓ pulmonary capillary wedge pressure
↓ peripheral edema
↓ left ventricular mass
Improvement of left ventricular diastolic dysfunction
Improvement of left ventricular systolic dysfunction
↓ Resting oxygen consumption
↓ Systemic arterial pressure
↓ Filling pressures of the right and the left side of the heart
↓ or no change in systemic arterial resistance
↓ resting heart rate
↓ QT_c interval
↑ HRV

HRV, heart rate variability.

been placed on bodyweight reduction as a key objective of lifestyle intervention programs. However, in view of the importance of body fat distribution, one could argue that, instead of targeting bodyweight per se, one should pay more attention to the WC and conservation of lean mass as a critical goal in intervention programs [23]. In accordance, it was found in the Look AHEAD trial that, after adjusting for both age and BMI, higher WC was still independently associated with lower exercise capacity for both men and women with diabetes [116]. Finally, until recently, there have been no prospective trials to convincingly show changes in mortality with medically induced weight loss in obese patients [117]. However, it has been shown that bariatric surgery-induced weight loss was associated with decreased overall mortality and mortality from CVD and from cancer [118,119].

Summary

Without a doubt, obesity is a risk factor for CVD. Accurate diagnosis of obesity may entail more refined assessment of body fat composition and distribution. Although BMI has been useful in epidemiological studies in order to assess the presence of obesity, it fails to differentiate between differing body compositions. BMI does not characterize excess centrally distributed obesity, which is more consistently associated with adverse effects on metabolism, dyslipidemia, and insulin resistance. Thus, other clinical indices of adiposity such as WC and WHR should be incorporated into the clinical approach of the cardiologist in order to better target and manage "at risk" obesity. Prevention must begin early in life, because obesity in childhood, especially among older children and those with more severe obesity, is likely to persist into adulthood. With obesity occurring at younger ages, the children and young adults of today will carry and express obesity-related risks for more of their lifetime than previous generations. Unfortunately, the improvement in risk factor recognition and management that has developed through the last decades in modern cardiology may be counteracted by the greater incidence of obesity. From a public health perspective, increased physical activity early in life may become in the future the most cost-effective, non-pharmacological avenue to combat obesity. A combined intervention of behavior therapy, a low-calorie diet, and increased physical activity provides the most successful therapy for weight loss and weight maintenance. The establishment of permanent healthy lifestyle habits is a good outcome, regardless of weight change, because of the long-term health benefits of these behaviors.

References

1. Yusuf S, Hawken S, Ounpuu S, et al. Effect of potentially modifiable risk factors associated with myocardial infarction in 52 countries (the INTERHEART study): case-control study. *Lancet* 2004;364:937–52.
2. Poirier P, Giles TD, Bray GA, et al. Obesity and cardiovascular disease: pathophysiology, evaluation, and effect of weight loss: an update of the 1997 American Heart Association Scientific Statement on Obesity and Heart Disease from the Obesity Committee of the Council on Nutrition, Physical Activity, and Metabolism. *Circulation* 2006;113:898–918.
3. Barlow SE. Expert committee recommendations regarding the prevention, assessment, and treatment of child and adolescent overweight and obesity: summary report. *Pediatrics* 2007;120 Suppl 4:S164–92.
4. Poirier P, Alpert MA, Fleisher LA, et al. Cardiovascular evaluation and management of severely obese patients undergoing surgery: a science advisory from the American Heart Association. *Circulation* 2009;120:86–95.
5. Guidelines for reporting results in bariatric surgery. Standards Committee, American Society for Bariatric Surgery. *Obes Surg* 1997;7:521–2.
6. Sturm R. Increases in clinically severe obesity in the United States,1986–2000. *Arch Intern Med* 2003;163:2146–8.
7. Olshansky SJ, Passaro DJ, Hershow RC, et al. A potential decline in life expectancy in the United States in the 21st century. *N Engl J Med* 2005;352:1138–45.
8. Despres JP, Lemieux I. Abdominal obesity and metabolic syndrome. *Nature* 2006;444:881–7.

9. Eckel RH, Grundy SM, Zimmet PZ. The metabolic syndrome. *Lancet* 2005;365: 1415–28.

10. Poirier P, Despres JP. Waist circumference, visceral obesity, and cardiovascular risk. *J Cardiopulm Rehabil* 2003;23:161–9.

11. Kahn R, Buse J, Ferrannini E, Stern M. The metabolic syndrome: time for a critical appraisal: joint statement from the American Diabetes Association and the European Association for the Study of Diabetes. *Diabetes Care* 2005;28:2289–304.

12. Eckel RH, Krauss RM. American Heart Association call to action: obesity as a major risk factor for coronary heart disease. AHA Nutrition Committee. *Circulation* 1998;97:2099–100.

13. Krebs NF, Himes JH, Jacobson D, Nicklas TA, Guilday P, Styne D. Assessment of child and adolescent overweight and obesity. *Pediatrics* 2007;120 Suppl 4: S193–228.

14. Fontaine KR, Redden DT, Wang C, Westfall AO, Allison DB. Years of life lost due to obesity. *JAMA* 2003;289:187–93.

15. Snyder EE, Walts B, Perusse L, et al. The human obesity gene map: the 2003 update. *Obes Res* 2004;12:369–439.

16. Stunkard AJ, Foch TT, Hrubec Z. A twin study of human obesity. *JAMA* 1986;256:51–4.

17. Stunkard AJ, Sorensen TI, Hanis C, et al. An adoption study of human obesity. *N Engl J Med* 1986;314:193–8.

18. Vohl MC, Sladek R, Robitaille J, et al. A survey of genes differentially expressed in subcutaneous and visceral adipose tissue in men. *Obes Res* 2004;12:1217–22.

19. Bouchard L, Drapeau V, Provencher V, et al. Neuromedin beta: a strong candidate gene linking eating behaviors and susceptibility to obesity. *Am J Clin Nutr* 2004;80:1478–86.

20. Poirier P. Adiposity and cardiovascular disease: are we using the right definition of obesity? *Eur Heart J* 2007;28:2047–8.

21. Despres JP, Lemieux I, Bergeron J, et al. Abdominal obesity and the metabolic syndrome: contribution to global cardiometabolic risk. *Arterioscler Thromb Vasc Biol* 2008;28:1039–49.

22. Poirier P. Recurrent cardiovascular events in contemporary cardiology: obesity patients should not rest in PEACE. *Eur Heart J* 2006;27:1390–1.

23. Poirier P. Targeting abdominal obesity in cardiology: can we be effective? *Can J Cardiol* 2008;24 Suppl D:13–17D.

24. Alberti KGMM, Eckel RH, Grundy SM, et al. Harmonizing the metabolic syndrome: a joint interim statement of the International Diabetes Federation Task Force on Epidemiology and Prevention, National Heart Lung and Blood Institute, American Heart Association, World Heart Federation, International Atherosclerosis Society, and International Association for the Study of Obesity. *Circulation* 2009;120: 1640–45.

25. Kurth T, Gaziano JM, Berger K, et al. Body mass index and the risk of stroke in men. *Arch Intern Med* 2002;162:2557–62.

26. Hu G, Tuomilehto J, Silventoinen K, Sarti C, Mannisto S, Jousilahti P. Body mass index, waist circumference, and waist-hip ratio on the risk of total and type-specific stroke. *Arch Intern Med* 2007;167:1420–7.

27. Wang J, Ruotsalainen S, Moilanen L, Lepisto P, Laakso M, Kuusisto J. The metabolic syndrome predicts incident stroke: a 14-year follow-up study in elderly people in Finland. *Stroke* 2008;39:1078–83.

28. Olsen TS, Dehlendorff C, Petersen HG, Andersen KK. Body mass index and post-stroke mortality. *Neuroepidemiology* 2008;30:93–100.

29. Janssen I, Mark AE. Elevated body mass index and mortality risk in the elderly. *Obes Rev* 2007;8:41–59.

30. Mazza A, Zamboni S, Tikhonoff V, Schiavon L, Pessina AC, Casiglia E. Body mass index and mortality in elderly men and women from general population. The experience of Cardiovascular Study in the Elderly (CASTEL). *Gerontology* 2007;53:36–45.

31. Zhou M, Offer A, Yang G, et al. Body mass index, blood pressure, and mortality from stroke: a nationally representative prospective study of 212,000 Chinese men. *Stroke* 2008;39:753–9.

32. Whitmer RA, Gunderson EP, Barrett-Connor E, Quesenberry CP, Jr., Yaffe K. Obesity in middle age and future risk of dementia: a 27 year longitudinal population based study. *BMJ* 2005;330:1360.

33. Kivipelto M, Ngandu T, Fratiglioni L, et al. Obesity and vascular risk factors at midlife and the risk of dementia and Alzheimer disease. *Arch Neurol* 2005;62:1556–60.

34. Whitmer RA, Gunderson EP, Quesenberry CP, Jr., Zhou J, Yaffe K. Body mass index in midlife and risk of Alzheimer disease and vascular dementia. *Curr Alzheimer Res* 2007;4:103–9.

35. Whitmer RA, Gustafson DR, Barrett-Connor E, Haan MN, Gunderson EP, Yaffe K. Central obesity and increased risk of dementia more than three decades later. *Neurology* 2008;71:1057–64.

36. Yaffe K, Kanaya A, Lindquist K, et al. The metabolic syndrome, inflammation, and risk of cognitive decline. *JAMA* 2004;292:2237–42.

37. Gustafson D, Lissner L, Bengtsson C, Bjorkelund C, Skoog I. A 24-year follow-up of body mass index and cerebral atrophy. *Neurology* 2004;63:1876–81.

38. Gustafson DR, Steen B, Skoog I. Body mass index and white matter lesions in elderly women: an 18-year longitudinal study. *Int Psychogeriatr* 2004;16:327–36.

39. Rondinone CM. Adipocyte-derived hormones, cytokines, and mediators. *Endocrine* 2006;29:81–90.

40. Harvey J. Leptin: a multifaceted hormone in the central nervous system. *Mol Neurobiol* 2003;28:245–58.

41. Harvey J. Novel actions of leptin in the hippocampus. *Ann Med* 2003;35:197–206.

42. Fewlass DC, Noboa K, Pi-Sunyer FX, Johnston JM, Yan SD, Tezapsidis N. Obesity-related leptin regulates Alzheimer's Abeta. *FASEB J* 2004;18:1870–8.

43. Holden KF, Lindquist K, Tylavsky FA, Rosano C, Harris TB, Yaffe K. Serum leptin level and cognition in the elderly: Findings from the Health ABC Study. *Neurobiol Aging* 2009;30:1483–9.

44. McGill HC, Jr. Fatty streaks in the coronary arteries and aorta. *Lab Invest* 1968;18:560–4.

45. Skalen K, Gustafsson M, Rydberg EK, et al. Subendothelial retention of atherogenic lipoproteins in early atherosclerosis. *Nature* 2002;417:750–4.

46. Zieske AW, Malcom GT, Strong JP. Natural history and risk factors of atherosclerosis in children and youth: the PDAY study. *Pediatr Pathol Mol Med* 2002;21:213–37.

47. Kortelainen ML, Sarkioja T. Visceral fat and coronary pathology in male adolescents. *Int J Obes Relat Metab Disord* 2001;25:228–32.
48. Kondo I, Mizushige K, Hirao K, et al. Ultrasonographic assessment of coronary flow reserve and abdominal fat in obesity. *Ultrasound Med Biol* 2001;27: 1199–205.
49. Amano T, Matsubara T, Uetani T, et al. Impact of metabolic syndrome on tissue characteristics of angiographically mild to moderate coronary lesions integrated backscatter intravascular ultrasound study. *J Am Coll Cardiol* 2007;49:1149–56.
50. Rosito GA, Massaro JM, Hoffmann U, et al. Pericardial fat, visceral abdominal fat, cardiovascular disease risk factors, and vascular calcification in a community-based sample: the Framingham Heart Study. *Circulation* 2008;117:605–13.
51. Lakka TA, Lakka HM, Salonen R, Kaplan GA, Salonen JT. Abdominal obesity is associated with accelerated progression of carotid atherosclerosis in men. *Atherosclerosis* 2001;154:497–504.
52. Korpilahti K, Syvanne M, Engblom E, Hamalainen H, Puukka P, Ronnemaa T. Components of the insulin resistance syndrome are associated with progression of atherosclerosis in non-grafted arteries 5 years after coronary artery bypass surgery. *Eur Heart J* 1998;19:711–9.
53. Iacobellis G, Sharma AM. Epicardial adipose tissue as new cardio-metabolic risk marker and potential therapeutic target in the metabolic syndrome. *Curr Pharm Des* 2007;13:2180–4.
54. Sacks HS, Fain JN. Human epicardial adipose tissue: a review. *Am Heart J* 2007;153:907–17.
55. Iacobellis G, Corradi D, Sharma AM. Epicardial adipose tissue: anatomic, biomolecular and clinical relationships with the heart. *Nat Clin Pract Cardiovasc Med* 2005;2:536–43.
56. Iacobellis G, Barbaro G. The double role of epicardial adipose tissue as pro- and anti-inflammatory organ. *Horm Metab Res* 2008;40:442–5.
57. Vela D, Buja LM, Madjid M, et al. The role of periadventitial fat in atherosclerosis. *Arch Pathol Lab Med* 2007;131:481–7.
58. Ishii T, Asuwa N, Masuda S, Ishikawa Y. The effects of a myocardial bridge on coronary atherosclerosis and ischaemia. *J Pathol* 1998;185:4–9.
59. Jeong JW, Jeong MH, Yun KH, et al. Echocardiographic epicardial fat thickness and coronary artery disease. *Circ J* 2007;71:536–9.
60. Ishikawa Y, Ishii T, Asuwa N, Masuda S. Absence of atherosclerosis evolution in the coronary arterial segment covered by myocardial tissue in cholesterol-fed rabbits. *Virchows Arch* 1997;430:163–71.
61. Baker AR, Silva NF, Quinn DW, et al. Human epicardial adipose tissue expresses a pathogenic profile of adipocytokines in patients with cardiovascular disease. *Cardiovasc Diabetol* 2006;5:1.
62. Barandier C, Montani JP, Yang Z. Mature adipocytes and perivascular adipose tissue stimulate vascular smooth muscle cell proliferation: effects of aging and obesity. *Am J Physiol Heart Circ Physiol* 2005;289:H1807–13.
63. Otsuka Y, Miyazaki S, Okumura H, et al. Abnormal glucose tolerance, not small vessel diameter, is a determinant of long-term prognosis in patients treated with balloon coronary angioplasty. *Eur Heart J* 2000;21:1790–6.

64. St Pierre J, Lemieux I, Vohl MC, et al. Contribution of abdominal obesity and hypertriglyceridemia to impaired fasting glucose and coronary artery disease. *Am J Cardiol* 2002;90:15–18.

65. Rana JS, Monraats PS, Zwinderman AH, et al. Metabolic syndrome and risk of restenosis in patients undergoing percutaneous coronary intervention. *Diabetes Care* 2005;28:873–7.

66. Rana JS, Mittleman MA, Ho KK, Cutlip DE. Obesity and clinical restenosis after coronary stent placement. *Am Heart J* 2005;150:821–6.

67. Ascione R, Angelini GD. Is obesity still a risk factor for patients undergoing coronary surgery? *Ital Heart J* 2003;4:824–8.

68. Rockx MA, Fox SA, Stitt LW, et al. Is obesity a predictor of mortality, morbidity and readmission after cardiac surgery? *Can J Surg* 2004;47:34–8.

69. Moulton MJ, Creswell LL, Mackey ME, Cox JL, Rosenbloom M. Obesity is not a risk factor for significant adverse outcomes after cardiac surgery. *Circulation* 1996;94:II87–I92.

70. Birkmeyer NJ, Charlesworth DC, Hernandez F, et al. Obesity and risk of adverse outcomes associated with coronary artery bypass surgery. Northern New England Cardiovascular Disease Study Group. *Circulation* 1998;97:1689–94.

71. Kuduvalli M, Grayson AD, Oo AY, Fabri BM, Rashid A. Risk of morbidity and in-hospital mortality in obese patients undergoing coronary artery bypass surgery. *Eur J Cardiothorac Surg* 2002;22:787–93.

72. Maurer MS, Luchsinger JA, Wellner R, Kukuy E, Edwards NM. The effect of body mass index on complications from cardiac surgery in the oldest old. *J Am Geriatr Soc* 2002;50:988–94.

73. Wigfield CH, Lindsey JD, Munoz A, Chopra PS, Edwards NM, Love RB. Is extreme obesity a risk factor for cardiac surgery? An analysis of patients with a BMI > or = 40. *Eur J Cardiothorac Surg* 2006;29:434–40.

74. Villavicencio MA, Sundt TM, III, Daly RC, et al. Cardiac surgery in patients with body mass index of 50 or greater. *Ann Thorac Surg* 2007;83:1403–11.

75. Echahidi N, Pibarot P, Despres JP, et al. Metabolic syndrome increases operative mortality in patients undergoing coronary artery bypass grafting surgery. *J Am Coll Cardiol* 2007;50:843–51.

76. Echahidi N, Mohty D, Pibarot P, et al. Obesity and metabolic syndrome are independent risk factors for atrial fibrillation after coronary artery bypass graft surgery. *Circulation* 2007;116:I213–19.

77. Katz R, Wong ND, Kronmal R, et al. Features of the metabolic syndrome and diabetes mellitus as predictors of aortic valve calcification in the Multi-Ethnic Study of Atherosclerosis. *Circulation* 2006;113:2113–19.

78. Briand M, Lemieux I, Dumesnil JG, et al. Metabolic syndrome negatively influences disease progression and prognosis in aortic stenosis. *J Am Coll Cardiol* 2006;47:2229–36.

79. Briand M, Pibarot P, Despres JP, et al. Metabolic syndrome is associated with faster degeneration of bioprosthetic valves. *Circulation* 2006;114:I512–17.

80. Unger RH. Hyperleptinemia: protecting the heart from lipid overload. *Hypertension* 2005;45:1031–4.

81. Lopaschuk GD, Folmes CD, Stanley WC. Cardiac energy metabolism in obesity. *Circ Res* 2007;101:335–47.

82. McGavock JM, Victor RG, Unger RH, Szczepaniak LS. Adiposity of the heart, revisited. *Ann Intern Med* 2006;144:517–24.

83. van der Meer RW, Hammer S, Smit JW, et al. Short-term caloric restriction induces accumulation of myocardial triglycerides and decreases left ventricular diastolic function in healthy subjects. *Diabetes* 2007;56:2849–53.

84. Corbi GM, Carbone S, Ziccardi P, et al. FFAs and QT intervals in obese women with visceral adiposity: effects of sustained weight loss over 1 year. *J Clin Endocrinol Metab* 2002;87:2080–3.

85. Ector J, Dragusin O, Adriaenssens B, et al. Obesity is a major determinant of radiation dose in patients undergoing pulmonary vein isolation for atrial fibrillation. *J Am Coll Cardiol* 2007;50:234–42.

86. Watanabe H, Tanabe N, Watanabe T, et al. Metabolic syndrome and risk of development of atrial fibrillation: the Niigata preventive medicine study. *Circulation* 2008;117:1255–60.

87. Romero-Corral A, Montori VM, Somers VK, et al. Association of body weight with total mortality and with cardiovascular events in coronary artery disease: a systematic review of cohort studies. *Lancet* 2006;368:666–78.

88. Uretsky S, Messerli FH, Bangalore S, et al. Obesity paradox in patients with hypertension and coronary artery disease. *Am J Med* 2007;120:863–70.

89. Buettner HJ, Mueller C, Gick M, et al. The impact of obesity on mortality in UA/non-ST-segment elevation myocardial infarction. *Eur Heart J* 2007;28:1694–701.

90. Romero-Corral A, Lopez-Jimenez F, Sierra-Johnson J, Somers VK. Differentiating between body fat and lean mass-how should we measure obesity? *Nat Clin Pract Endocrinol Metab* 2008;4:322–3.

91. Romero-Corral A, Somers VK, Sierra-Johnson J, et al. Diagnostic performance of body mass index to detect obesity in patients with coronary artery disease. *Eur Heart J* 2007;28:2087–93.

92. Dagenais GR, Yi Q, Mann JF, Bosch J, Pogue J, Yusuf S. Prognostic impact of body weight and abdominal obesity in women and men with cardiovascular disease. *Am Heart J* 2005;149:54–60.

93. Kragelund C, Hassager C, Hildebrandt P, Torp-Pedersen C, Kober L. Impact of obesity on long-term prognosis following acute myocardial infarction. *Int J Cardiol* 2005;98:123–31.

94. Rexrode KM, Carey VJ, Hennekens CH, et al. Abdominal adiposity and coronary heart disease in women. *JAMA* 1998;280:1843–8.

95. Oppert JM, Charles MA, Thibult N, Guy-Grand B, Eschwege E, Ducimetiere P. Anthropometric estimates of muscle and fat mass in relation to cardiac and cancer mortality in men: the Paris Prospective Study. *Am J Clin Nutr* 2002;75:1107–13.

96. Kanaya AM, Vittinghoff E, Shlipak MG, et al. Association of total and central obesity with mortality in postmenopausal women with coronary heart disease. *Am J Epidemiol* 2003;158:1161–70.

97. Rubinshtein R, Halon DA, Jaffe R, Shahla J, Lewis BS. Relation between obesity and severity of coronary artery disease in patients undergoing coronary angiography. *Am J Cardiol* 2006;97:1277–80.

98. Mohamed-Ali V, Goodrick S, Bulmer K, Holly JM, Yudkin JS, Coppack SW. Production of soluble tumor necrosis factor receptors by human subcutaneous adipose tissue in vivo. *Am J Physiol* 1999;277:E971–5.

99. Beddhu S, Pappas LM, Ramkumar N, Samore M. Effects of body size and body composition on survival in hemodialysis patients. *J Am Soc Nephrol* 2003;14:2366–72.

100. Kakiya R, Shoji T, Tsujimoto Y, et al. Body fat mass and lean mass as predictors of survival in hemodialysis patients. *Kidney Int* 2006;70:549–56.

101. Baik I, Ascherio A, Rimm EB, et al. Adiposity and mortality in men. *Am J Epidemiol* 2000;152:264–71.

102. Visscher TL, Seidell JC, Molarius A, van der KD, Hofman A, Witteman JC. A comparison of body mass index, waist-hip ratio and waist circumference as predictors of all-cause mortality among the elderly: the Rotterdam study. *Int J Obes Relat Metab Disord* 2001;25:1730–5.

103. Price GM, Uauy R, Breeze E, Bulpitt CJ, Fletcher AE. Weight, shape, and mortality risk in older persons: elevated waist-hip ratio, not high body mass index, is associated with a greater risk of death. *Am J Clin Nutr* 2006;84:449–60.

104. Janssen I, Katzmarzyk PT, Ross R. Body mass index is inversely related to mortality in older people after adjustment for waist circumference. *J Am Geriatr Soc* 2005;53:2112–18.

105. Yusuf S, Hawken S, Ounpuu S, et al. Obesity and the risk of myocardial infarction in 27,000 participants from 52 countries: a case-control study. *Lancet* 2005;366:1640–9.

106. Poirier P. Healthy lifestyle: even if you are doing everything right, extra weight carries an excess risk of acute coronary events. *Circulation* 2008;117:3057–9.

107. Balkau B, Deanfield JE, Despres JP, et al. International Day for the Evaluation of Abdominal Obesity (IDEA): a study of waist circumference, cardiovascular disease, and diabetes mellitus in 168,000 primary care patients in 63 countries. *Circulation* 2007;116:1942–51.

108. Lopez-Jimenez F, Malinski M, Gutt M, et al. Recognition, diagnosis and management of obesity after myocardial infarction. *Int J Obes (Lond)* 2005;29:137–41.

109. Wang F, Schultz AB, Musich S, McDonald T, Hirschland D, Edington DW. The relationship between National Heart, Lung, and Blood Institute Weight Guidelines and concurrent medical costs in a manufacturing population. *Am J Health Promot* 2003;17:183–9.

110. Cornier MA, Tate CW, Grunwald GK, Bessesen DH. Relationship between waist circumference, body mass index, and medical care costs. *Obes Res* 2002;10:1167–72.

111. Poirier P, Despres JP. Exercise in weight management of obesity. *Cardiol Clin* 2001;19:459–70.

112. Kraus WE, Houmard JA, Duscha BD, et al. Effects of the amount and intensity of exercise on plasma lipoproteins. *N Engl J Med* 2002;347:1483–92.

113. Klein S, Burke LE, Bray GA, et al. Clinical implications of obesity with specific focus on cardiovascular disease: a statement for professionals from the American Heart Association Council on Nutrition, Physical Activity, and Metabolism: endorsed by the American College of Cardiology Foundation. *Circulation* 2004;110:2952–67.

114. Drolet B, Simard C, Poirier P. Impact of weight-loss medications on the cardiovascular system: focus on current and future anti-obesity drugs. *Am J Cardiovasc Drugs* 2007;7:273–88.

115. Ryan DH, Espeland MA, Foster GD, et al. Look AHEAD (Action for Health in Diabetes): design and methods for a clinical trial of weight loss for the prevention of cardiovascular disease in type 2 diabetes. *Control Clin Trials* 2003;24:610–28.

116. Ribisl PM, Lang W, Jaramillo SA, et al. Exercise capacity and cardiovascular/ metabolic characteristics of overweight and obese individuals with type 2 diabetes: the Look AHEAD clinical trial. *Diabetes Care* 2007;30:2679–84.

117. Bray GA. The missing link – lose weight, live longer. *N Engl J Med* 2007;357:818–20.

118. Sjostrom L, Narbro K, Sjostrom CD, et al. Effects of bariatric surgery on mortality in Swedish obese subjects. *N Engl J Med* 2007;357:741–52.

119. Adams TD, Gress RE, Smith SC, et al. Long-term mortality after gastric bypass surgery. *N Engl J Med* 2007;357:753–61.

Chapter 7

Insulin resistance, the metabolic syndrome, and cardiovascular risk

Stanley S. Wang and Sidney C. Smith, Jr

Introduction

Cardiovascular disease (CVD) arises frequently in patients with selected metabolic derangements, including insulin resistance (IR) syndromes such as type 2 diabetes mellitus. IR is frequently associated with additional metabolic derangements collectively referred to as the metabolic syndrome (MetS). Better understanding of IR and MetS has given rise to the concept of cardiometabolic risk, which has gained increasing recognition as an important and modifiable cause of CVD [1]. Because IR (and particularly MetS) is related to adiposity, the worldwide obesity epidemic detailed in the previous chapter has thrust IR and MetS into the forefront of discussions on preventive and therapeutic strategies to reduce CVD risk.

The current definition of MetS in the United States was promulgated by the National Cholesterol Education Program – Adult Treatment Panel III (NCEP-ATP III) in 2001 [2] and revised by the American Heart Association (AHA) and National Heart, Lung, and Blood Institute (NHLBI) in 2005 [3]. Under this definition, a patient is diagnosed with MetS by meeting at least three of five criteria reflecting blood pressure dysregulation, adiposity, dysglycemia, and dyslipidemia (Table 7.1).

Of note, several other criteria for diagnosing MetS had been used clinically and in research, including those published by the World Health Organization (WHO) [4], European Group for the Study of Insulin Resistance [5], American Association of Clinical Endocrinologists [6], International Diabetes Federation (IDF) [7], and others [8]. Notably, the WHO criteria for diagnosing MetS required a finding of IR inferred from elevated glucose levels or direct measurements of

Metabolic Risk for Cardiovascular Disease, 1st edition. Edited by R. H. Eckel.
© 2011 American Heart Association. By Blackwell Publishing Ltd.

Table 7.1 AHA/NHLBI criteria for diagnosing metabolic syndrome

1 Blood pressure $\geq 130/85$ mm Hg*

2 Waist circumference ≥ 102 cm in men or ≥ 88 cm in women**

3 Fasting glucose ≥ 100 mg/dL*

4 Triglycerides ≥ 150 mg/dL*

5 HDL-C < 40 mg/dL in men or < 50 mg/dL in women*

A patient has metabolic syndrome if three of these five criteria are met [3].
*Each criterion is also considered to be met if the patient is on drug therapy for the criterion.
**The waist circumference criterion is more stringent in Asian American patients, in whom the waist circumference criteria are ≥ 90 cm in men or ≥ 80 cm in women.

insulin levels [9]. On the other hand, the IDF criteria shifted the emphasis from insulin resistance to its presumed manifestations of increased body size (as defined by specific racial/ethnic criteria) and elevated glucose.

Recently, the AHA, NHLBI, IDF, World Heart Federation, International Atherosclerosis Society, and International Association for the Study of Obesity produced a joint interim statement that represents an effort to adopt a common clinical definition for MetS [10]. While the blood pressure and laboratory parameters (glucose, triglycerides, high-density lipoprotein cholesterol; HDL-C) remain the same, the waist circumference (WC) criterion will vary depending on the country and ethnic population. In the US, the current WC criteria are unchanged (although stricter WC cut-offs of ≥ 94 cm in men and ≥ 80 cm in women portend greater CVD risk), pending the discussions associated with the release of updated guidelines in 2010.

Epidemiology

The incidence of IR is uncertain, but its associated clinical presentations, especially MetS, are highly prevalent. Data from 1999–2000 suggest that nearly one-third of adults in the US have MetS [11]. Moreover, the incidence of MetS is increasing along with that of obesity [12]. Worldwide, the prevalence of MetS ranges from roughly 10% in East Asia [13] to 25% in Europe and Latin America [12], with more exact estimates made difficult by variations in the criteria used to define MetS.

MetS appears to have a greater impact in African-American [14] and especially Mexican-American populations, in whom the highest age-adjusted prevalence of MetS is found [15]. Among younger populations, however, the prevalence of MetS and its risk factors appears to be lower in African-American populations [16]. Gender seems to play a lesser role with MetS, being similarly prevalent in men and women, but women also suffer from polycystic ovary syndrome [17].

While MetS is more prevalent in older populations, and approximately 40% of adults over age 60 meet diagnostic criteria [15], there have been troublesome increases in prevalence among younger populations [18].

There are additional clinical manifestations of IR such as polycystic ovary syndrome, which affects 6.5–8.0% of women of reproductive age (an estimated 4–5 million women in the US) [19].

Pathophysiology

Underlying insulin resistance appears to play a significant role in the clustering of the individual components of the metabolic syndrome, and may contribute to their synergistic impact on CVD risk [20], although there remains some controversy regarding its "causative pathogenesis" and clinical implications [8].

The etiology of IR is thought to be multifactorial, with both genetic and environmental components. Insulin is secreted by pancreatic β-cells in proportion to circulating glucose and amino acid levels, and acts as an anabolic hormone that plays a key role in glucose regulation [21]. It affects numerous target organs, including the liver, where it inhibits gluconeogenesis and glycolysis, thus reducing glucose production. It also promotes glucose uptake into skeletal muscle and adipose tissue through a complex process leading to translocation of transmembrane glucose transporters (Figure 7.1) [22].

In addition, insulin is important in lipid regulation as it promotes lipid production in hepatocytes and adipocytes, while inhibiting fatty acid secretion from the latter. As IR develops, these organs become less responsive to normal circulating levels of insulin, and metabolic dysregulation ensues.

The mechanisms by which tissues become resistant to insulin have been studied intensively, and many potential sites along the complicated pathway of insulin activity (Figure 7.1) may be involved, ranging from the insulin receptor modifications [23] to signal transduction pathway changes [23]. In addition, a number of inflammatory cytokines have been implicated in the genesis of IR [24].

The development of a "lipotoxic" state, with inappropriate accumulation of lipids in hepatocytes and skeletal myocytes and elevated plasma free fatty acid levels [25], is thought to induce IR and contribute to the development of MetS [21]. Free fatty acids may worsen hyperglycemia by reducing skeletal muscle responsiveness to insulin and inhibiting glucose uptake [26,27], and also by stimulating hepatic glucose production.

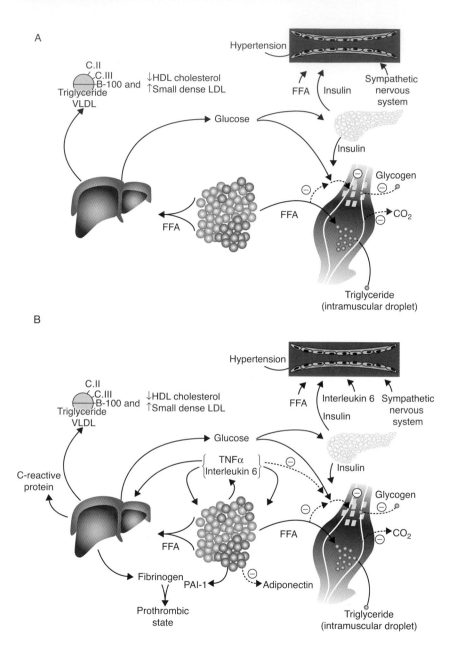

While IR is associated with MetS, it is not the sole cause and other factors play a role, which explains the absence of obesity, hypertension, or dyslipidemia in patients with dysfunctional insulin receptors or insulin receptor antibodies [28]. Rather, it is believed that the secondary effects of persistent hyperglycemia, compensatory hyperinsulinemia, and imbalance of intracellular insulin signaling pathways give rise to some of the features of MetS [29].

Metabolic syndrome and cardiovascular risk

Whether the collective diagnosis of MetS adds additional prognostic value has been the subject of some debate [8,30]. In a study of older populations (ages 60–82), MetS did not predict incident diabetes more than fasting glucose alone, and three of the MetS criteria (elevated triglycerides, elevated glucose, increased waist circumference) did not predict CVD outcomes [31], raising concern that MetS may not imply independent risk but rather is a product of confounding. Some of the controversy over MetS has centered over dispute regarding definitional problems, uncertainty regarding pathogenesis, and doubt regarding its

----

Figure 7.1 Pathophysiology of the metabolic syndrome and insulin resistance. A. FFA are released in abundance from an expanded adipose tissue mass. In the liver, FFA result in increased production of glucose and triglyceridesand secretion of VLDL. Associated lipid/lipoprotein abnormalities include reductions in HDL-C and increased density of LDL. FFA also reduce insulin sensitivity in muscle by inhibiting insulin-mediated glucose update. Associated defects include a reduction in glucose partitioning to glycogen and increased lipid accumulation. Elevated circulating glucose and to some extent FFA increase pancreatic insulin secretion, resulting in hyperinsulinemia. Hyperinsulinemia may result in enhanced sodium reabsorption and increased sympathetic nervous system activity and may contribute to hypertension, as might increased levels of FFA. B. Superimposed and contributory to the insulin resistance produced by excessive FFA is the paracrine and endocrine effect of the proinflammatory state. Produced by a variety of cells in adipose tissue, including adipocytes and monocyte-derived macrophages, the enhanced secretion of IL-6 and TNF-α among others results in more insulin resistance and lipolysis of adipose tissue triglyceride stores, resulting in increased circulating FFA. IL-6 and other cytokines also are increased in the circulation and may enhance hepatic glucose production, the production of VLDL by the liver, and insulin resistance in muscle. Cytokines and FFA also increase the production of fibrinogen and PAI-1 by the liver, complementing the overproduction of PAI-1 by adipose tissue. This results in a prothrombotic state. Reductions in the production of the antiinflammatory and insulin-sensitizing cytokine adiponectin are also associated with the metabolic syndrome and insulin resistance. FFA, free fatty acids; HDL-C, high-density lipoprotein cholesterol; IL-6, interleukin 6; LDL, low-density lipoprotein; PAI-1, plasminogen activator inhibitor 1; TNF-α, tumor necrosis factor-alpha; VLDL, very-low-density lipoprotein. Reproduced from Eckel et al., *Lancet* 2005;365:1415–28 with permission from Elsevier.

additive value in predicting CVD risk [32,33]. Each of these concerns is being addressed. As discussed above, the recent multi-society joint statement represents important progress toward an eventual common clinical definition of MetS.

In addition, ongoing research continues to detail plausible pathophysiological mechanisms through which MetS may contribute additional CVD risk beyond that conferred by its component abnormalities. MetS is associated with greater arterial stiffness [34] as well as microvascular dysfunction, which in turn may exacerbate insulin resistance and hypertension [35]. In addition, patients with MetS may be more likely to have endothelial dysfunction and elevated levels of adipokines and plasminogen activator type 1, all of which promote thrombogenicity [36].

Not surprisingly, a multitude of studies have shown that the presence of MetS leads to an approximate doubling of CVD risk even in the absence of diabetes [3,37]. Age-adjusted Framingham data suggest that MetS confers a relative risk for CVD events as high as 2.88 in men and 2.25 in women [38]. Importantly, a meta-analysis of longitudinal studies estimated the overall relative risk to be 1.78 (95% CI, 1.58–2.00) with excess CVD risk present *even after controlling for the traditional CVD risk factors* (relative risk of 1.54 with 95% CI 1.32–1.79) [39]. When compared to Framingham-based risk estimation, the diagnosis of MetS appeared to add independent prognostic value in some [40,41], but not all [31,42], studies [8].

In addition to coronary CVD, studies have suggested that MetS is also associated with greater risks of incident diabetes [43] and many forms of non-coronary CVD, including atrial fibrillation [44], heart failure, aortic stenosis [45], and ischemic stroke [46,47]. MetS also may be related to certain sleep-related breathing disorders, particularly obstructive sleep apnea (OSA), whose potential role in CVD has been recognized by the AHA/NHLBI [48]. Recent evidence suggests that OSA can cause or worsen inflammation [49] and abnormalities in glucose metabolism [50]. In addition, OSA has been linked with obesity [51] and hypertension [52,53], raising the possibility of an independent link between OSA and MetS [54,55]. Peripheral studies have linked MetS to other important, non-cardiovascular diseases including non-alcoholic fatty liver disease [56], psoriasis [57], accelerated cognitive aging [58], and cancers of the breast [59], colon, kidney, gallbladder, and possibly the prostate gland [60].

Diagnosis and evaluation

History and physical examination

MetS is defined by clusters of established metabolic derangements (Table 7.1), and the presence of one of these derangements should prompt consideration of further evaluation for the others. Symptoms suggesting a component disorder, such as polyuria, polydipsia, or polyphagia suggesting hyperglycemia, or relevant signs, such as elevated blood pressure or waist circumference, deserve careful attention as potential clues to underlying MetS. Similarly, laboratory features including elevated triglycerides and decreased HDL levels should lead to consideration of MetS.

Assessment of associated risk factors for MetS (and for CVD) is a crucial component of the clinical evaluation of a patient with suspected MetS. A thorough family history may reveal the presence of MetS in other family members as there is thought to be a genetic component to MetS, although specific genes have not been consistently identified, suggesting an important environmental impact on the genesis of the disease [61]. The patient's social history should include not only surveillance for traditional CVD risk factors such as tobacco, alcohol, and illicit drug use, but also an examination of the patient's diet and exercise habits because of the potential impact these have on the development – and treatment – of MetS.

Additional questions should be directed at the patient's sleep history, as patients with unrefreshing sleep, daytime drowsiness, and a history of snoring may have a sleep-related breathing disorder such as OSA.

Routine physical examination should include measurements of blood pressure and waist circumference, as well as thorough evaluation for stigmata of metabolic dysfunction (retinopathy, acanthosis nigricans, hirsutism, xanthomas, xanthelasmas) and CVD (cardiac gallops, peripheral bruits).

Diagnostic testing

Laboratory work-up for MetS should begin with standard chemistries to determine fasting glucose levels and check for evidence of renal or hepatic dysfunction. In addition, fasting lipids should be checked for evidence of elevated triglyceride or low HDL levels, as well as to guide potential LDL and non-HDL cholesterol-based therapies. In selected clinical situations, additional blood testing for markers of inflammation and cardiovascular risk may be appropriate, such as uric acid (commonly elevated in MetS [62]) or C-reactive protein.

No specific imaging studies are necessary for MetS but should be considered as symptoms warrant. Given the association of MetS with CVD risk, appropriate electrocardiographic, ultrasonographic, and nuclear imaging should be pursued for complaints suggestive of ischemia, such as chest pain, dyspnea, or claudication. In addition, patients with sleep complaints may benefit from polysomnography to guide potential therapy of an underlying sleep-related breathing disorder.

Treatment

Non-pharmacological treatment

Front-line therapy for MetS involves diet and physical activity. Evidence suggests that Westernized diets are associated with an increased risk of developing

MetS [63], while diets rich in fish, cereal grains, and dairy products may be associated with a decreased risk [64]. Mediterranean-style diets are associated with not only decreased risk of developing MetS but also possible resolution of the disease in patients with the diagnosis, especially when adopted in conjunction with adequate physical activity [65].

Physical inactivity has been associated with pathophysiological changes seen in MetS [66], whereas moderate and vigorous exercise may be associated with a reduced risk of being diagnosed with MetS [67]. Experimental and animal models have suggested that exercise results in numerous favorable biochemical changes that may be beneficial in patients with MetS [68].

Emerging evidence suggests that mechanical treatment of an underlying sleep-related breathing disorder (especially OSA) with continuous positive airway pressure (CPAP) may provide valuable benefits in IR syndromes. There is theoretical support for CPAP therapy based on shared pathophysiological mechanisms between OSA and MetS [69], and preliminary data suggest that CPAP therapy in patients with severe OSA may improve insulin sensitivity and reduce CVD risk [70].

Pharmacological treatment

Pharmacological treatment for MetS should be directed toward treatment of the component abnormalities when diet and exercise fail to achieve target goals. Hypertension should be treated according to the guidelines of the 7th Report of the Joint National Committee on Prevention, Detection, Evaluation, and Treatment of High Blood Pressure (JNC-7) [71], although there is growing support for a more stringent treatment goal as well as for the preferential use of angiotensin-converting enzyme inhibitors or angiotensin receptor blockers in MetS patients [72]. Lipid abnormalities should be treated according to the guidelines of the National Cholesterol Education Program Expert Panel on Detection, Evaluation, and Treatment of High Blood Cholesterol in Adults (NCEP-ATP III) [73], which were updated in 2004 [74]. Of note, revisions of both guidelines are expected in late 2009/early 2010.

Treatment of hyperglycemia in MetS patients typically includes an insulin sensitizing agent such as metformin, which may counteract some of the underlying metabolic derangements in MetS. Metformin has shown promise in conjunction with intensive lifestyle intervention [75] as well as with peroxisome proliferator-activated receptor agonists [76], such as the thiazoladinediones [77] and the fibrates [78].

In patients with elevated triglycerides and decreased HDL refractory to therapeutic lifestyle interventions, consideration may be given to drug therapy. The American College of Cardiology Foundation and the American Diabetes Association have released a consensus conference report dealing with advanced lipoprotein management [79]. There is some evidence suggesting that nicotinic acid reduces CVD risk and total mortality [80], but further studies are needed to support a strong recommendation [81]. Fibrates may reduce CVD risk, but studies demonstrating mortality reduction are still lacking [82].

Empiric 3-hydroxy-3-methylglutaryl-CoA reductase inhibitor (statin) therapy may be beneficial in suppressing related inflammation in MetS patients [83], although there is some uncertainty regarding potential dysglycemic effects with specific statins [84].

The use of pharmaceutical agents, such as sibutramine and orlistat, to achieve weight loss holds promise for ameliorating the components of MetS, but further studies are needed to determine the long-term clinical implications [85].

Surgical treatment

Bariatric surgery is emerging as a potentially effective treatment for MetS [86]. While data are limited, a recent retrospective study suggested that Roux-en-Y gastric bypass was associated in improvements in all parameters of MetS, particularly in patients who achieved at least a 5% weight loss [87]. This association has also been reported in laparoscopic gastric bypass procedures [88].

Conclusion

Insulin resistance and the metabolic syndrome appear to be associated with elevated CVD risk. The prevalence of MetS is rising along with the obesity epidemic, providing impetus for better understanding of the pathophysiology and clinical management of the condition. Treatment of the underlying components of MetS should be pursued according to established guidelines, with additional evidence favoring the use of therapeutic lifestyle interventions and possibly insulin sensitizing agents in patients with MetS. Surgical therapy aimed at reducing obesity holds promise, but as with many aspects of MetS and CVD risk, more robust data are needed to clarify potential clinical ramifications.

References

1. Brunzell JD, Davidson M, Furberg CD, Goldberg RB, Howard BV, Stein JH, Witztum JL. Lipoprotein management in patients with cardiometabolic risk: consensus conference report from the American Diabetes Association and the American College of Cardiology Foundation. *J Am Coll Cardiol* 2008;51:1512–24.
2. Expert Panel on Detection, Evaluation, and Treatment of High Blood Cholesterol in Adults. Executive Summary of The Third Report of The National Cholesterol Education Program (NCEP) Expert Panel on Detection, Evaluation, And Treatment of High Blood Cholesterol In Adults (Adult Treatment Panel III). *JAMA* 2001;285(19):2486–97.
3. Grundy SM, Cleeman JI, Daniels SR, Donato KA, Eckel RH, Franklin BA, Gordon DJ, Krauss RM, Savage PJ, Smith SC Jr, Spertus JA, Costa F; American Heart Association; National Heart, Lung, and Blood Institute. Diagnosis and management of the metabolic syndrome: an American Heart Association/National Heart, Lung,

and Blood Institute Scientific Statement. *Circulation* 2005;112(17):2735–52. [Erratum in: *Circulation* 2005;112(17):e297. *Circulation* 2005;112(17):e298.]

4. Alberti KG, Zimmet PZ. Definition, diagnosis and classification of diabetes mellitus and its complications. Part 1: diagnosis and classification of diabetes mellitus provisional report of a WHO consultation. *Diabet Med* 1998;15(7):539–53.

5. Balkau B, Charles MA. Comment on the provisional report from the WHO consultation. European Group for the Study of Insulin Resistance (EGIR). *Diabet Med* 1999;16(5):442–3.

6. Bloomgarden ZT. American Association of Clinical Endocrinologists (AACE) consensus conference on the insulin resistance syndrome: 25–26 August 2002, Washington, DC. *Diabetes Care* 2003;26(4):1297–303.

7. Alberti KG, Zimmet P, Shaw J. Metabolic syndrome – a new world-wide definition. A Consensus Statement from the International Diabetes Federation. *Diabet Med* 2006;23(5):469–80.

8. Cornier MA, Dabelea D, Hernandez TL, Lindstrom RC, Steig AJ, Stob NR, Van Pelt RE, Wang H, Eckel RH. The metabolic syndrome. *Endocr Rev* 2008;29(7):777–822.

9. Miranda PJ, DeFronzo RA, Califf RM, Guyton JR. Metabolic syndrome: definition, pathophysiology, and mechanisms. *Am Heart J* 2005;149(1):33–45.

10. Harmonizing the metabolic syndrome: a joint interim statement of the International Diabetes Federation Task Force on Epidemiology and Prevention; National Heart, Lung, and Blood Institute; American Heart Association; World Heart Federation; International Atherosclerosis Society; and International Association for the Study of Obesity. Alberti KG, Eckel RH, Grundy SM et al; International Diabetes Federation Task Force on Epidemiology and Prevention; National Heart, Lung, and Blood Institute; American Heart Association; World Heart Federation; International Atherosclerosis Society; International Association for the Study of Obesity. *Circulation* 2009 Oct 20;120(16):1640–5. Epub 2009 Oct 5.

11. Ford ES, Giles WH, Mokdad AH. Increasing prevalence of the metabolic syndrome among U.S. adults. *Diabetes Care* 2004;27(10):2444–9.

12. Grundy SM. Metabolic syndrome pandemic. *Arterioscler Thromb Vasc Biol* 2008;28(4):629–36.

13. Hoang KC, Le TV, Wong ND. The metabolic syndrome in East Asians. *J Cardiometab Syndr* 2007;2(4):276–82.

14. Clark LT, El-Atat F. Metabolic syndrome in African Americans: implications for preventing coronary heart disease. *Clin Cardiol* 2007;30(4):161–4.

15. Ford ES, Giles WH, Dietz WH. Prevalence of the metabolic syndrome among US adults: findings from the third National Health and Nutrition Examination Survey. *JAMA* 2002;287(3):356–9.

16. Johnson WD, Kroon JJ, Greenway FL, Bouchard C, Ryan D, Katzmarzyk PT. Prevalence of risk factors for metabolic syndrome in adolescents: National Health and Nutrition Examination Survey (NHANES), 2001–2006. *Arch Pediatr Adolesc Med* 2009;163(4):371–7.

17. Bentley-Lewis R, Koruda K, Seely EW. The metabolic syndrome in women. *Nat Clin Pract Endocrinol Metab* 2007;3(10):696–704.

18. De Ferranti SD, Osganian SK. Epidemiology of paediatric metabolic syndrome and type 2 diabetes mellitus. *Diab Vasc Dis Res* 2007;4(4):285–96.

19. Goodarzi MO, Azziz R. Diagnosis, epidemiology, and genetics of the polycystic ovary syndrome. *Best Pract Res Clin Endocrinol Metab* 2006;20(2):193–205.

20. Yip J, Facchini FS, Reaven GM. Resistance to insulin-mediated glucose disposal as a predictor of cardiovascular disease. *J Clin Endocrinol Metab* 1998;83(8):2773–6.

21. Sesti G. Pathophysiology of insulin resistance. *Best Pract Res Clin Endocrinol Metab* 2006;20(4):665–79.

22. Federici M, Porzio O, Zucaro L, Giovannone B, Borboni P, Marini MA, Lauro D, Sesti G. Increased abundance of insulin/IGF-I hybrid receptors in adipose tissue from NIDDM patients. *Mol Cell Endocrinol* 1997;135(1):41–7.

23. Arner P, Pollare T, Lithell H, Livingston JN. Defective insulin receptor tyrosine kinase in human skeletal muscle in obesity and type 2 (non-insulin-dependent) diabetes mellitus. *Diabetologia* 1987;30(6):437–40.

24. Kern PA, Ranganathan S, Li C, Wood L, Ranganathan G. Adipose tissue tumor necrosis factor and interleukin-6 expression in human obesity and insulin resistance. *Am J Physiol Endocrinol Metab* 2001;280(5):E745–51.

25. Shulman GI. Cellular mechanisms of insulin resistance. *J Clin Invest* 2000;106(2):171–176.

26. Delarue J, Magnan C. Free fatty acids and insulin resistance. *Curr Opin Clin Nutr Metab Care* 2007;10(2):142–8.

27. Kraegen EW, Cooney GJ. Free fatty acids and skeletal muscle insulin resistance. *Curr Opin Lipidol* 2008;19(3):235–41.

28. Kahn CR, Flier JS, Bar RS, Archer JA, Gorden P, Martin MM, Roth J. The syndromes of insulin resistance and acanthosis nigricans. Insulin-receptor disorders in man. *N Engl J Med* 1976;294(14):739–45.

29. Miranda PJ, DeFronzo RA, Califf RM, Guyton JR. Metabolic syndrome: definition, pathophysiology, and mechanisms. *Am Heart J* 2005;149(1):33–45.

30. Nilsson PM. Cardiovascular risk in the metabolic syndrome: fact or fiction? *Curr Cardiol Rep* 2007;9(6):479–85.

31. Sattar N, McConnachie A, Shaper AG, Blauw GJ, Buckley BM, de Craen AJ, Ford I, Forouhi NG, Freeman DJ, Jukema JW, Lennon L, Macfarlane PW, Murphy MB, Packard CJ, Stott DJ, Westendorp RG, Whincup PH, Shepherd J, Wannamethee SG. Can metabolic syndrome usefully predict cardiovascular disease and diabetes? Outcome data from two prospective studies. *Lancet* 2008;371(9628):1927–35.

32. Kahn R, Buse J, Ferrannini E, Stern M; American Diabetes Association; European Association for the Study of Diabetes. The metabolic syndrome: time for a critical appraisal: joint statement from the American Diabetes Association and the European Association for the Study of Diabetes. *Diabetes Care* 2005;28(9):2289–304.

33. Grundy SM. Metabolic syndrome: connecting and reconciling cardiovascular and diabetes worlds. *J Am Coll Cardiol* 2006;47(6):1093–100.

34. Stehouwer CD, Henry RM, Ferreira I. Arterial stiffness in diabetes and the metabolic syndrome: a pathway to cardiovascular disease. *Diabetologia* 2008;51(4):527–39.

35. Serné EH, de Jongh RT, Eringa EC, Ijzerman RG, Stehouwer CD. Microvascular dysfunction: a potential pathophysiological role in the metabolic syndrome. *Hypertension* 2007;50(1):204–11.

36. Alessi MC, Juhan-Vague I. Metabolic syndrome, haemostasis and thrombosis. *Thromb Haemost* 2008;99:995–1000.

37. Grundy SM. Metabolic syndrome: a multiplex cardiovascular risk factor. *J Clin Endocrinol Metab* 2007;92(2):399–404.

38. Wilson PW, D'Agostino RB, Parise H, Sullivan L, Meigs JB. Metabolic syndrome as a precursor of cardiovascular disease and type 2 diabetes mellitus. *Circulation* 2005;112(20):3066–72.

39. Gami AS, Witt BJ, Howard DE, Erwin PJ, Gami LA, Somers VK, Montori VM. Metabolic syndrome and risk of incident cardiovascular events and death: a systematic review and meta-analysis of longitudinal studies. *J Am Coll Cardiol* 2007;49(4):403–14.

40. Girman CJ, Rhodes T, Mercuri M, Pyörälä K, Kjekshus J, Pedersen TR, Beere PA, Gotto AM, Clearfield M; 4S Group and the AFCAPS/TexCAPS Research Group. The metabolic syndrome and risk of major coronary events in the Scandinavian Simvastatin Survival Study (4S) and the Air Force/Texas Coronary Atherosclerosis Prevention Study (AFCAPS/TexCAPS). *Am J Cardiol* 2004;93(2):136–41.

41. Wannamethee SG, Shaper AG, Lennon L, Morris RW. Metabolic syndrome vs Framingham Risk Score for prediction of coronary heart disease, stroke, and type 2 diabetes mellitus. *Arch Intern Med* 2005;165(22):2644–50.

42. McNeill AM, Rosamond WD, Girman CJ, Golden SH, Schmidt MI, East HE, Ballantyne CM, Heiss G. The metabolic syndrome and 11-year risk of incident cardiovascular disease in the atherosclerosis risk in communities study. *Diabetes Care* 2005;28(2):385–90.

43. Hanley AJ, Karter AJ, Williams K, Festa A, D'Agostino RB Jr, Wagenknecht LE, Haffner SM. Prediction of type 2 diabetes mellitus with alternative definitions of the metabolic syndrome: the Insulin Resistance Atherosclerosis Study. *Circulation* 2005;112:3713–21.

44. Umetani K, Kodama Y, Nakamura T, Mende A, Kitta Y, Kawabata K, Obata JE, Takano H, Kugiyama K. High prevalence of paroxysmal atrial fibrillation and/or atrial flutter in metabolic syndrome. *Circ J* 2007;71(2):252–5.

45. Obunai K, Jani S, Dangas GD. Cardiovascular morbidity and mortality of the metabolic syndrome. *Med Clin North Am* 2007;91(6):1169–84, x.

46. Air EL, Kissela BM. Diabetes, the metabolic syndrome, and ischemic stroke: epidemiology and possible mechanisms. *Diabetes Care* 2007;30(12):3131–40.

47. Li W, Ma D, Liu M, Liu H, Feng S, Hao Z, Wu B, Zhang S. Association between metabolic syndrome and risk of stroke: a meta-analysis of cohort studies. *Cerebrovasc Dis* 2008;25(6):539–47.

48. Somers VK, White DP, Amin R, Abraham WT, Costa F, Culebras A, Daniels S, Floras JS, Hunt CE, Olson LJ, Pickering TG, Russell R, Woo M, Young T. Sleep apnea and cardiovascular disease: an American Heart Association/American College of Cardiology Foundation Scientific Statement from the American Heart Association Council for High Blood Pressure Research Professional Education Committee, Council on Clinical Cardiology, Stroke Council, and Council on Cardiovascular Nursing. *J Am Coll Cardiol* 2008;52(8):686–717.

49. Alam I, Lewis K, Stephens JW, Baxter JN. Obesity, metabolic syndrome and sleep apnoea: all pro-inflammatory states. *Obes Rev* 2007;8(2):119–27.

50. Tasali E, Ip MS. Obstructive sleep apnea and metabolic syndrome: alterations in glucose metabolism and inflammation. *Proc Am Thorac Soc* 2008;5(2):207–17.

51. Schwartz AR, Patil SP, Laffan AM, Polotsky V, Schneider H, Smith PL. Obesity and obstructive sleep apnea: pathogenic mechanisms and therapeutic approaches. *Proc Am Thorac Soc* 2008;5(2):185–92.

52. Peppard PE, Young T, Palta M, Skatrud J. Prospective study of the association between sleep-disordered breathing and hypertension. *N Engl J Med* 2000;342(19):1378–84.

53. Nieto FJ, Young TB, Lind BK, Shahar E, Samet JM, Redline S, D'Agostino RB, Newman AB, Lebowitz MD, Pickering TG. Association of sleep-disordered breathing, sleep apnea, and hypertension in a large community-based study. Sleep Heart Health Study. *JAMA* 2000;283(14):1829–36.

54. Vgontzas AN, Bixler EO, Chrousos GP. Sleep apnea is a manifestation of the metabolic syndrome. *Sleep Med Rev* 2005;9(3):211–24.

55. Tasali E, Ip MS. Obstructive sleep apnea and metabolic syndrome: alterations in glucose metabolism and inflammation. *Proc Am Thorac Soc* 2008;5(2):207–17.

56. Lidofsky SD. Nonalcoholic fatty liver disease: diagnosis and relation to metabolic syndrome and approach to treatment. *Curr Diab Rep* 2008;8(1):25–30.

57. Cohen AD, Sherf M, Vidavsky L, Vardy DA, Shapiro J, Meyerovitch J. Association between psoriasis and the metabolic syndrome. A cross-sectional study. *Dermatology* 2008;216(2):152–5.

58. Yaffe K. Metabolic syndrome and cognitive decline. *Curr Alzheimer Res* 2007;4(2):123–6.

59. Beaulieu LM, Whitley BR, Wiesner TF, Rehault SM, Palmieri D, Elkahloun AG, Church FC. Breast cancer and metabolic syndrome linked through the plasminogen activator inhibitor-1 cycle. *Bioessays* 2007;29(10):1029–38

60. Hsing AW, Sakoda LC, Chua S Jr. Obesity, metabolic syndrome, and prostate cancer. *Am J Clin Nutr* 2007;86(3):s843–57.

61. Joy T, Lahiry P, Pollex RL, Hegele RA. Genetics of metabolic syndrome. *Curr Diab Rep* 2008;8(2):141–8.

62. Puig JG, Martínez MA. Hyperuricemia, gout and the metabolic syndrome. *Curr Opin Rheumatol* 2008;20(2):187–91.

63. Yoneda M, Yamane K, Jitsuiki K, Nakanishi S, Kamei N, Watanabe H, Kohno N. Prevalence of metabolic syndrome compared between native Japanese and Japanese-Americans. *Diabetes Res Clin Pract* 2008;79(3):518–22.

64. Ruidavets JB, Bongard V, Dallongeville J, Arveiler D, Ducimetière P, Perret B, Simon C, Amouyel P, Ferrières J. High consumptions of grain, fish, dairy products and combinations of these are associated with a low prevalence of metabolic syndrome. *J Epidemiol Community Health* 2007;61(9):810–17.

65. Esposito K, Ciotola M, Giugliano D. Mediterranean diet and the metabolic syndrome. *Mol Nutr Food Res* 2007;51(10):1268–74.

66. Hamilton MT, Hamilton DG, Zderic TW. Role of low energy expenditure and sitting in obesity, metabolic syndrome, type 2 diabetes, and cardiovascular disease. *Diabetes* 2007;56(11):2655–67.

67. Rennie KL, McCarthy N, Yazdgerdi S, Marmot M, Brunner E. Association of the metabolic syndrome with both vigorous and moderate physical activity. *Int J Epidemiol* 2003;32(4):600–6.

68. Yung LM, Laher I, Yao X, Chen ZY, Huang Y, Leung FP. Exercise, vascular wall and cardiovascular diseases: an update (part 2). *Sports Med* 2009;39(1):45–63.

69. Bonsignore MR, Zito A. Metabolic effects of the obstructive sleep apnea syndrome and cardiovascular risk. *Arch Physiol Biochem* 2008;114(4):255–60.

70. Dorkova Z, Petrasova D, Molcanyiova A, Popovnakova M, Tkacova R. Effects of continuous positive airway pressure on cardiovascular risk profile in patients

with severe obstructive sleep apnea and metabolic syndrome. *Chest* 2008;134(4):686–92.

71. Chobanian AV, Bakris GL, Black HR, Cushman WC, Green LA, Izzo JL Jr, Jones DW, Materson BJ, Oparil S, Wright JT Jr, Roccella EJ; Joint National Committee on Prevention, Detection, Evaluation, and Treatment of High Blood Pressure. National Heart, Lung, and Blood Institute; National High Blood Pressure Education Program Coordinating Committee. Seventh report of the Joint National Committee on Prevention, Detection, Evaluation, and Treatment of High Blood Pressure. *Hypertension* 2003;42(6):1206–52.

72. Suzuki T, Homma S. Treatment of hypertension and other cardiovascular risk factors in patients with metabolic syndrome. *Med Clin North Am* 2007;91(6):1211–23, x.

73. National Cholesterol Education Program (NCEP) Expert Panel on Detection, Evaluation, and Treatment of High Blood Cholesterol in Adults (Adult Treatment Panel III). Third Report of the National Cholesterol Education Program (NCEP) Expert Panel on Detection, Evaluation, and Treatment of High Blood Cholesterol in Adults (Adult Treatment Panel III) final report. *Circulation* 2002;106(25):3143–421.

74. Grundy SM, Cleeman JI, Merz CN, Brewer HB Jr, Clark LT, Hunninghake DB, Pasternak RC, Smith SC Jr, Stone NJ; National Heart, Lung, and Blood Institute; American College of Cardiology Foundation; American Heart Association.Implications of recent clinical trials for the National Cholesterol Education Program Adult Treatment Panel III guidelines. *Circulation* 2004;110(2):227–39. [Erratum in: *Circulation* 2004;110(6):763].

75. Orchard TJ, Temprosa M, Goldberg R, Haffner S, Ratner R, Marcovina S, Fowler S; Diabetes Prevention Program Research Group. The effect of metformin and intensive lifestyle intervention on the metabolic syndrome: the Diabetes Prevention Program randomized trial. *Ann Intern Med* 2005;142(8):611–19.

76. Bragt MC, Popeijus HE. Peroxisome proliferator-activated receptors and the metabolic syndrome. *Physiol Behav* 2008;94(2):187–97.

77. Derosa G, D'Angelo A, Ragonesi PD, Ciccarelli L, Piccinni MN, Pricolo F, Salvadeo SA, Montagna L, Gravina A, Ferrari I, Paniga S, Cicero AF. Metabolic effects of pioglitazone and rosiglitazone in patients with diabetes and metabolic syndrome treated with metformin. *Intern Med J* 2007;37(2):79–86.

78. Nieuwdorp M, Stroes ES, Kastelein JJ; Fenofibrate/Metformin Study Group. Normalization of metabolic syndrome using fenofibrate, metformin or their combination. *Diabetes Obes Metab* 2007;9(6):869–78.

79. Brunzell JD, Davidson M, Furberg CD, Goldberg RB, Howard BV, Stein JH, Witztum JL. Lipoprotein management in patients with cardiometabolic risk: consensus conference report from the American Diabetes Association and the American College of Cardiology Foundation. *J Am Coll Cardiol* 2008;51(15):1512–24.

80. Canner PL, Berge KG, Wenger NK, Stamler J, Friedman L, Prineas RJ, Friedewald W. Fifteen year mortality in Coronary Drug Project patients: long-term benefit with niacin. *J Am Coll Cardiol* 1986;8(6):1245–55.

81. Ito MK. The metabolic syndrome: pathophysiology, clinical relevance, and use of niacin. *Ann Pharmacother* 2004;38(2):277–85.

82. Barter PJ, Rye KA. Is there a role for fibrates in the management of dyslipidemia in the metabolic syndrome? *Arterioscler Thromb Vasc Biol* 2008;28(1):39–46.

83. Bulcão C, Ribeiro-Filho FF, Sañudo A, Roberta Ferreira SG. Effects of simvastatin and metformin on inflammation and insulin resistance in individuals with mild metabolic syndrome. *Am J Cardiovasc Drugs* 2007;7(3):219–24.
84. Ridker PM, Danielson E, Fonseca FA, Genest J, Gotto AM Jr, Kastelein JJ, Koenig W, Libby P, Lorenzatti AJ, MacFadyen JG, Nordestgaard BG, Shepherd J, Willerson JT, Glynn RJ; JUPITER Study Group. Rosuvastatin to prevent vascular events in men and women with elevated C-reactive protein. *N Engl J Med* 2008;359(21):2195–207.
85. Bray GA, Greenway FL. Pharmacological treatment of the overweight patient. *Pharmacol Rev* 2007;59(2):151–84.
86. Kini S, Herron DM, Yanagisawa RT. Bariatric surgery for morbid obesity – a cure for metabolic syndrome? *Med Clin North Am* 2007;91(6):1255–71, xi.
87. Batsis JA, Romero-Corral A, Collazo-Clavell ML, Sarr MG, Somers VK, Lopez-Jimenez F. Effect of bariatric surgery on the metabolic syndrome: a population-based, long-term controlled study. *Mayo Clin Proc* 2008;83(8):897 907.
88. Nugent C, Bai C, Elariny H, Gopalakrishnan P, Quigley C, Garone M Jr, Afendy M, Chan O, Wheeler A, Afendy A, Younossi ZM. Metabolic syndrome after laparoscopic bariatric surgery. *Obes Surg* 2008;18(10):1278–86.

Chapter 8

Diabetes mellitus and cardiovascular risk

Peter W.F. Wilson

Although coronary heart disease (CHD) mortality has decreased in the USA since the 1960s, a commensurate decline in non-fatal CHD events has not occurred, and the population risk for CHD continues to be high in the USA and around the world [1]. Over the past two decades the prevalence of obesity and diabetes mellitus has increased dramatically [2], and these trends fuel the development of atherosclerotic cardiovascular disease (CVD). The discussion in this chapter focuses on CHD and CVD reported for diabetic participants in cohort studies and surveys. The content is generally weighted toward information relating to type 2 diabetes mellitus (T2DM), although some information is provided concerning cardiovascular risk in persons with type 1 diabetes mellitus (T1DM).

Diabetes prevalence

The prevalence of diabetes mellitus in the USA has been assessed at intervals with the National Health and Nutrition Examination Surveys (NHANES) [3,4]. The frequency of diabetes is similar in men and women and is positively associated with age. Criteria for diabetes mellitus have evolved over the last 40 years. In 1979 a fasting glucose $\geq 140\,\text{mg}/\text{dL}$ was diagnostic for diabetes mellitus, and the threshold was lowered to $\geq 26\,\text{mg}/\text{dL}$ in 1997 [5,6]. The lower fasting glucose cut-off value, increasing prevalence of obesity, and lack of physical activity are believed to be important reasons underlying the increased prevalence of diabetes in the USA over the past decade.

Metabolic Risk for Cardiovascular Disease, 1st edition. Edited by R. H. Eckel.
© 2011 American Heart Association. By Blackwell Publishing Ltd.

Self-reported diabetes mellitus is often used in studies, but that approach underestimates the true prevalence of diabetes mellitus, and may misclassify a sizable fraction of the participants. It is preferred to have glucose testing or glycosylated hemoglobin levels measured to identify persons with diabetes mellitus [7]. Oral glucose tolerance information may also be used to identify persons with diabetes mellitus with greater precision. For example, in the 1990s an oral glucose tolerance test was administered to middle-aged Framingham Offspring who had a mean age of approximately 50 years. Overall there were 4% with known diabetes who did not take the glucose tolerance test, 4% with newly diagnosed diabetes mellitus, and 12% with impaired glucose tolerance (2-hour glucose levels 140–200 mg/dL) [8]. Many persons with non-diabetic hyperglycemia go on to develop diabetes mellitus, and it has been estimated that the lifetime risk of T2DM for persons born in the USA in 2000 is approximately 33% for men and 39% for women [9].

Diabetes and death

Adults with diabetes mellitus are more likely to die prematurely and risk has been reported to be related to the level of HbA1c [10]. Risk of death from CVD was shown to be increased in diabetic individuals after adjustment for smoking habit, hypertension, and cholesterol level in more than 347 000 male screenees in the Multiple Risk Factor Intervention Trial; the CVD death rate was approximately twice the rate observed in non-diabetic men [11]. In a 25-year incidence study of Olmsted County, Minnesota, the 10-year mortality was approximately 40% among diabetics versus 30% among age- and sex-matched controls; coronary mortality was the key reason for the different rates [12]. Similarly, Rancho Bernardo investigators in southern California reported in a 14-year incidence study that CHD death rates were greater among diabetic patients and the risk factor adjusted odds ratio was 3.3 in men and 1.9 in women [13].

Summary analyses have reported that about 65% of deaths among diabetic patients are from vascular or heart disease, 13% are from diabetes itself, 13% are from neoplasms, and the rest are from other causes [14]. Most data concerning diabetes and death in adults are concerned with T2DM, and the limited data on mortality associated with type 1 diabetes mellitus have suggested that approximately one-third are from diabetes itself, one-third are from kidney disease, and one-third are from cardiovascular disease [15,16].

Researchers have investigated the effect of diabetes on life expectancy. An Iowa study showed that estimated life expectancy was 59.7 years at birth for diabetic men and 69.8 years in diabetic women, and it was estimated that diabetes reduced the lifespan by 9.1 years in diabetic men and 6.7 years in diabetic women [17]. From US national survey data it has been estimated that men known to have diabetes at age 40 years will lose 11.6 life-years and similarly affected women will lose 14.3 life-years [9].

Coronary mortality has generally declined in the USA since the late 1960s and investigators have compared the experience of persons with diabetes mellitus versus those without diabetes. In a 1999 US study that compared time trends in mortality in persons with diabetes and those without diabetes, the investigators identified a decrease in risk for all-cause mortality, heart disease mortality, and ischemic heart disease mortality in men with diabetes and men without diabetes. Although a decline in all three of these mortality classifications was observed for men with diabetes mellitus, increased rates for each of these mortality groupings was identified for women with diabetes [18]. It has been estimated that the incidence of CVD death has decreased approximately 50% in the past few decades in the USA, and that non-diabetic men and women along with diabetic men experienced this improvement, but the decline was more modest in diabetic women [19].

Cardiovascular disease morbidity

The Centers for Disease Control reported that there were 8 million diabetic American adults with CVD in 1997 and the number increased to more than 11 million in 2007 (Figure 8.1) [20]. Approximately half of the diabetic persons with CVD reported a history of clinical CHD, a diagnostic category with a prevalence of 4 million in 1997 and nearly 6 million in 2007. Self-reported prevalence of

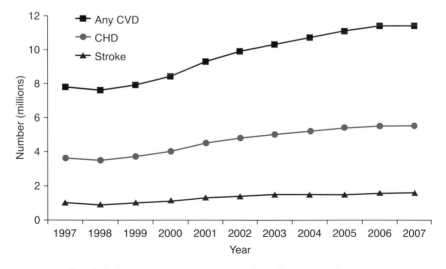

Figure 8.1 Trends in the prevalence of self-reported cardiovascular disease among adults with diabetes mellitus in the USA, age > 35 years. CVD = cardiovascular disease, CHD = coronary heart disease. Redrawn from Centers for Disease Control [20].

stroke did not change appreciably over the 10-year interval. Coupled with incidence data concerning the overall risk of CVD, these reports suggest that diabetic patients continue to experience CVD at a high rate and are surviving, which has resulted in an increased prevalence of diabetic patients with CVD [21].

Angina pectoris

Diabetes is associated with an increased risk of angina pectoris [22]. Framingham investigators reported that approximately 30% to 50% of ischemic CHD episodes occurred without clinical symptoms, and that sort of presentation occurred with equal frequency in persons with diabetes and those without diabetes [23]. Painless ischemic CHD has been generally reported for persons with diabetes mellitus in studies from Rancho Bernardo, San Luis Valley, and King County [14]. It has been suggested that coronary vasodilatation is reduced in diabetic persons after submaximal exercise and increased myocardial demand. Such physiological changes may help to account for why diabetic patients with CHD may have clinical presentations that differ from non-diabetic individuals [24].

Myocardial infarction

Compared to persons without diabetes mellitus, myocardial infarction rates are greater in diabetic patients at all ages. Among diabetic individuals 35–64 years of age, the rates of myocardial infarction in diabetic patients are typically twice the observed rates for non-diabetic individuals among men and triple the rate observed for those without diabetes (Figure 8.2). Therapeutic concerns at the

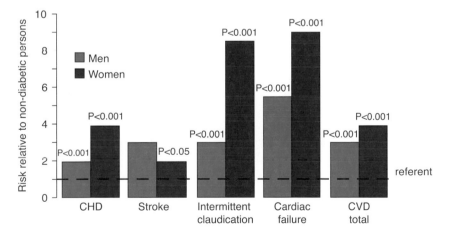

Figure 8.2 Relative risk over 30 years of follow-up for various cardiovascular events in the Framingham Study participants with diabetes compared to those without diabetes in adults aged 35–64 years at baseline. CHD = coronary heart disease, CVD = cardiovascular disease. Redrawn from Wilson [22].

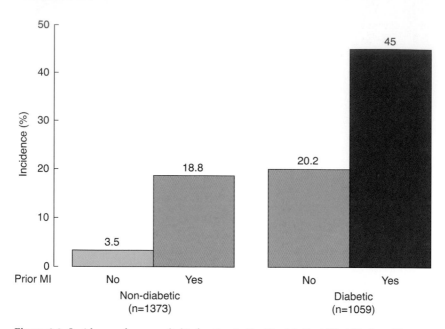

Figure 8.3 Incidence of myocardial infarction in the Finnish East-West Study with comparisons according to diabetes status and history of prior myocardial infarction (MI). Redrawn from Haffner et al. [25].

time of a myocardial infarction should include control of glycemia, acidosis, potassium, and elevated triglycerides.

A publication in the late 1990s compared the risk of myocardial infarction among Finns according to their diabetes status and history of a previous myocardial infarction (Figure 8.3) [25]. The authors identified the lowest risk for a myocardial infarction among persons without diabetes and the highest risk among persons with a history of both diabetes mellitus and a prior myocardial infarction. At an intermediate risk were myocardial infarction survivors without diabetes mellitus and persons with diabetes but without heart disease. This manuscript introduced the concept that diabetes mellitus is a CHD risk equivalent. Subsequent investigations have not definitively confirmed the findings that diabetes is a coronary risk equivalent [26], but the concept that diabetes mellitus greatly increases the risk of CVD became firmly ingrained with this report.

The size of a myocardial infarction is usually not increased in diabetic compared to non-diabetic patients, but complications are more common among persons with diabetes, including early mortality, shock, myocardial rupture, and arrhythmias [27–30]. Historically, the location of the myocardial infarction appeared to affect outcomes in a Duke study, and greater mortality was observed for men and women with an anterior myocardial infarction compared with other sites (47% vs. 13%) over 12 years of follow-up, fatalities were more common among those with diabetes, and 60-day mortality after myocardial infarction was greater in diabetic (55%) than in non-diabetic patients (31%) [31]. Overall 1-, 2-, and 5-year survival after myocardial infarction in a population-based Swedish cohort was 94%, 92%, and 82%, respectively, in non-diabetic patients and 82%, 78%, and 58%, respectively, in diabetic patients. The corresponding re-infarction rates were 12%, 17%, and 27% in non-diabetic individuals and 18%, 28%, and 46% in those with diabetes [32]. In Framingham participants with diabetes mellitus a recurrent MI was more likely if the patient had experience congestive heart failure (CHF) following the initial myocardial infarction [33].

Short-term glycemic control in known or newly diagnosed diabetic individuals at the time of a myocardial infarction or acute coronary syndrome is an area of research interest. Such investigations are usually based on glucose levels when the patient is first admitted and glucose determinations over the time course of the hospitalization for the ischemic episode. Higher glycemic levels in this setting have generally been associated with worse prognosis, and relatively low glucose levels (< 90 mg/dL) have also been shown to adversely affect outcomes in observational studies [34,35]. Initial trials with insulin infusions are under way to rigorously assess the role of glycemic control on outcomes in this setting.

Subclinical cardiovascular disease in diabetic patients

A variety of reports have described increased prevalence of subclinical atherosclerotic cardiovascular disease in persons with T2DM. For example, the Insulin Resistance Atherosclerosis Study identified greater intima-media thickening in persons with T2DM compared to non-diabetic individuals [36]. Investigating vascular disease calcification, Framingham scientists described greater coronary artery calcification in terms of median Agatston scores among persons with previously known diabetes mellitus or those with newly diagnosed diabetes mellitus in comparison to persons with normal glucose tolerance, as shown in Figure 8.4 [37]. In comparisons of coronary calcification in T1DM and T2DM patients it has been reported that T2DM patients are more likely to have more extensive coronary artery disease and more non-calcified plaques [38].

Cardiac failure and cardiomyopathy

Diabetes is an important precursor of cardiac failure and among Framingham participants aged 45–74 years the frequency was increased twofold for men with diabetes and fivefold for women with diabetes [39]. Myocardial infarction in diabetic women was especially associated with an increased risk of cardiac

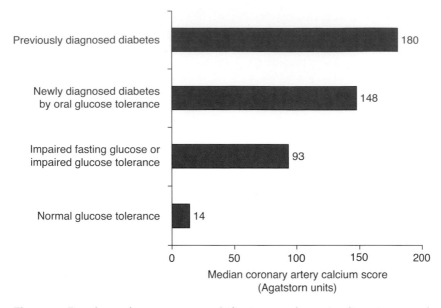

Figure 8.4 Prevalence of coronary artery calcification according to insulin resistance and glycemic status in Framingham Offspring. Redrawn from Meigs et al. with permission [37].

failure in the Framingham cohort [33,40]. Factors such as hypertension and clinical coronary artery disease contribute to the causation of heart failure and multiple causes no doubt contribute to the increased incidence and prevalence of this condition in diabetic patients [41]. The pathophysiological effects of microvascular disease on CHF in diabetes are not well characterized, but pathological studies in diabetic persons dying of CHF have shown myocardial lesions such as arteriolar thickening, microaneurysms, and basement membrane thickening [42].

Diastolic dysfunction is characterized by increased left ventricular end-diastolic pressure, reduced left ventricular end-diastolic volume, and a normal ejection fraction. These abnormalities appear to be more common in diabetic individuals [30]. Metabolic alterations in cardiac myosin isozyme content, myocardial cell calcium homeostasis, sarcolemma sodium exchange, and a decrease in Na^+,K^+-ATPase activity have been described with diabetic cardiomyopathy, and insulin resistance has been suggested as a possible mechanism [43].

Conduction disorders, atrial fibrillation, heart rate variability, and autonomic changes in the vascular system

Cardiac conduction abnormalities such as left bundle branch block and cardiac rhythm disturbance like atrial fibrillation occur more commonly in persons with diabetes [44,45]. A large number of cardiac autonomic abnormalities, such as increased heart rate after resting, less beat-to-beat variation in the heart rate, and orthostatic hypotension, are also more common in persons with diabetes. The presence of autonomic abnormalities in persons with diabetes has been associated with reduced survival [46,47].

Risk factors in diabetic patients

Long-term glycemic control

The advent of hemoglobin A1c (HbA1c) measurements in the 1970s provided a summary measure of glucose control to gauge effects on CVD risk [48]. For example, investigators followed a cohort of type 1 diabetic patients and found that a single HbA1c determination was not associated with greater CHD risk over 4 years [49], and investigations carried out in middle-aged and elderly Finns with T2DM showed that higher HbA1c levels were associated with greater risk for CHD [50].

The Diabetes Complications and Control Trial (DCCT) focused on glycemic control in persons with T1DM, and found little evidence that long-term glycemic control affected risk for CHD events in relatively young adults at the conclusion of the trial. The participants were subsequently followed several years longer as part of an observational cohort in the Epidemiology of Diabetes Interventions and Complications (EDIC) study. After 17 years of follow-up, more than a decade after the trial ended, the investigators reported that assignment to the aggressive glycemic arm in the clinical trial was associated with a 57% lower

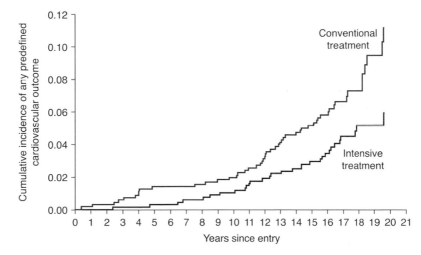

Figure 8.5 Long-term follow-up experience for cardiovascular events in the DCCT/EDIC cohort with comparison of conventional and intensive treatment arms. Redrawn from Nathan et al. [51], with permission. Copyright © [2005] Massachusetts Medical Society. All rights reserved.

risk for CHD (Figure 8.5) [51]. The authors used the term "metabolic memory" to describe the cardioprotective effect of smaller exposure to glucose over time. A similar CVD benefit for tighter glycemic control was observed for participants in the observational phase of the United Kingdom Prospective Diabetes Study when data were analyzed that examined the outcome experience 10 years after the trial ended [52].

Blood pressure, kidney disease, and microalbuminuria

Hypertension in diabetic patients is associated with greater risk of small vessel disease of the kidney and eye, and the prevalence of hypertension in persons with T2DM is more than twice the prevalence in non-diabetic individuals [53,54]. Hypertension especially acts synergistically with other risk factors to increase risk of cardiomyopathy and microalbuminuria. The list of risk factors that cluster with microalbuminuria is long: central obesity, insulin resistance, abnormal HDL-C and triglycerides, systolic hypertension, absent nocturnal drop in blood pressure, salt sensitivity, male sex, increased cardiovascular oxidative stress, impaired endothelial function, and abnormal coagulation [53].

Observational studies have generally demonstrated that risk for CVD in diabetic patients is positively related to blood pressure levels. As described in the Seventh Report of the Joint National Committee for blood pressure management, a general rule is that CVD risk approximately doubles for each 20 mmHg increment of systolic BP and 10 mmHg increment of diastolic BP above 115/75 mmHg [55]. Current recommendations generally follow the pattern of lowering blood pressure more aggressively in persons with diabetes (Table 8.1). The most recent recommendations include using angiotensin-converting enzyme inhibiting drugs or angiotensin receptor blockers in diabetics with hypertension and proteinuria, and the guidelines show a preference for low-dose diuretics in persons with T2DM.

Treatment of diabetic hypertensive patients has been associated with less microalbuminuria and a slower decline in renal function compared with less aggressively treated diabetics [56]. The blood pressure target for diabetic individuals is typically < 130/80 mmHg and even lower blood pressure levels are targeted if there is evidence of kidney disease [57].

Lipids

Blood lipid levels have been compared in several studies of T1DM and T2DM patients [58–62]. Mean total cholesterol and low-density lipoprotein cholesterol (LDL-C) concentrations often do not differ in diabetic and non diabetic patients, but high-density lipoprotein cholesterol (HDL-C) levels are usually lower in diabetic individuals and triglycerides are usually higher. The frequencies of lipid abnormalities in men and women with T2DM compared to non-diabetic controls in the Framingham Study are shown in Figure 8.6 for men and

Table 8.1 Blood pressure goals in diabetic patients

Blood pressure level	Intervention
Systolic 130–139 mmHg or Diastolic 80–89 mmHg (confirm BP level on separate day)	• Lifestyle and behavioral therapy for up to 3 months, then drug therapy if not at target
Systolic > 140 mmHg or Diastolic 80–89 mmHg (confirm BP level on separate day)	• Lifestyle and behavioral therapy • Drug therapy included with initial treatment • Drug regimen should include ACE inhibitor or ARB • Monitor renal function and serum potassium over first 3 months (if on ACE inhibitor, ARB, or diuretic), then every 6 months as needed • Will generally require multiple drugs to achieve control

ACE, angiotensin-converting enzyme; ARB, angiotensin II receptor blocker.
Source: Buse et al. [57].

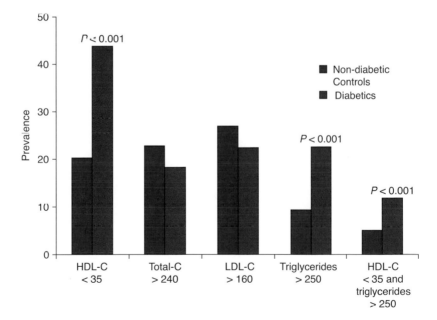

Figure 8.6 Frequency of lipid extremes in diabetic and non-diabetic men in the Framingham Offspring. All units mg/dL. HDL-C = high density lipoprotein cholestrol; LDL-C = low density lipoprotein cholestrol. Redrawn from Siegel et al. with permission [64].

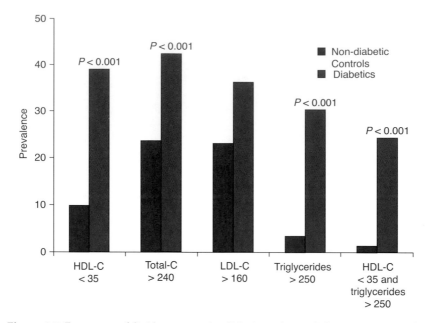

Figure 8.7 Frequency of lipid extremes in diabetic and non-diabetic women in the Framingham Offspring. All units mg/dL. HDL-C = high density lipoprotein cholestrol; LDL-C = low density lipoprotein cholestrol. Redrawn from Siegel et al. with permission [64].

Figure 8.7 for women. In both sexes the mean cholesterol and LDL-C levels tend to be relatively similar in T2DM and non-diabetic subjects. On the other hand, low HDL-C and elevated triglyceride levels occurred more commonly in diabetic individuals, especially in women with diabetes. Recent data show that lipid abnormalities are common in diabetic women who have experienced CVD. A report from the Translating Research Into Action for Diabetes study, a multicenter study of diabetes in managed care in diabetic patients with CVD, reported that LDL-C levels were less likely to be at target levels in diabetic women, and the authors believed that the difference in reaching target lipid goals may contribute to the sex disparity in CVD mortality trends [63].

Apolipoprotein levels tend to parallel the results for the cholesterol fractions. Apolipoprotein B, largely contained in low- and very-low-density lipoprotein particles, is often increased in diabetics, but not always. On the other hand, apolipoprotein A, found in HDL particles, is typically decreased in most diabetics [64,65]. Lipoprotein(a) – Lp(a) – is another potentially atherogenic particle, and it is composed of an LDL moiety that is attached to apoprotein(a). Concentration of Lp(a) has been reported to vary according to glycemic control in type 1 diabetes and not to differ in type 2 diabetic subjects compared with non-diabetic controls [66]. In diabetic persons the data suggest that Lp(a) levels and apo(a) polymorphism variants are related to the severity of CAD at the time of cardiac catheterization [67]. In a separate study of diabetic patients with coronary disease the authors reported that Lp(a) levels were not related to the incidence of future vascular events [68].

The size and number of LDL particles vary in plasma. Originally characterized as pattern B (small, dense) and pattern A (large, buoyant) [69], it is now apparent that several LDL particles of different size are present in plasma [70–72]. Patients with T2DM typically have an increased concentration of the small, dense LDL particles and the same patients usually have elevated triglyceride concentrations in the plasma [73].

Current recommendations for lipid levels in adult diabetic patients were put forward by the National Cholesterol Education Panel Adult Treatment Panel (NCEP ATP-III) in 2001 [74]. These recommendations were updated in 2004 with the suggestion to treat diabetic patients to a target LDL-C < 100 mg/dL on therapy and diabetic patients at high risk for vascular disease or with diagnosed vascular disease even more aggressively to a target LDL-C of < 70 mg/dL [75]. Summary analyses with the endpoint CHD death that included participants from the Atherosclerotic Risk in Communities Study, Framingham, and the Multiple Risk Factor Intervention Trial reported that non-HDL cholesterol was an important risk factor for CHD death even with LDL-C < 100 mg/dL in both diabetic patients and non-diabetic individuals (Figure 8.8) [76]. There is great interest in lipid optimization in persons with diabetes and concern that meeting LDL-C goals will not adequately lower CVD risk. The American Diabetes Association and the American College of Cardiology issued a joint statement for

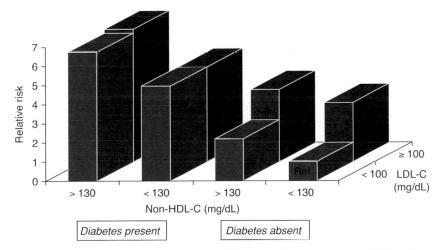

Figure 8.8 Risk of CHD death according to difference lipid measures in ARIC, Framingham, and MRFIT Usual Care. HDL-C = high density lipoprotein cholestrol; LDL-C = low density lipoprotein cholestrol. Redrawn from Liu et al. with permission [76].

Table 8.2 American Diabetes Association–American College of Cardiology 2008 Consensus: suggested treatment goals in patients with cardiometabolic risk and lipoprotein abnormalities

Risk category	LDL-C	Goals (mg/dL) Non-HDL-C	apoB
Highest-risk including those with (1) known CVD or (2) diabetes plus one or more additional major CVD risk factors*	< 70	< 100	< 80
High-risk patients including those with (1) no diabetes or known clinical CVD but two or more additional major CVD risk factors* or (2) diabetes but not other major CVD risk factors	< 100	< 130	< 90

*Other major risk factors (beyond lipids) include smoking, hypertension, and family history of premature coronary artery disease.
apoB, apolipoprotein B; CVD, cardiovascular disease; LDL-C, low-density lipoprotein cholesterol; non-HDL-C, non-high-density lipoprotein cholesterol.
Source: Brunzell et al. with permission [77].

lipid lowering in diabetics, and they recommended LDL-C, non-HDL-C, and apolipoprotein B target levels to reduce CVD risk (Table 8.2) [77].

Hypoglycemic therapy has the potential to affect blood lipid levels. A meta-analysis drawn from 41 studies reported that metformin was generally associated with small effects, but significantly lower levels of total cholesterol and LDL-C in comparison to other hypoglycemic agents [78]. Thiazolidinediones have been investigated for their metabolic effects on blood lipids, and in a head-to-head comparison of pioglitazone versus rosiglitazone the former was reported to have more favorable effects on triglycerides, HDL-C, non-HDL-C, and LDL-C, although HbA1c effects were not different for the thiazolidinediones that were compared [79].

Obesity

Increased adiposity typically precedes the development of T2DM and persists throughout the rest of life for affected patients. Increased adiposity is positively associated with lower HDL-C levels and higher blood pressure levels [80], but greater adiposity has not been highly associated with the development of CHD events over 12 years of follow-up after statistical adjustment with traditional cardiovascular risk factors [81]. An investigation by Fox and colleagues showed that higher body mass index was highly associated with the development of

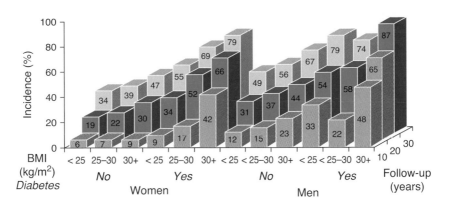

Figure 8.9 Long-term risk of cardiovascular disease according to diabetes status and BMI in Framingham men and women according to diabetes status at baseline. Redrawn from Fox et al. [82].

CVD in both sexes and in persons with diabetes mellitus (Figure 8.9) [82]. The trends were especially evident in persons with diabetes mellitus who were followed 20 years or more.

Other biological markers and factors

Microvascular disease that affects the retina has been associated with greater risk of CHD among persons with T2DM [83]. Elevated levels of inflammatory markers, leukocyte count, and fibrinogen [84–86], as well as C-reactive protein [87,88], and increased platelet adhesiveness[89,90] have been associated with diabetes, pre-diabetes, and greater risk of atherosclerotic risk in population studies. Higher glucose concentrations in the plasma can lead to glycosylation of proteins in the artery wall, and greater concentrations of the circulating soluble receptor for advanced glycation end products has been described in diabetic persons with coronary atherosclerosis [91].

Total risk factor burden and risk of vascular events

Lamentably, risk factor control for HbA1c, blood pressure < 130/80 mmHg, and total cholesterol < 200 mg/dL has not been very good in the USA (Figure 8.10). A report that compared control of these risk factors in diabetic patients in the NHANES III and NHANES 1999–2000 studies described only minimal improvement in control for each factor. Overall, only 7% of American diabetic patients had HbA1c, blood pressure, and total cholesterol at target values at the turn of the century [92].

Observational studies with more baseline information have been used to develop CHD risk prediction algorithms, and the effect of risk factors

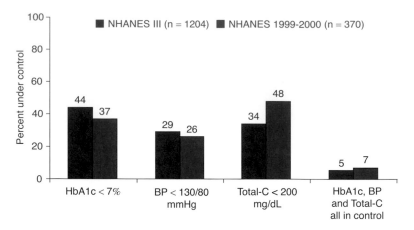

Figure 8.10 Frequency of risk factor control among NHANES participants with diabetes in 1988–1994 and 1999–2000. Measure include HbA1c < 7%, blood pressure < 130/80 mmHg, and cholesterol < 200 mg/dL. All rights reserved. HbA1c = glycosylated hemoglobin; BP = blood pressure; Total-C = total cholesterol. Redrawn from Saydah SH, Fradkin J, Cowie CC. Poor control of risk factors for vascular disease among adults with previously diagnosed diabetes. JAMA 2004;291:335–42, with permission. Copyright © (2009) American Medical Association.

and diabetes on CHD and CVD has been estimated from the experience of observational studies such as the Framingham Study and the placebo arm of the UKPDS clinical trial [81,93,94]. These studies measured risk factors in persons with diabetes who were free of CVD at baseline and tracked them for the development of atherosclerotic events. Using multivariable formulations the authors have estimated risk of CHD for diabetic patients with various combinations of risk factors.

Figure 8.11 estimated risk for CVD outcomes in men and women according to various risk factors used in the UKPDS risk engine, which includes age, diabetes duration, presence of atrial fibrillation, HbA1c, systolic blood pressure level, total cholesterol concentration, HDL-C concentration, race, and smoking status [95]. Investigators from the EPIC-Norfolk Observational Study tested the utility of CHD risk prediction with the UKPDS risk engine and Framingham prediction algorithms in persons with normoglycemia, non-diabetic hyperglycemia, or known to have diabetes mellitus [96]. They found that both Framingham and UKPDS were good at ranking individuals according their risk, but absolute risk for an event was typically overestimated.

Fewer diabetes complications such as mortality, renal failure, and neuropathy have been observed for adult T1DM patients in the Pittsburgh Epidemiology of Diabetes Complications Study over recent years. On the other hand, risk of proliferative retinopathy, overt nephropathy, and clinical CAD have not declined over the long-term follow-up interval of 30 years [97].

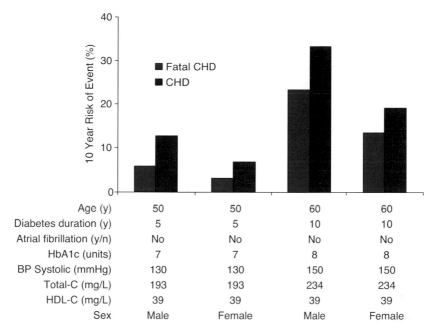

Age (y)	50	50	60	60
Diabetes duration (y)	5	5	10	10
Atrial fibrillation (y/n)	No	No	No	No
HbA1c (units)	7	7	8	8
BP Systolic (mmHg)	130	130	150	150
Total-C (mg/L)	193	193	234	234
HDL-C (mg/L)	39	39	39	39
Sex	Male	Female	Male	Female

Figure 8.11 Estimation of risk for vascular events in diabetic patients using Oxford Risk Engine Prediction. HbA1c = glycosylated hemoglobin; BP = blood pressure; Total-C = total cholesterol; HDL-C = high density lipoprotein cholestrol. Estimates derived from Stevens et al. [93].

Although attention has particularly focused on glycemic control in diabetes clinics, practitioners and patients should work together to reduce the overall burden of risk factors associated with diabetes. Diet and exercise programs, smoking cessation, blood pressure control, and lipid reductions are all important in an effort to lower the risk of initial and recurrent CVD events in diabetic patients, and a blueprint for how to carry this out is contained in a joint publication from the American Heart Association and the American Diabetes Association [57].

Summary

The prevalence of diabetes mellitus has increased greatly over the past two decades in the USA and in other regions of the world. In middle-aged and older diabetic adults the most common cause of death is cardiovascular disease. Observational data have generally showed that greater adiposity, glycemia, atherogenic lipid measures, and blood pressure are the key determinants of cardiovascular risk in diabetic persons.

References

1. Engelgau MM, Geiss LS, Saaddine JB, et al. The evolving diabetes burden in the United States. *Ann Intern Med* 2004;140:945–50.
2. Gregg EW, Cheng YJ, Cadwell BL, et al. Secular trends in cardiovascular disease risk factors according to body mass index in US adults. *JAMA* 2005;293:1868–74.
3. Harris MI, Hadden WC, Knowler WC, Bennett PH. Prevalence of diabetes and impaired glucose tolerance and plasma glucose levels in US population aged 20–74 yr. *Diabetes* 1987;36:523–34.
4. Resnick HE, Harris MI, Brock DB, Harris TB. American Diabetes Association diabetes diagnostic criteria, advancing age, and cardiovascular disease risk profiles: results from the Third National Health and Nutrition Examination Survey. *Diabetes Care* 2000;23:176–80.
5. National Diabetes Data Group. Classification and diagnosis of diabetes mellitus and other categories of glucose intolerance. *Diabetes* 1979;28:1039–57.
6. Report of the Expert Committee on the Diagnosis and Classification of Diabetes Mellitus. *Diabetes Care* 1997;20:1183–97.
7. International Expert Committee report on the role of the A1C assay in the diagnosis of diabetes. *Diabetes Care* 2009;32:1327–34. PMCID:PMC2699715.
8. Meigs JB, Nathan DM, Wilson PW, Cupples LA, Singer DE. Metabolic risk factors worsen continuously across the spectrum of nondiabetic glucose tolerance. The Framingham Offspring Study. *Ann Intern Med* 1998;128:524–33.
9. Narayan KM, Boyle JP, Thompson TJ, Sorensen SW, Williamson DF. Lifetime risk for diabetes mellitus in the United States. *JAMA* 2003;290:1884–90.
10. Saydah S, Tao M, Imperatore G, Gregg E. GHb level and subsequent mortality among adults in the US. *Diabetes Care* 2009;32:1440–6. PMCID:PMC2713636.
11. Stamler J, Vaccaro O, Neaton JD, Wentworth D. Diabetes, other risk factors, and 12-yr cardiovascular mortality for men screened in the Multiple Risk Factor Intervention Trial. *Diabetes Care* 1993;16:434–44.
12. Palumbo PJ, Elveback LR, Chu CP, Connolly DC, Kurland LT. Diabetes mellitus: incidence, prevalence, survivorship, and causes of death in Rochester, Minnesota, 1945–1970. *Diabetes* 1976;25:566–73.
13. Barrett-Connor EL, Cohn BA, Wingard DL, Edelstein SL. Why is diabetes mellitus a stronger risk factor for fatal ischemic heart disease in women than in men? *JAMA* 1991;265:627–32.
14. Wingard DL, Barrett-Connor EL. Heart disease and diabetes. In: Harris MI, editor. *Diabetes in America*, 2nd edn. Bethesda: National Institutes of Health, 1995; pp. 429–48.
15. Krolewski AS, Kosinski EJ, Warram JH, et al. Magnitude and determinants of coronary artery disease in juvenile-onset, insulin-dependent diabetes mellitus. *Am J Cardiol* 1987;59:750–5.
16. Krolewski AS, Warram JH, Rand LI, Kahn CR. Epidemiologic approach to the etiology of type I diabetes mellitus and its complications. *N Engl J Med* 1987;317:1390–8.
17. Bale GS, Entmacher PS. Estimated life expectancy of diabetics. *Diabetes* 1977;26:434–8.
18. Gu K, Cowie CC, Harris MI. Diabetes and decline in heart disease mortality in US adults. *JAMA* 1999;281:1291–7.
19. Fox CS, Coady S, Sorlie PD, et al. Trends in cardiovascular complications of diabetes. *JAMA* 2004;292:2495–9.

20. Centers for Disease Control. Diabetes Data and Trends 2009. Available from http://www.cdc.gov/diabetes/statistics/cvd.
21. Buse JB, Ginsberg HN, Bakris GL, et al. Primary prevention of cardiovascular diseases in people with diabetes mellitus: a scientific statement from the American Heart Association and the American Diabetes Association. *Circulation* 2007;115:114–26.
22. Wilson PW. Diabetes mellitus and coronary heart disease. *Am J Kidney Dis* 1998;32(5 Suppl 3):S89–100.
23. Kannel WB, Abbott RD. Incidence and prognosis of unrecognized myocardial infarction. An update on the Framingham Study. *N Engl J Med* 1984;311:1144–7.
24. Nahser PJ, Jr., Brown RE, Oskarsson H, Winniford MD, Rossen JD. Maximal coronary flow reserve and metabolic coronary vasodilation in patients with diabetes mellitus. *Circulation* 1995;91:635–40.
25. Haffner SM, Lehto S, Ronnemaa T, Pyorala K, Laakso M. Mortality from coronary heart disease in subjects with type 2 diabetes and in nondiabetic subjects with and without prior myocardial infarction. *N Engl J Med* 1998;339:229–34.
26. Bulugahapitiya U, Siyambalapitiya S, Sithole J, Idris I. Is diabetes a coronary risk equivalent? Systematic review and meta-analysis. *Diabet Med* 2009;26:142–8.
27. Herlitz J, Malmberg K, Karlson BW, Ryden L, Hjalmarson A. Mortality and morbidity during a five-year follow-up of diabetics with myocardial infarction. *Acta Med Scand* 1988;224:31–8.
28. Woods KL, Samanta A, Burden AC. Diabetes mellitus as a risk factor for acute myocardial infarction in Asians and Europeans. *Br Heart J* 1989;62:118–22.
29. Hands ME, Rutherford JD, Muller JE, et al. The in-hospital development of cardiogenic shock after myocardial infarction: incidence, predictors of occurrence, outcome and prognostic factors. The MILIS Study Group. *J Am Coll Cardiol* 1989;14:40–6; discussion 47–8.
30. Stone PH, Muller JE, Hartwell T, et al. The effect of diabetes mellitus on prognosis and serial left ventricular function after acute myocardial infarction: contribution of both coronary disease and diastolic left ventricular dysfunction to the adverse prognosis. The MILIS Study Group. *J Am Coll Cardiol* 1989;14:49–57.
31. Weitzman S, Wagner GS, Heiss G, Haney TL, Slome C. Myocardial infarction site and mortality in diabetes. *Diabetes Care* 1982;5:31–5.
32. Ulvenstam G, Aberg A, Bergstrand R, et al. Long-term prognosis after myocardial infarction in men with diabetes. *Diabetes* 1985;34:787–92.
33. Abbott RD, Donahue RP, Kannel WB, Wilson PWF. The impact of diabetes on survival following myocardial infarction in men versus women: The Framingham Study. *JAMA* 1988;260:3456–60.
34. Goyal A, Petersen JL, Mahaffey KW. The evaluation and management of dyslipidemia and impaired glucose metabolism during acute coronary syndromes. *Curr Cardiol Rep* 2004;6:300–7.
35. Svensson AM, McGuire DK, Abrahamsson P, Dellborg M. Association between hyper- and hypoglycaemia and 2 year all-cause mortality risk in diabetic patients with acute coronary events. *Eur Heart J* 2005;26:1255–61.
36. Haffner SM, Agostino RD, Jr., Saad MF, et al. Carotid artery atherosclerosis in type-2 diabetic and nondiabetic subjects with and without symptomatic coronary artery disease (The Insulin Resistance Atherosclerosis Study). *Am J Cardiol* 2000;85:1395–400.

37. Meigs JB, Larson MG, D'Agostino RB, et al. Coronary artery calcification in type 2 diabetes and insulin resistance: The Framingham Offspring Study. *Diabetes Care* 2002;25:1313–19.
38. Djaberi R, Schuijf JD, Boersma E, et al. Differences in atherosclerotic plaque burden and morphology between type 1 and 2 diabetes as assessed by multislice computed tomography. *Diabetes Care* 2009;32:1507–12. PMCID:PMC2713641.
39. Kannel WB, Hjortland MC, Castelli WP. Role of diabetes in congestive heart failure. The Framingham Study. *Am J Cardiol* 1974;34:29–34.
40. Langer A, Freeman MR, Josse RG, Steiner G, Armstrong PW. Detection of silent myocardial ischemia in diabetes mellitus. *Am J Cardiol* 1991;67:1073–8.
41. Schaffer SW. Cardiomyopathy associated with noninsulin-dependent diabetes. *Mol Cell Biochem* 1991;107:1–20.
42. Yarom R, Zirkin H, Stammler G, Rose AG. Human coronary microvessels in diabetes and ischaemia. Morphometric study of autopsy material. *J Pathol* 1992;166:265–70.
43. Malhotra A, Reich D, Reich D, Nakouzi A, Sanghi V, Geenen DL, Buttrick PM. Experimental diabetes is associated with functional activation of protein kinase C epsilon and phosphorylation of troponin I in the heart, which are prevented by angiotensin II receptor blockade. *Circ Res* 1997;81:1027–33.
44. Pfeffer MA, Braunwald E, Moye LA, et al. Effect of captopril on mortality and morbidity in patients with left ventricular dysfunction after myocardial infarction. Results of the survival and ventricular enlargement trial. The SAVE Investigators. *N Engl J Med* 1992;327:669–77.
45. Schneider JF, Thomas HE, Jr., Sorlie PD, Kreger BE, McNamara PM, Kannel WB. Comparative features of newly acquired left and right bundle branch block in the general population: The Framingham Study. *Am J Cardiol* 1981;47:931–40.
46. Benjamin EJ, Levy D, Vaziri SM, D'Agostino RB, Belanger AJ, Wolf PA. Independent risk factors for atrial fibrillation in a population-based cohort. The Framingham Heart Study. *JAMA* 1994;271:840–4.
47. Ewing DJ, Borsey DQ, Travis P, Bellavere F, Neilson JMM, Clarke BF. Abnormalites of ambulatory 24-hour heart rate in diabetes mellitus. *Diabetes* 1983;32:101–5.
48. Knatterud GL, Klimt CR, Levin ME, Jacobson ME, Goldner MG. Effects of hypoglycemic agents on vascular complications in patients with adult-onset diabetes. VII. Mortality and selected nonfatal events with insulin treatment. *JAMA* 1978;240:37–42.
49. Nathan DM, Singer DE, Hurxthal K, Goodson JD. The clinical information value of the glycosylated hemoglobin assay. *N Engl J Med* 1984;310:341–6.
50. Laakso M. Glycemic control and the risk for coronary heart disease in patients with non-insulin-dependent diabetes mellitus: the Finnish Studies. *Ann Intern Med* 1996;124:127–30.
51. Nathan DM, Cleary PA, Backlund JY, et al. Intensive diabetes treatment and cardiovascular disease in patients with type 1 diabetes. *N Engl J Med* 2005;353:2643–53.
52. Holman RR, Paul SK, Bethel MA, Matthews DR, Neil HA. 10-year follow-up of intensive glucose control in type 2 diabetes. *N Engl J Med* 2008;359:1577–89.
53. Sowers JR, Epstein M, Frohlich ED. Diabetes, hypertension, and cardiovascular disease: an update. *Hypertension* 2001;37:1053–9.
54. Sowers JR, Frohlich ED. Insulin and insulin resistance: impact on blood pressure and cardiovascular disease. *Med Clin N Am* 2004;88:63–82.

55. Chobanian AV, Bakris GL, Black HR, et al. The Seventh report of the Joint National Committee on Prevention, Detection, Evaluation, and Treatment of High Blood Pressure: the JNC 7 report. *JAMA* 2003;289:2560–72.

56. Whaley-Connell A, Sowers JR. Hypertension management in type 2 diabetes mellitus: recommendations of the Joint National Committee VII. *Endocrinol Metab Clin N Am* 2005;34:63–75.

57. Buse JB, Ginsberg HN, Bakris GL, et al. Primary prevention of cardiovascular diseases in people with diabetes mellitus: a scientific statement from the American Heart Association and the American Diabetes Association. *Diabetes Care* 2007;30: 162–72.

58. Howard BV, Lee ET, Cowan LD, et al. Coronary heart disease prevalence and its relation to risk factors in American Indians. The Strong Heart Study. *Am J Epidemiol* 1995;142:254–68.

59. Laakso M, Ronnemaa T, Pyorala K, Kallio V, Puska P, Penttila I. Atherosclerotic vascular disease and its risk factors in non-insulin-dependent diabetic and nondiabetic subjects in Finland. *Diabetes Care* 1988;11:449–63.

60. Haffner SM, Stern MP, Hazuda HP, Mitchell BD, Patterson JK. Cardiovascular risk factors in confirmed prediabetic individuals: Does the clock for coronary heart disease start ticking before the onset of clinical diabetes? *JAMA* 1990;263:2893–8.

61. Cowie CC, Harris MI. Physical and metabolic characteristics of persons with diabetes. In: Harris MI (ed.) *Diabetes in America*, 2nd edn. Bethesda: National Institutes of Health, 1995. pp. 117–64.

62. Guy J, Ogden L, Wadwa RP, et al. Lipid and lipoprotein profiles in youth with and without type 1 diabetes: the SEARCH for Diabetes in Youth case-control study. *Diabetes Care* 2009;32:416–20. PMCID:PMC2646019

63. Ferrara A, Mangione CM, Kim C, et al. Sex disparities in control and treatment of modifiable cardiovascular disease risk factors among patients with diabetes: Translating Research Into Action for Diabetes (TRIAD) Study. *Diabetes Care* 2008;31:69–74.

64. Siegel RD, Cupples A, Schaefer EJ, Wilson PW. Lipoproteins, apolipoproteins, and low-density lipoprotein size among diabetics in the Framingham offspring study. *Metabolism* 1996;45:1267–72.

65. Adiels M, Olofsson SO, Taskinen MR, Boren J. Diabetic dyslipidaemia. *Curr Opin Lipidol* 2006;17:238–46.

66. Haffner SM. Lipoprotein(a) and diabetes. An update. *Diabetes Care* 1993;16:835–40.

67. Gazzaruso C, Bruno R, Pujia A, et al. Lipoprotein(a), apolipoprotein(a) polymorphism and coronary atherosclerosis severity in type 2 diabetic patients. *Int J Cardiol* 2006;108:354–8.

68. Saely CH, Koch L, Schmid F, et al. Lipoprotein(a), type 2 diabetes and vascular risk in coronary patients. *Eur J Clin Invest* 2006;36:91–7.

69. Krauss RM, Burke DJ. Identification of multiple subclasses of plasma low density lipoproteins in normal humans. *J Lipid Res* 1982;23:97–104.

70. Campos H, Genest JJ, Jr., Blijlevens E, et al. Low density lipoprotein particle size and coronary artery disease. *Arterioscler Thromb* 1992;12:187–95.

71. Williams PT, Superko HR, Haskell WL, et al. Smallest LDL particles are most strongly related to coronary disease progression in men. *Arterioscler Thromb Vasc Biol* 2003;23:314–21.

72. Cromwell W, Otvos JD, Keyes MJ, et al. LDL particle number and risk of future cardiovascular disease in the Framingham Offspring Study – Implications for LDL management. *J Clin Lipidol* 2007;1:583–92.

73. Cromwell WC, Otvos JD. Heterogeneity of low-density lipoprotein particle number in patients with type 2 diabetes mellitus and low-density lipoprotein cholesterol <100 mg/dl. *Am J Cardiol* 2006;98:1599–602.

74. Executive Summary of the Third Report of The National Cholesterol Education Program (NCEP) Expert Panel on Detection, Evaluation, and Treatment of High Blood Cholesterol In Adults (Adult Treatment Panel III). *JAMA* 2001;285:2486–97.

75. Grundy SM, Cleeman JI, Merz CN, et al. Implications of recent clinical trials for the National Cholesterol Education Program Adult Treatment Panel III guidelines. *Circulation* 2004;110:227–39.

76. Liu J, Sempos C, Donahue RP, Dorn J, Trevisan M, Grundy SM. Joint distribution of non-HDL and LDL cholesterol and coronary heart disease risk prediction among individuals with and without diabetes. *Diabetes Care* 2005;28:1916–21.

77. Brunzell JD, Davidson M, Furberg CD, et al. Lipoprotein management in patients with cardiometabolic risk: consensus conference report from the American Diabetes Association and the American College of Cardiology Foundation. *J Am Coll Cardiol* 2008;51:1512–24.

78. Wulffele MG, Kooy A, de Zeeuw D, Stehouwer CD, Gansevoort RT. The effect of metformin on blood pressure, plasma cholesterol and triglycerides in type 2 diabetes mellitus: a systematic review. *J Intern Med* 2004;256:1–14.

79. Goldberg RB, Kendall DM, Deeg MA, et al. A comparison of lipid and glycemic effects of pioglitazone and rosiglitazone in patients with type 2 diabetes and dyslipidemia. *Diabetes Care* 2005;28:1547–54.

80. Lamon-Fava S, Wilson PW, Schaefer EJ. Impact of body mass index on coronary heart disease risk factors in men and women. The Framingham Offspring Study. *Arterioscler Thromb Vasc Biol* 1996;16:1509–15.

81. Wilson PW, D'Agostino RB, Levy D, Belanger AM, Silbershatz H, Kannel WB. Prediction of coronary heart disease using risk factor categories. *Circulation* 1998;97:1837–47.

82. Fox CS, Pencina MJ, Wilson PW, Paynter NP, Vasan RS, D'Agostino RB, Sr. Lifetime risk of cardiovascular disease among individuals with and without diabetes stratified by obesity status in the Framingham heart study. *Diabetes Care* 2008;31:1582–4. PMCID:PMC2494632.

83. Hiller R, Sperduto RD, Podgor MJ, Ferris FLI, Wilson PWF. Diabetic retinopathy and cardiovascular disease in Type II diabetics. The Framingham Heart Study and the Framingham Eye Study. *Am J Epidemiol* 1988;128:402–9.

84. Kannel WB, D'Agostino RB, Wilson PWF, Belanger AJ, Gagnon DR. Diabetes, fibrinogen, and risk of cardiovascular disease: The Framingham experience. *Am Heart J* 1990;120:672–6.

85. Danesh J, Lewington S, Thompson SG, et al. Plasma fibrinogen level and the risk of major cardiovascular diseases and nonvascular mortality: an individual participant meta-analysis. *JAMA* 2005;294:1799–809.

86. Meigs JB, Mittleman MA, Nathan DM, et al. Hyperinsulinemia, hyperglycemia, and impaired hemostasis: the Framingham Offspring Study. *JAMA* 2000;283:221–8.

87. Haffner SM. Insulin resistance, inflammation, and the prediabetic state. *Am J Cardiol* 2003;92(4A):18–26J.

88. Wilson PW, Meigs JB, Sullivan L, Fox CS, Nathan DM, D'Agostino RB, Sr. Prediction of Incident Diabetes Mellitus in Middle-aged Adults: The Framingham Offspring Study. *Arch Intern Med* 2007;167:1068–74.

89. Colwell JA. Antiplatelet agents for the prevention of cardiovascular disease in diabetes mellitus. *Am J Cardiovasc Drugs* 2004;4:87–106.

90. Colwell JA. Aspirin for primary prevention of cardiovascular events in diabetes. *Diabetes Care* 2003;26:3349–50.

91. Lindsey JB, de Lemos JA, Cipollone F, et al. Association between circulating soluble receptor for advanced glycation end products and atherosclerosis: observations from the Dallas Heart Study. *Diabetes Care* 2009;32:1218–20. PMCID:PMC2699719.

92. Saydah SH, Fradkin J, Cowie CC. Poor control of risk factors for vascular disease among adults with previously diagnosed diabetes. *JAMA* 2004;291:335–42.

93. Stevens RJ, Kothari V, Adler AI, Stratton IM. The UKPDS risk engine: a model for the risk of coronary heart disease in Type II diabetes (UKPDS 56). *Clin Sci (Lond)* 2001;101:671–9.

94. D'Agostino RB, Sr., Vasan RS, Pencina MJ, et al. General cardiovascular risk profile for use in primary care: the Framingham Heart Study. *Circulation* 2008;117:743–53.

95. Diabetes Trials Units Risk Engine, v 2.0 2008 Available from http://www.dtu.ox.ac.uk.

96. Simmons RK, Coleman RL, Price HC, et al. Performance of the UK Prospective Diabetes Study Risk Engine and the Framingham Risk Equations in Estimating Cardiovascular Disease in the. *Diabetes Care* 2009;32:708–13. PMCID:PMC2660447.

97. Pambianco G, Costacou T, Ellis D, Becker DJ, Klein R, Orchard TJ. The 30-year natural history of type 1 diabetes complications: the Pittsburgh Epidemiology of Diabetes Complications Study experience. *Diabetes* 2006;55:1463–9.

Chapter 9

Lipid management and cardiovascular risk reduction

Antonio M. Gotto, Jr. and John A. Farmer

During the past three decades, the industrialized world has witnessed an encouraging reduction in age-adjusted morbidity and mortality in cardiovascular disease (CVD). The significant decline in the incidence of myocardial infarction and stroke reflects a complex interplay between refinements in hygienic (diet and exercise) measures, medical therapy, diagnostic imaging, and revascularization techniques. However, medical therapy and surgical procedures like coronary artery bypass and percutaneous angioplasty are not curative measures, and the absolute prevalence of atherosclerosis is increasing since patients with established vascular disease are surviving longer. The initiation and progression of atherosclerosis results from the interaction of various genetic and environmental factors, and effective therapy requires a multifactorial approach to global risk reduction.

Evidence for lipid management

The lipid hypothesis was proposed over 100 years ago to explain the central role of cholesterol in atherosclerosis, and data from epidemiological, experimental, pathological, and genetic studies have now confirmed the primary role of dyslipidemia in the atherosclerotic process. Epidemiologic studies such as the Framingham Heart Study and the Multiple Risk Factor Intervention Trial provided initial, incontrovertible evidence establishing a strong statistical correlation between cholesterol levels and the risk of developing atherosclerosis [1,2]. However, the results of early cholesterol-lowering prospective trials such as the Lipid Research Clinics Coronary Primary Prevention Trial (LRC-CPPT)

Metabolic Risk for Cardiovascular Disease, 1st edition. Edited by R. H. Eckel.
© 2011 American Heart Association. By Blackwell Publishing Ltd.

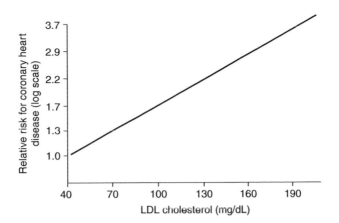

Figure 9.1 Log-linear relationship between LDL cholesterol levels and relative risk for coronary heart disease. Epidemiological and clinical trial data indicate that for every 30 mg/dL reduction in LDL cholesterol, the relative risk for coronary heart disease decreases by about 30%. The relative risk is set at 1.0 when the LDL cholesterol level is 40 mg/dL. Reproduced from Grundy et al. [16] with permission from Elsevier.

and the Helsinki Heart Study (HHS) were statistically significant but demonstrated minimal absolute reductions in coronary events, possibly due to flaws in study design [3,4]. Additionally, total mortality was not reduced, which implied that lipid reduction could have a potentially adverse effect. The advent of statin therapy, however, not only legitimized pharmacological interventions to lower CVD risk, but also provided confirmation of the lipid hypothesis (Figure 9.1). The primary effect of the statins is to lower low-density lipoprotein cholesterol (LDL-C) through partial inhibition of the rate-limiting enzyme in cholesterol synthesis (3-hydroxy-3-methylglutaryl Coenzyme A reductase; HMG-CoA reductase) [5]. Clinical trials comparing the administration of statin therapy to placebo have demonstrated that statins reduce CVD risk across the spectrum of vascular disease.

Five large-scale trials in the 1990s first established the efficacy and safety of statin therapy in primary and secondary prevention. The Scandinavian Simvastatin Survival Study (4S) was the first trial to show that lipid lowering was associated with a significant reduction in total mortality. In individuals with a history of myocardial infarction or angina, simvastatin at 20 mg/day was associated with a 36% reduction in LDL-C, which translated into a 30% reduction in all-cause mortality and a 42% reduction in coronary heart disease (CHD) deaths [6]. The West of Scotland Coronary Prevention Study (WOSCOPS), a primary prevention trial, examined 6595 men with elevated cholesterol and no history of myocardial infarction and found that 40 mg/day of pravastatin was associated with a 26% reduction in LDL-C and a 31% reduction in the risk for non-fatal myocardial infarction or CHD death, compared to placebo [7].

The Cholesterol and Recurrent Events (CARE) trial and the Long-Term Intervention with Pravastatin in Ischemic Disease (LIPID) trial were secondary prevention trials with pravastatin in patients with "average" cholesterol levels, and both demonstrated significant reductions in the rate of recurrent events [8,9]. LIPID was the second trial to achieve a reduction in all-cause mortality (22%). The Air Force/Texas Coronary Atherosclerosis Prevention Study (AFCAPS/TexCAPS) was the first primary prevention trial to show cardiovascular risk reduction in patients with average total cholesterol (TC) and LDL-C, but below-average high-density lipoprotein cholesterol (HDL-C) levels [10].

A group of five subsequent trials extended the benefit of statin therapy to high-risk subgroups underrepresented in earlier trials, including women, the elderly, diabetic and hypertensive patients, and those with below average LDL-C [11–15]. These trials formed the basis for the 2004 update of the Adult Treatment Panel of the National Cholesterol Education Program (ATP-III), which recommended more intensive LDL-C treatment targets for high-risk patients [16]. The Heart Protection Study (HPS) was the largest of these trials and included 20 536 patients with coronary disease, diabetes, occlusive arterial disease, or treated hypertension, but with a mean baseline LDL-C of 131 mg/dL [11]. The HPS and the other "second-generation" statin trials helped extend the body of clinical trial data to include a larger proportion of the general population.

More recent clinical trials have examined the effects of intensive statin therapy aimed at low LDL-C targets in patients following acute coronary syndromes (ACS) or with stable CHD. For example, the Treating to New Targets (TNT) study examined 10 001 patients with stable CHD and LDL-C < 130 mg/dL, who were randomized to atorvastatin 80 mg/day or 10 mg/day with the goal of lowering LDL-C to below the recommended target of 100 mg/dL. After a median follow-up of 4.9 years, patients treated with intensive therapy achieved a mean LDL-C of 77 mg/dL, as compared to 101 mg/dL in the standard dose group, and experienced a 22% relative reduction in the risk of a first major cardiovascular event, with no increase in adverse events [17].

Meta-analyses of the large statin trials demonstrate that there is a linear relation between cholesterol reduction and decreased CHD risk. The Cholesterol Treatment Trialists' Collaborators found that each 1 mmol/L ($\sim$ 40 mg/dL) reduction in LDL-C resulted in a relative 12% reduction in all-cause mortality, a 19% reduction in coronary mortality, and a 21% reduction in any major vascular event [18]. While the body of evidence is greatest for statin therapy, it appears that LDL-C reduction decreases cardiovascular risk regardless of the mechanism used. Another meta-analysis of 19 lipid-lowering trials, which included five dietary trials, three trials with bile acid resins, one ileal bypass study, and 10 statin trials, found a linear relationship between percent reductions in LDL-C and relative risk reductions in non-fatal myocardial infarction and CHD death over 5 years of treatment (Figure 9.2) [19].

Current evidence does not indicate a lower threshold beyond which LDL-C reduction ceases to be beneficial. The recent Justification for the Use of Statins in

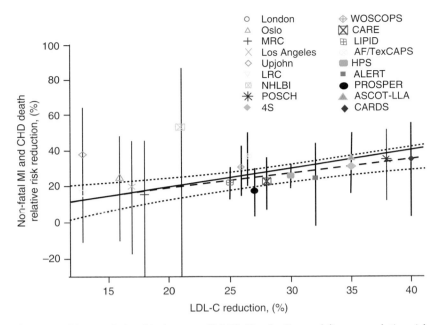

Figure 9.2 Linear relationship between % LDL-C reduction and five-year relative risk for nonfatal MI and CHD death maintained across a variety of lipid-lowering trials. The solid line has a slope = 1. The crude risk estimates from the individual studies are plotted along with their associated 95% confidence intervals. CHD, coronary heart disease; MI, myocardial infarction. Reproduced from Robinson et al. [19] with permission from Elsevier.

Primary Prevention: an Intervention Trial Evaluating Rosuvastatin (JUPITER) confirms that LDL-C reduction to very low levels, even in healthy adults, confers substantial benefit, and it indicates that C-reactive protein (CRP), a marker of systemic inflammation, may possibly also be a useful therapeutic target. In this trial, 17 802 healthy, middle-aged adults with LDL-C < 130 mg/dL and elevated CRP (> 2 mg/L) were randomized to rosuvastatin at 20 mg/day or placebo. After 1.9 years, the trial was stopped due to early evidence of efficacy. The rosuvastatin group achieved a median LDL-C of 55 mg/dL, which was associated with a 44% relative reduction in the rate of a major cardiovascular event and a 20% reduction in all-cause mortality, with no increase in adverse events [20]. Individuals who achieved the greatest reductions in both LDL-C (< 70 mg/dL) and CRP (< 1 mg/L) experienced the greatest benefit, with an observed 79% relative reduction in the rate of a major cardiovascular event [21]. These strong results suggest that dual targets for LDL-C and CRP may yield maximal benefit in low-risk primary prevention, although it remains to be seen how JUPITER affects future practice guidelines. Further research is also necessary to determine whether CRP is a marker or a mediator of atherosclerosis and CVD.

Diagnosis of dyslipidemia

Early efforts to manage dyslipidemia focused on modification of total choles-terol; however, this measurement has significant practical limitations since a significant overlap exists between subjects with and without atherosclerosis. Total cholesterol is measured in the fasting state to exclude the contribution of chylomicrons, which are formed within the gastrointestinal tract following in-gestion of a fatty meal and cleared relatively rapidly. Cholesterol is distributed in a variety of circulating lipoproteins that have variable impact on CVD risk.

Low-density lipoprotein

Low-density lipoprotein (LDL) is a metabolic end-product and is most closely linked to the risk of developing atherosclerosis. LDL exists as a family of cir-culating particles that vary in size, density, and cholesterol content. Epidemi-ological studies have suggested that small, dense LDL may increase the risk of atherosclerosis due to an enhanced ability to penetrate the endothelium, increased cytotoxicity, and greater susceptibility to oxidation.

Very-low-density lipoprotein

Very-low-density lipoprotein (VLDL) is the major endogenously (hepatic) pro-duced particle and is relatively enriched in triglycerides. The role that VLDL plays as an independent contributor to CVD risk is controversial since ele-vated triglycerides are frequently found in patients with diabetes, obesity, the metabolic syndrome, and low high-density lipoprotein cholesterol (HDL-C). Early epidemiological studies minimized the independent role that triglyceride-rich lipoproteins play in the atherosclerotic process, although increasing evi-dence suggests a more substantial contribution [22]. Fasting triglyceride levels may not accurately reflect the cumulative effects of exposure to potentially atherogenic lipoproteins on the vascular endothelium over a 24-hour period. Postprandial lipemia, or the inability to clear triglyceride-rich and cytotoxic VLDL remnant particles (ß-VLDL) following a meal, is common in subjects with diabetes, obesity, and physical inactivity, and it has been correlated with increased CVD risk.

High-density lipoprotein

High-density lipoprotein (HDL) is produced within the liver and ileum, and it circulates in multiple subforms. Increased circulating levels of HDL-C are thought to confer protection in the development of atherosclerosis [23]. Al-though the precise mechanism is controversial, it is postulated that HDL low-ers CVD risk through reverse cholesterol transport, decreased LDL oxidation, prostacyclin metabolism, and a complex metabolic interaction with triglyceride-rich particles. Although population studies demonstrate a clear inverse rela-tionship between levels of HDL-C and CVD risk, genetic syndromes that are characterized by low levels of circulating HDL-C (e.g., ApoA-I Milano mutation) do not appear to confer increased risk for premature atherosclerosis [24]. When exposed to increased oxidative or inflammatory stress, the HDL particle may become dysfunctional and its protective capacity reduced, even at normal or high circulating levels [25].

Lipoprotein(a)

Lipoprotein(a) is a complex lipoprotein that is composed of an LDL particle attached to apoprotein(a) via a sulfhydryl linkage [26]. Apoprotein(a) is homologous to plasminogen but lacks serine protease activity and may interfere with thrombolysis due to competition for receptor binding. Circulating levels of lipoprotein(a) are mostly genetically determined, and clinical trials have not demonstrated benefit with its modification.

Identification of the at-risk patient

Optimal screening for dyslipidemia includes a thorough history (with emphasis on the prevalence of premature atherosclerosis in the family), physical examination, and laboratory measurement of lipid subfractions. Although physical examination is insensitive for dyslipidemia, relatively specific markers of genetic lipid abnormalities can be discerned. In white subjects under the age of 35, the presence of corneal arcus is frequently a marker of genetic dyslipidemia, but it is non-specific in African-Americans and subjects over the age of 45. Cutaneous xanthelasmas, which are generally periorbital in location, are not specific for the diagnosis of dyslipidemia, as roughly 50% of subjects with this dermatological condition have normal lipid profiles, but their presence should still prompt the determination of a full lipid profile. In contrast, the presence of tendinous xanthomas on extensor tendons (e.g., Achilles) is virtually specific for diagnosis of familial hypercholesterolemia. Familial hypercholesterolemia is relatively common (1/500 white subjects) and is associated with severe premature atherosclerosis, accounting for approximately 10% of premature myocardial infarction [27]. Lipemia retinalis, which is characterized by orange discoloration of the retina, is associated with severe hypertriglyceridemia, as are eruptive and planar xanthomas. The presence of peripheral vascular disease coexistent with dyslipidemia should be determined by a careful arterial examination for bruits and for trophic changes of the nails.

Dyslipidemia can be associated with a variety of secondary causes that should be excluded prior to the initiation of pharmacological therapy. Borderline hypothyroidism or frank myxedema is associated with an increase in circulating levels of LDL-C, and a thyroid profile should be obtained in dyslipidemic subjects whose LDL-C level exceeds 160 mg/dL. Renal insufficiency associated with nephrotic-range proteinuria is also characterized by elevated LDL-C.

Obstructive liver disease is associated with a therapeutically challenging form of dyslipidemia that includes the presence of lipoprotein X, which contains a high proportion of unesterified cholesterol [28]. Concomitant drug therapy may also alter the lipid profile. Treatment for hypertension with non-cardioselective beta-blockers and high-dose thiazide diuretics adversely affects the lipid profile. Conversely, calcium channel blockers are metabolically neutral, and modulators of the renin–angiotensin system may increase insulin sensitivity. Treatment with antiretroviral therapy (ART) has dramatically altered the morbidity and mortality associated with HIV, but it can also lead to lipid abnormalities that increase CVD risk, including dyslipidemia, increased visceral fat, insulin resistance, and diabetes [29]. On the other hand, ART may also decrease cardiovascular risk by controlling HIV-associated inflammation, immune activation, and endothelial dysfunction [30]. The link between HIV and increased CVD risk may be further complicated by a higher prevalence of traditional risk factors, such as smoking, among HIV-infected patients as compared to the general population [31].

Lipid guidelines

The successful clinical management of dyslipidemia requires a multifactorial approach, including proper diagnosis, identification of secondary causes of dyslipidemia, and risk stratification. Initial risk stratification should be based on a basic lipid profile obtained in the fasting state. ATP-III has established guidelines for the identification of subjects with dyslipidemia and appropriate treatment goals [32] (Tables 9.1, 9.2, and 9.3).

Therapeutic lifestyle changes

Lifestyle modification (therapeutic lifestyle changes or TLC) including diet and exercise should always be the mainstay of therapy. Consumption of saturated fat should be less than 7% of total caloric intake. Dietary studies have demonstrated that for each 1% of calories derived from saturated fatty acids, serum LDL-C increases by approximately 2% [32]. Consumption of *trans* fatty acids can be reduced through substitution of liquid vegetable oils and soft margarine. Dietary cholesterol should not exceed 200 mg/day, and total fat should be restricted to 25 to 35% of total calories. Monounsaturated fats, which are the mainstay of the Mediterranean diet, may include up to 20% of total calories. Carbohydrate intake should be 50 to 60% of total calories, as high-carbohydrate diets can increase circulating triglyceride levels, particularly in subjects with metabolic syndrome, obesity, and diabetes. Complex carbohydrates should be consumed in the form of whole grains, vegetables, and fruits containing viscous fiber. Approximately 20 to 30 g/day of soluble fiber may reduce the level of cholesterol absorption.

Table 9.1 National Cholesterol Education Program Adult Treatment Panel III lipid classifications [32]

Lipid	Value (mg/dL)	Classification
Total cholesterol	< 200	Desirable
	200–239	Borderline high
	≥ 240	High
LDL-C	< 100	Optimal
	100–129	Near or above optimal
	130–159	Borderline high
	160–189	High
	≥ 190	Very high
HDL-C	< 40	Low
	≥ 60	High
Fasting triglycerides	< 150	Normal
	150–199	Borderline high
	200–499	High
	≥ 500	Very high

Table 9.2 Major risk factors (exclusive of LDL-C) that modify LDL goals in patients without CHD or CHD risk equivalents [32]

Risk factor	Definition
Cigarette smoking	Any
Hypertension	BP ≥ 140/90 mmHg; or on antihypertensive medication
Low HDL-C*	< 40 mg/dL
Family history of premature CHD	CHD in male first-degree relative < 55 years; CHD in female first-degree relative < 65 years
Age	Men ≥ 45 years; women ≥ 55 years

*HDL-C ≥ 60 mg/dL is a "negative" risk factor that removes one risk factor from the total count.

Table 9.3 LDL-C goals according to categories of risk [16]

Risk category	LDL-C goal (mg/dL)
High risk: CHD and CHD risk equivalents (clinical atherosclerotic disease, diabetes mellitus, 10-year CHD risk > 20%)	< 100
Very high risk	Optional goal of < 70
Moderately high risk: ≥ 2 risk factors (10-yearr risk 10–20%)	< 130 (optional goal of < 100)
Moderate risk: ≥ 2 risk factors (10-year risk < 10%)	< 130
Low risk: ≤ 1 risk factor	< 160

Pharmacological management of dyslipidemia

Therapeutic lifestyle changes should always be initiated as the first step in the management of dyslipidemia, but when dietary therapy alone may be insufficient, as in a variety of genetic lipid disorders, early commencement of pharmacological therapy is warranted. Additionally, in high-risk individuals following an acute coronary syndrome, aggressive and prompt lipid-lowering therapy has been shown unequivocally to reduce the risk of subsequent CVD events. The choice of pharmacological agent is determined by the predominant lipid phenotype, which is either characterized by elevated LDL-C or by abnormalities involving triglycerides or HDL-C (Table 9.4).

Table 9.4 Effects of drug classes on serum lipids [82]

Drug class	Total cholesterol	LDL-C	HDL-C	Triglycerides
Statins	↓ 15%–60%	↓ 15%–60%	↑ 5%–15%	↓ 15%–25%
Bile acid resins	↓ 20%	↓ 15%–25%	↑ 3%–5%	Variable
Cholesterol absorption inhibitors	↓ 13%	↓ 17–20%	↑ 3%	↓ 8%
Nicotinic acid	↓ 25%	↓ 5%–25%	↑ 15%–35%	↓ 20%–50%
Fibric acid derivatives	↓ 15%	Variable	↑ 10%–20%	↓ 20%–50%
Omega-3 fatty acids	N/A	N/A	N/A	↓ 35% – 50%

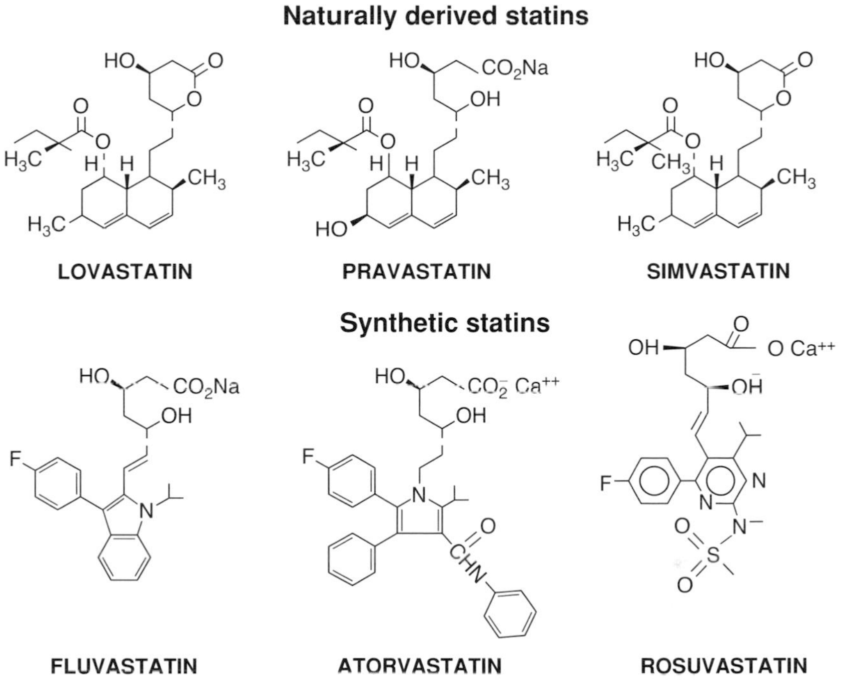

Naturally derived statins

LOVASTATIN   PRAVASTATIN   SIMVASTATIN

Synthetic statins

FLUVASTATIN   ATORVASTATIN   ROSUVASTATIN

Figure 9.3 Structure of naturally derived and synthetic statins.

Lipid phenotype predominantly characterized by elevated LDL-C

Statin therapy

In clinical studies, statin therapy, either alone or in combination, has been demonstrated to reduce CVD risk in patients across various stages of the atherosclerotic spectrum. Angiographic trials with statins have shown both regression of atherosclerosis and reduced progression of coronary luminal occlusion, as compared to control populations. The statins are a class of hypolipidemic agents with differing chemical structures that are either derived as primary fungal metabolites or are chemically synthesized (Figure 9.3). Lovastatin, pravastatin, and simvastatin were the first agents to be released and are fungal derivatives. Atorvastatin, fluvastatin, and rosuvastatin are synthetic compounds that retain the same basic properties despite considerable differences in chemical structure.

Mechanism of action

The statins differ in terms of chemical structure, efficacy of lipid reduction, lipophilicity, metabolic pathways, and pharmacokinetics, yet they share a common mechanism in which the primary effect is a partial and reversible reduction in the activity of the rate-limiting enzyme in cholesterol synthesis (HMG CoA reductase), leading to an overall reduction in LDL-C [33]. Within the liver, the level of cholesterol is tightly regulated and remains constant due to a dual mechanism that balances cholesterol synthesis with receptor-mediated clearance of cholesterol-rich lipoproteins. Reduction of intrahepatic cholesterol leads to a subsequent upregulation of the LDL (apoB/E) receptor. The upregulation of the number or function of LDL receptors results in increased recognition and binding of lipoproteins that express apoB or E particles on their surface. LDL contains only apoB on its surface, while VLDL and intermediate-density lipoprotein (IDL) express both apoB and E. The receptor-mediated removal of circulating lipoproteins thus partially explains the reduction of triglycerides with statin therapy, as both IDL and VLDL are relatively rich in triglycerides.

Lipophilic statins such as simvastatin may also reduce the hepatic synthesis of VLDL [34]. The effect of atorvastatin on VLDL synthesis has been inferred by studies performed on subjects with homozygous familial hypercholesterolemia undergoing lipoprotein apheresis [35]. Subjects with familial hypercholesterolemia (FH) have fewer LDL receptors or reduced functioning of LDL receptors, and they are defective in clearing apoB-containing particles from the circulation. In receptor-negative FH patients, the administration of atorvastatin decreased the hepatic production rates of VLDL by 20–25% as compared to placebo, without an increase in the fractional clearance rate. LDL is formed by the catabolism of VLDL, which acts as a precursor in the endogenous lipid cascade, so the reduction of hepatic VLDL synthesis results in a secondary decrease in LDL-C, even in the absence of LDL receptors. In addition to its effects on lipoprotein metabolism, statin therapy is postulated to have a variety of non-lipid, or pleiotropic, effects, including improvements in endothelial function and fibrinolysis, as well as anti-inflammatory and antithrombotic effects [36]. Although the clinical relevance of these pleiotropic effects is controversial, they appear to be present in all currently available statins, albeit at differing magnitudes.

The primary effect of statin monotherapy is LDL-C reduction. The response is variable depending on the dose and the agent employed, but will generally lead to reductions in circulating LDL-C levels of 15 to 60%. Statin therapy may lead to modest increases in HDL-C although the mechanism is controversial and not well characterized. Additionally, reductions in triglycerides of 15 to 25% may be noted with statin therapy.

Side effects
The statins have been closely monitored in both post-marketing studies and prospective clinical trials for the induction of adverse side effects. Initial concerns regarding ocular safety, sleep disturbance, increased risk of malignancy, and other side effects have not been verified in multiple studies. The major

clinically relevant side effects of statin therapy are related to induction of muscle and hepatic toxicity [37].

The potential for hepatic abnormalities secondary to statin therapy was recognized in early clinical studies, and increases in serum alanine aminotransferase and aspartate aminotransferase were among the first statin-related side effects noted. Clinically relevant elevations of hepatic enzymes are defined as a sustained increase in circulating levels that exceed three times the upper limit of normal; such elevations can be found in approximately 1% of treated subjects. The clinical relevance of asymptomatic, mild elevations in hepatic enzymes is difficult to interpret due to frequent variability in circulating levels. Lipophilic statins were initially felt to demonstrate a propensity for elevation of hepatic enzymes due to increased tissue penetration mediated by an enhanced capacity for diffusion. However, the transport of statins into hepatic tissue is also mediated by the organic ion transporter (OAT), and pure diffusion in the liver is not the sole mechanism of drug transport [38]. Elevations of circulating levels of hepatic enzymes have been demonstrated with all of the currently available statins and appear to represent a class effect. A recent meta-analysis evaluating 49 275 statin recipients found a relatively similar rate of alteration in hepatic enzymes across the different statins [39]. Increases in levels of hepatic enzymes generally occur within the first three to four months of therapy. The National Lipid Association does not recommend repetitive routine screening of liver enzymes in asymptomatic subjects [40].

Statin-related myotoxicity is a spectrum ranging from non-specific myalgias to life-threatening rhabdomyolysis [41]. Myositis is an intermediate form of muscle toxicity that is defined as a statin-related increase in creatine kinase, in addition to the presence of an associated symptom complex. Rhabdomyolysis is the most serious statin-mediated side effect and is relatively uncommon with statin monotherapy [42]. It is characterized clinically by diffuse muscle destruction and is accompanied by myoglobinuria and the potential for irreversible renal failure. The release of myoglobin from muscle beds may be confirmed by specific immunoassay. The risk of muscle toxicity has been found with all of the statins and appears to be a class effect. Metabolic myopathies such as deficiencies of phosphorylase, phosphofructokinase, carnitine palmitoyltransferase, etc. are associated with an increased risk for the development of statin-mediated myotoxicity [43]. In vitro studies suggest that statin-induced depletion of metabolic intermediates in the cholesterol synthetic pathway (mevalonate, farnesyl pyrophosphate, and geranylgeraniol) may play a causal role in the induction of statin-related myopathy. Farnesyl pyrophosphate is an intermediate in the production of ubiquinone (coenzyme Q), and anecdotal reports have supported the prophylactic administration of coenzyme Q with statin therapy. However, a recent literature review found insignificant evidence to demonstrate an etiological role for coenzyme Q deficiency in statin-associated myopathy [44], and the National Lipid Association does not currently recommend routine coenzyme Q

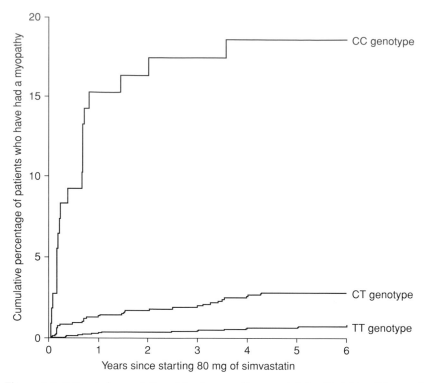

Figure 9.4 Estimated cumulative risk of myopathy associated with taking 80 mg of simvastatin daily, according to 3 common genotypes for *SLCO1B1*, the gene that encodes OATP1B1, an organic anion-transporting polypeptide that regulates the hepatic uptake of statins. Reproduced from (Study of the Effectiveness of Additional Reductions in Cholesterol and Homocysteine) SEARCH Collaborative Group [45] with permission of the publisher. © 2008 Massachusetts Medical Society. All rights reserved.

administration until prospective clinical trial evidence demonstrating its benefit is available. In addition, a recent genome-wide association study suggests that common variants in the gene encoding OAT polypeptide 1B1 (OATP1B1), which is thought to regulate the hepatic uptake of statins, are strongly associated with increased risk of statin-induced myopathy (Figure 9.4) [45].

Rhabdomyolysis, defined as a compatible clinical syndrome coupled with creatine kinase elevation in excess of 1000 international units, occurs with an incidence of 0.1 to 0.5% with statin monotherapy. The risk is increased in subjects with advanced age, renal impairment, or concurrent therapy with medications that inhibit the cytochrome P450 (3A4) isoforms, such as cyclosporine, erythromycin, certain antifungal agents, and fibrates. Pravastatin is the only currently available statin that is not metabolized by the cytochrome P450 enzyme system.

Bile acid resins
The bile acid sequestrants were initially utilized as therapeutic agents to decrease the severity of pruritic symptoms in subjects with obstructive liver disease. They interrupt the enterohepatic circulation of cholesterol-rich bile acids by binding to them and increasing their rate of excretion. In clinical trials such as LRC-CPPT, they have been shown to reduce LDL-C and the risk of coronary events.

Mechanism of action
The bile acids are synthesized in the liver from cholesterol and stored in the gallbladder [46]. The increased excretion of the bile acid pool following the administration of resin therapy stimulates the conversion of cholesterol into bile acids via activation of the rate-limiting enzyme 7α-hydroxylase, with a resultant decrease in intrahepatic cholesterol levels. This reduction then stimulates the activity of the apoB/E receptor and leads secondarily to increased clearance of LDL from the circulation. The major source of cholesterol utilized in hepatic bile acid synthesis is delivered to the liver by HDL in reverse cholesterol transport, a process that may in turn be upregulated as bile acid production is increased [47]. In normal physiology, approximately 95% of the bile acids are reabsorbed in the distal ileum, and this recycling occurs 5–10 times per day. The 5% of bile acids normally excreted in the feces is counterbalanced by a secondary increase in synthesis within the liver, resulting in a relatively constant concentration. The administration of bile acid sequestrants at the maximal dose lowers LDL-C by 15 to 25%, and HDL-C may be minimally increased. Generally, triglyceride concentrations are not significantly altered although increased circulating levels following treatment have been found in patients with diabetes, metabolic syndrome, and obesity.

Side effects
Due to their side effect profile, the bile acid sequestrants have limited usage. In the USA, cholestyramine and colestipol are administered in powder form, while colesevelam is a tablet. Despite differences in administration and chemical structure, side effects are roughly similar, although colesevelam may be more tolerable [48]. In part because of their large molecular weight, the bile acid resins are not absorbed into the systemic circulation, and systemic side effects are minimal, although transient elevation of hepatic enzymes may be noted. However, bile acid resins are associated with multiple gastrointestinal problems and, in particular, with an increased frequency of constipation that can be severe, due to a prolongation in bile acid transit time through the gastrointestinal tract. Subjects enrolled in the LRC-CPPT reported a 39% prevalence of moderate to severe constipation [49]. Constipation can be minimized by the co-administration of soluble fiber and stool softeners, but is frequently a limiting factor in compliance. Due to molecular structural modifications that increase bile acid affinity

and binding capacity, colesevelam may induce fewer gastrointestinal side effects [50]. Despite concerns over increased carcinogenicity with resin therapy, multiple clinical trials with colestipol and cholestyramine have not supported these claims [51]. The bile acid sequestrants are non-specific ion exchangers and may bind any negatively charged compound that is co-administered. They have been found to reduce the absorption of digitalis, warfarin, beta-blockers, thyroxine, furosemide, statins, and fibrates. The minimization of drug interactions may be achieved by ingesting co-administered medications at least one hour before bile acid sequestrants.

Cholesterol absorption inhibitors

The bulk of cholesterol presented to the gastrointestinal tract is derived from the bile acid pool as opposed to dietary sources, and dietary changes have little effect on overall intrahepatic cholesterol levels. Cholesterol absorption from the gastrointestinal tract occurs in part through passive diffusion across a concentration gradient. Additionally, Niemann-Pick C1 Like 1 (NPC1L1) is a transport protein that modulates cholesterol absorption [52]. Genetically engineered, experimental animals lacking the NPC1L1 protein express a dramatically decreased ability to absorb free cholesterol [53]. Ezetimibe is a pharmacological antagonist to this protein that acts as a specific cholesterol absorption blocker [54]. As opposed to the bile acid sequestrants, ezetimibe does not interfere with the intestinal absorption of fat-soluble vitamins or other co-administered drugs, and bile acid metabolism is not altered. The degree of cholesterol absorption from the gastrointestinal tract is at least partially genetically mediated and follows a Gaussian distribution, with normal subjects absorbing approximately 55% of the available free cholesterol [55]. The efficacy of ezetimibe therapy depends on individual absorptive capacity, although subjects with a normal capacity for cholesterol absorption can expect an approximately 17 to 20% reduction in LDL-C. Minimal, albeit statistically significant, beneficial alterations in circulating triglyceride and HDL-C levels may also be observed.

Results from the ENHANCE (Effect of Combination Ezetimibe and High-Dose Simvastatin vs. Simvastatin Alone on the Atherosclerotic Process in Patients with Heterozygous Familial Hypercholesterolemia) trial indicate that in patients with familial hypercholesterolemia, treatment with ezetimibe and simvastatin did not improve atherosclerotic plaque regression, despite a greater degree of LDL-C lowering than with simvastatin alone [56]. In the Simvastatin and Ezetimibe in Aortic Stenosis (SEAS) trial, the ezetimibe/simvastatin combination did not reduce aortic valve and ischemic events in patients with mild-to-moderate asymptomatic aortic stenosis [57]. The results from SEAS also suggested that ezetimibe might be associated with increased risk of cancer, although a separate analysis of SEAS and two ongoing trials with simvastatin/ezetimibe, IMPROVE-IT and SHARP, indicated that the increase in cancer incidence was due to chance [58]. The results of the large-scale IMPROVE-IT (Improved Reduction of Outcomes: Vytorin Efficacy International Trial) in patients with ACS and SHARP (Study of Heart and Renal Protection) in patients with chronic kidney disease will provide further clarification on the effects on clinical outcomes of LDL-C lowering with the ezetimibe/simvastatin combination.

Primary triglyceride-lowering agents

Elevated triglyceride levels ($\geq 150\,mg/dL$) are an independent risk factor for CVD. Weight reduction and physical activity are recommended for borderline high triglycerides, while elevations $\geq 200\,mg/dL$ generally call for pharmacotherapy to a target of $< 150\,mg/dL$. In patients with high triglycerides, non-HDL-C, which includes VLDL-C, may be a secondary target for lipid lowering after LDL-C targets are achieved. A VLDL-C of $\geq 30\,mg/dL$ is considered normal, so non-HDL-C goals for each risk category are set at $30\,mg/dL$ higher than the corresponding LDL-C goal. Nicotinic acid, the fibric acid derivatives, and fish oil have been shown to have significant effects on circulating triglyceride and HDL-C levels. The primary triglyceride-lowering agents have a long clinical history with well-established efficacy and safety.

Nicotinic acid

Nicotinic acid is an essential water-soluble B vitamin that was initially used to prevent the deficiency disease, pellagra. However, it was subsequently found that nicotinic acid improves the lipid profile at doses far exceeding those necessary to prevent pellagra. Nicotinic acid is available in crystalline form and in a variety of slow-release preparations that are designed to minimize cutaneous side effects. In the Coronary Drug Project (CDP), nicotinic acid effectively lowered LDL-C and was associated with long-term benefit [59]. The ongoing AIM-HIGH (Atherothrombosis Intervention in Metabolic Syndrome with Low HDL/High Triglycerides and Impact on Global Health Outcomes) and HPS-2 THRIVE (Heart Protection Study-2 Treatment of HDL to Reduce the Incidence of Vascular Events) trials are designed to assess nicotinic acid's HDL-raising capacity in combination with statin therapy.

Mechanism of action

Nicotinic acid has a complex mechanism of action involving multiple metabolic pathways, and its administration has been shown to decrease the degree of lipolysis within the adipocyte [60]. Nicotinic acid recognizes and binds to G-coupled cell surface proteins [61]; its pharmacologically active receptors are HM74A and PUMA-G (protein upregulated in macrophages by interferon-gamma), which are concentrated in adipose tissue. Activation of the niacin receptors results in the inhibition of adenyl cyclase, with a resultant decrease in the rate of lipolysis. This reduction in lipolysis decreases both the rate of production of free fatty acids (FFAs) and their release into the circulation. Since FFAs are the metabolic substrate for the synthesis of VLDL, the hepatic production of triglyceride-rich particles is then decreased. Nicotinic acid may also inhibit the formation of triglycerides by decreasing the activity of hepatic diacylglycerol acyltransferase (DGAT, a key enzyme in triglyceride production) and increasing the degradation of apolipoprotein B (required for VLDL synthesis) [62]. Nicotinic acid is the only commonly used pharmacological agent that has been demonstrated to exert beneficial effects on all lipoprotein fractions including lipoprotein(a). The administration of nicotinic acid results in reductions in total cholesterol, LDL-C, triglycerides, and lipoprotein(a), as well as a significant increase in HDL-C levels [63]. Although the mechanism is controversial, nicotinic acid may increase HDL-C by either reducing the catabolic rate or increasing the synthesis of ApoA-I. It is hypothesized that nicotinic acid inhibits the hepatic-mediated removal of HDL/ApoA-I particles without interfering with the removal of cholesterol carried within HDL, potentially resulting in an enhancement of reverse cholesterol transport [64]. It is unclear how nicotinic acid favorably affects circulating levels of lipoprotein(a). Clinical studies have not shown a reduction in the catabolic rate of the lipoprotein(a) fraction, which implies that nicotinic acid may perhaps reduce the synthesis of Lp(a) by decreasing the synthesis of apoB [65]. Nicotinic acid can also exhibit non-lipid effects, including beneficial alterations in the total fibrinolytic activity in dyslipidemic patients [60].

Side effects

The most common side effect associated with immediate-release nicotinic acid is an intense cutaneous flushing and pruritus. It was recently shown that nicotinic acid-induced flushing is mediated by prostaglandin D2 and other dermal eicosanoids [66]. Flushing may be reduced by co-administration of aspirin, and an experimental compound, laropiprant, that acts as a selective antagonist to the prostaglandin D2 receptor subtype 1 (DP1) and minimizes nicotinic acid-induced flushing, is in development [67]. Hepatotoxicity with nicotinic acid is a clinical concern, and sustained-release preparations of nicotinic acid that minimize dermal side effects may have increased hepatotoxicity relative to crystalline niacin. Hepatic toxicity induced by sustained-released nicotinic acid occurs mainly at doses in excess of 1500 mg/day, and the incidence of abnormal hepatic enzymes with such preparations is less than 0.5% [68].

Additionally, nicotinic acid has been demonstrated to adversely affect glucose tolerance. Insulin sensitivity may be decreased by approximately 20% following a relatively short duration of therapy, and these effects may be more significant in older subjects [69]. However, the induction of insulin resistance is manageable with close monitoring and adjustment of other medical therapies. The CDP found benefit with nicotinic acid in diabetic patients [70]. Nicotinic acid has also been associated with the induction of peptic ulcer disease, precipitation of gout, and acanthosis nigricans.

Fibric acid derivatives

The fibric acid derivatives have a long history in the clinical management of dyslipidemia, and their efficacy and safety are well established. Clofibrate was the first fibric acid derivative employed in clinical practice, although current use has declined due to safety concerns. Gemfibrozil and fenofibrate are the fibric acid derivatives currently utilized in the USA. Clinical trials such as the secondary prevention Veteran Affairs Cooperative Studies Program High-density Lipoprotein Cholesterol Intervention Trial (VA-HIT) and the primary prevention HHS provide the strongest evidence of benefit with fibric acid derivatives in high-risk and healthy patients [4,71]. The recent Fenofibrate Intervention and Event Lowering in Diabetes (FIELD) study demonstrated trends in benefit in diabetic subjects, although findings were inconclusive [72].

Mechanisms of action
Fibric acid derivatives activate transcriptional factors expressed in the liver, leading to alterations in both the synthesis and catabolism of triglyceride-rich lipoproteins. The peroxisome proliferator-activated receptor-α (PPAR-α) is a member of the nuclear hormone receptor superfamily that regulates the translation of genes involved in lipid metabolism [73]. The activation of PPAR-α by gemfibrozil and fenofibrate increases the activity of lipoprotein lipase with a resultant enhanced degradation of triglyceride-rich lipoproteins, including chylomicrons and VLDL, and increases in HDL-C. Additionally, fibrates enhance the oxidation of FFAs in the liver and in myocytes at the periphery, and the influx of FFAs from the peripheral adipocyte to the liver is thus reduced. This reduction in the precursor molecules for triglyceride synthesis results in a decrease in the hepatic synthesis of VLDL. The fibric acid derivatives increase the synthesis of the major apolipoproteins of HDL (ApoA-I and ApoA-II) and have been demonstrated to reduce the activity of cholesteryl ester transfer protein, leading to secondary increases in HDL-C [74]. Additionally, compositional changes in LDL with a reduction in the levels of small, dense LDL have been observed; it is hypothesized that these changes may decrease CVD risk [75].

The fibrates exhibit a variety of non-lipid, or pleiotropic, effects, including direct anti-atherogenic effects on vascular tissue. In atherosclerosis, tumor necrosis factor-α increases the expression of vascular cellular adhesion molecules produced by the endothelium and may be inhibited by fibrates [76]. Thus, fibrates may reduce both the binding of monocytes to inflammatory cells and their subsequent transmigration from the plasma compartment. PPAR-α agonists have been shown to decrease the activity of vascular smooth muscle cells and may help reduce plaque cellularity. Fibrates may also improve vascular reactivity. Coagulation markers are considered emerging risk factors in the prediction of coronary events, and fibrinogen has been linked with coronary events in a variety of epidemiological studies. Levels of fibrinogen are variably reduced

(12 to 25%) by fibric acid derivatives, although the clinical relevance of this modification remains controversial [77].

Side effects

Clinically significant side effects occur in approximately 5–10% of subjects, but are generally not of sufficient severity to warrant drug discontinuation. The most commonly encountered side effect is an increased prevalence of non-specific gastrointestinal symptoms. Clofibrate has been found to increase the incidence of gallstones, but is infrequently utilized. Liver function abnormalities have been observed, but are generally not associated with significant hepatic dysfunction. Mixed dyslipidemia, which is characterized by elevated LDL-C and VLDL-C, is an appropriate phenotype for combination therapy with a statin and a fibric acid derivative; however, this combination is associated with an increased risk of rhabdomyolysis. Gemfibrozil interferes with the glucuronidation of statins and reduces their rate of excretion [78]. The risk of rhabdomyolysis may be less if a statin is combined with fenofibrate.

Fish oil

Epidemiological observations indicate that consuming a diet rich in marine-derived omega-3 fatty acids is inversely correlated with the incidence of coronary and cerebrovascular disease [79]. Omega-3 fatty acids, in particular eicosapentaenoic acid (EPA) and docosahexaenoic acid (DHA), have multiple, potentially beneficial cardiovascular effects, including reductions in platelet aggregation, inflammation, and vasoconstriction. Additionally, they significantly improve the lipid profile, primarily by reducing circulating triglyceride levels, although modest increases in HDL-C can also be observed [80]. Reductions in VLDL-C may be caused by reductions in FFA availability, decreased FFA transport to the liver, or decreased activity of triglyceride synthetic pathways and associated enzyme systems. Marine-derived omega-3 fatty acids inhibit a key gene transcription factor, sterol regulatory element binding protein 1-C (SREBP 1-C), which results in a subsequent decrease in the hepatic synthesis of triglyceride-rich lipoproteins, although other mechanisms are also involved. The reduction of circulating triglycerides by omega-3 fatty acids ranges from 20 to 50% and is at least partially a function of pretreatment levels. In 2002, the American Heart Association approved the use of fish oil supplementation in patients with coronary heart disease [81]. Prescription-strength fish oil (Lovaza) is approved by the FDA to decrease triglycerides ≥ 500 mg/dL at a dose of 4 g/day. The general public is recommended to consume two fatty fish meals a week. Patients with CHD should have 1 g/day of EPA/DHA, while patients with hypertriglyceridemia require 3–5 g/day of EPA/DHA while under a physician's supervision.

Summary

The lipid hypothesis was proposed as a mechanism for the initiation and progression of atherosclerosis over 100 years ago. Since then, the central role of dyslipidemia in atherosclerosis has been confirmed by a large body of epidemiological, genetic, and pathological evidence. The advent of statin therapy justified aggressive lipid-lowering strategies and clearly demonstrated CVD benefit in primary and secondary prevention among numerous patient populations. Current strategies for lipid management can be classified as those that primarily affect LDL-C levels and those that primarily modify triglycerides and HDL. In general, the statins, bile acid resins, cholesterol absorption inhibitor, nicotinic acid, fibrates, and omega-3 fatty acids are safe and effective treatments for the management of dyslipidemia and CVD risk reduction.

References

1. Gordon T, Kannel WB, Castelli WP, Dawber TR. Lipoproteins, cardiovascular disease, and death. The Framingham study. *Arch Intern Med* 1981;141:1128–31.
2. The multiple risk factor intervention trial (MRFIT). A national study of primary prevention of coronary heart disease. *JAMA* 1976;235:825–7.
3. The Lipid Research Clinics Coronary Primary Prevention Trial results. I. Reduction in incidence of coronary heart disease. *JAMA* 1984;251:351–64.
4. Frick MH, Elo O, Haapa K, et al. Helsinki Heart Study: primary-prevention trial with gemfibrozil in middle-aged men with dyslipidemia. Safety of treatment, changes in risk factors, and incidence of coronary heart disease. *N Engl J Med* 1987;317:1237–45.
5. Endo A, Kuroda M, Tanzawa K. Competitive inhibition of 3-hydroxy-3-methylglutaryl coenzyme A reductase by ML-236A and ML-236B fungal metabolites, having hypocholesterolemic activity. *FEBS Lett* 1976;72:323–6.
6. Randomised trial of cholesterol lowering in 4444 patients with coronary heart disease: the Scandinavian Simvastatin Survival Study (4S). *Lancet* 1994;344:1383–9.
7. Shepherd J, Cobbe SM, Ford I, et al. Prevention of coronary heart disease with pravastatin in men with hypercholesterolemia. West of Scotland Coronary Prevention Study Group. *N Engl J Med* 1995;333:1301–7.
8. Sacks FM, Pfeffer MA, Moye LA, et al. The effect of pravastatin on coronary events after myocardial infarction in patients with average cholesterol levels. Cholesterol and Recurrent Events Trial investigators. *N Engl J Med* 1996;335:1001–9.
9. Prevention of cardiovascular events and death with pravastatin in patients with coronary heart disease and a broad range of initial cholesterol levels. The Long-Term Intervention with Pravastatin in Ischemic Disease (LIPID) Study Group. *N Engl J Med* 1998;339:1349–57.
10. Downs JR, Clearfield M, Weis S et al. Primary prevention of acute coronary events with lovastatin in men and women with average cholesterol levels: Results of AFCAPS/TexCAPS. Air Force/Texas Coronary Atherosclerosis Prevention Study. *JAMA* 1998;279:1615–22.

11. Heart Protection Study Collaborative Group: MRC/BHF Heart Protection Study of cholesterol lowering with simvastatin in 20,536 high-risk individuals: a randomised placebo-controlled trial. *Lancet* 2002;360:7–22.

12. Cannon CP, Braunwald E, McCabe CH, et al. Intensive versus moderate lipid lowering with statins after acute coronary syndromes. *N Engl J Med* 2004;350:1495–1504.

13. Sever PS, Dahlöf B, Poulter NR, et al. Prevention of coronary and stroke events with atorvastatin in hypertensive patients who have average or lower-than-average cholesterol concentrations, in the Anglo-Scandinavian Cardiac Outcomes Trial – Lipid Lowering Arm (ASCOT-LLA): a multicentre randomised controlled trial. *Lancet* 2003;361:1149–58.

14. Major outcomes in moderately hypercholesterolemic, hypertensive patients randomized to pravastatin vs usual care: The Antihypertensive and Lipid-Lowering Treatment to Prevent Heart Attack Trial (ALLHAT-LLT). *JAMA* 2002;288:2998–3007.

15. Shepherd J, Blauw GJ, Murphy MB, et al. Pravastatin in elderly individuals at risk of vascular disease (PROSPER): a randomised controlled trial. *Lancet* 2002;360:1623–30.

16. Grundy SM, Cleeman JI, Merz CN, et al. Implications of recent clinical trials for the National Cholesterol Education Program Adult Treatment Panel III Guidelines. *Circulation* 2004;110:227–239.

17. LaRosa JC, Grunday SM, Waters DD, et al. Intensive lipid lowering with atorvastatin in patients with stable coronary disease. *N Engl J Med* 2005;352:1425–35.

18. Baigent C, Keech A, Kearney PM, et al. Efficacy and safety of cholesterol-lowering treatment: prospective meta-analysis of data from 90,056 participants in 14 randomised trials of statins. *Lancet* 2005;366:1267–78.

19. Robinson JG, Smith B, Maheshwari N, Schrott H. Pleiotropic effects of statins: benefit beyond cholesterol reduction? A meta-regression analysis. *J Am Coll Cardiol* 2005;46:1855–62.

20. Ridker PM, Danielson E, Fonseca FA, et al. Rosuvastatin to prevent vascular events in men and women with elevated C-reactive protein. *N Engl J Med* 2008;359(21): 2195–2207.

21. Ridker PM, Danielson E, Fonseca FA, et al.; JUPITER Trial Study Group. Reduction in C-reactive protein and LDL cholesterol and cardiovascular event rates after initiation of rosuvastatin: a prospective study of the JUPITER trial. *Lancet* 2009;373:1175–82.

22. Austin MA. Triglyceride, small, dense low-density lipoprotein, and the atherogenic lipoprotein phenotype. *Curr Atheroscler Rep* 2000;2:200–7.

23. Toth PP. High-density lipoprotein as a therapeutic target: clinical evidence and treatment strategies. *Am J Cardiol* 2005;96(9A): 50–8K; discussion 34–5K.

24. Nissen SE, Tsunoda T, Tuzcu EM, et al. Effect of recombinant ApoA-I Milano on coronary atherosclerosis in patients with acute coronary syndromes: a randomized controlled trial. *JAMA* 2003;290:2292–300.

25. Watson KE, Ansell BJ, Watson AD, Fonarow GC. HDL function as a target of lipid-modifying therapy. *Rev Cardiovasc Med* 2007;8:1–8.

26. Scanu AM, Lawn RM, Berg K. Lipoprotein(a) and atherosclerosis. *Ann Intern Med* 1991;115:209–18.

27. Brown MS, Goldstein JL. Familial hypercholesterolemia: genetic, biochemical and pathophysiologic considerations. *Adv Intern Med* 1975;20:273–96.

28. Ross A, Murphy GM, Wilkinson PA, Mills GL, Sherlock S. Occurrence of an abnormal lipoprotein in patients with liver disease. *Gut* 1970;11:1035–7.

29. Penzak SR, Chuck SK. Hyperlipidemia associated with HIV protease inhibitor use: pathophysiology, prevalence, risk factors and treatment. *Scand J Infect Dis* 2000;32:111–23.

30. Currier JS, Lundgren JD, Carr A, et al.; Working Group 2. Epidemiological evidence for cardiovascular disease in HIV-infected patients and relationship to highly active antiretroviral therapy. *Circulation* 2008;118:29–35.

31. Pere D, Ignacio SL, Ramón T, et al. Dyslipidemia and cardiovascular disease risk factor management in HIV-1 infected subjects treated with HAART in the Spanish VACH cohort. *Open AIDS J* 2008;2:26–38.

32. Third Report of the National Cholesterol Education Program (NCEP) Expert Panel on Detection, Evaluation, and Treatment of High Blood Cholesterol in Adults (Adult Treatment Panel III) final report. *Circulation* 2002;106:3143–421.

33. Sirtori CR. Pharmacology and mechanism of action of the new HMG-CoA reductase inhibitors. *Pharmacol Res* 1990;22:555–63.

34. Burnett JR, Wilcox LJ, Telford DE, et al. Inhibition of HMG-CoA reductase by atorvastatin decreases both VLDL and LDL apolipoprotein B production in miniature pigs. *Arterioscler Thromb Vasc Biol* 1997;17:2589–600.

35. Yamamoto A, Harada-Shiba M, Kawaguchi A, et al. The effect of atorvastatin on serum lipids and lipoproteins in patients with homozyous familial hypercholesterolemia undergoing LDL-apheresis therapy. *Atherosclerosis* 2000;153:89–98.

36. Liao JK, Laufs U. Pleiotropic effects of statins. *Ann Rev Pharmacol Toxicol* 2005;45:89–118.

37. McKenney JM, Davidson MH, Jacobson TA, Guyton JR; National Lipid Association Statin Safety Assessment Task Force. Final conclusions and recommendations of the National Lipid Association Statin Safety Assessment Task Force. *Am J Cardiol* 2006;97(8A):89–94C.

38. Yamazaki M, Tokui T, Ishigami M, Sugiyama Y. Tissue-selective uptake of pravastatin in rats: contribution of a specific carrier-mediated uptake system. *Biopharm Drug Dispos* 1996;17:775–89.

39. de Denus S, Spinler SA, Miller K, Peterson AM. Statins and liver toxicity: a meta-analysis. *Pharmacotherapy* 2004;24:584–91.

40. Cohen DE, Anania FA, Chalasani N; National Lipid Association Statin Safety Assessment Task Force Liver Expert Panel. An assessment of statin safety by hepatologists. *Am J Cardiol* 2006;97(8A):77–81C.

41. Thompson PD, Clarkson PM, Rosenson RS; National Lipid Association Statin Safety Assessment Task Force Muscle Safety Expert Panel. An assessment of statin safety by muscle experts. *Am J Cardiol* 2006;97(8A):69–76C.

42. Schreiber DH, Anderson TR. Statin-induced rhabdomyolysis. *J Emerg Med* 2006;31:177–80.

43. Farmer JA, Torre-Amione G. Comparative tolerability of the HMG-CoA reductase inhibitors. *Drug Saf* 2000;23:197–213.

44. Marcoff L, Thompson PD. The role of coenzyme Q10 in statin-associated myopathy: a systematic review. *J Am Coll Cardiol* 2007;49:2231–7.

45. SEARCH Collaborative Group. *SLCO1B1* variants and statin-induced myopathy – a genomewide study. *N Engl J Med* 2008;359:789–99.

46. Chiang JY. Bile acid regulation of gene expression: roles of nuclear hormone receptors. *Endocr Rev* 2002;23:443–63.

47. Schwartz CC, Halloran LG, Vlahcevic ZR, Gregory DH, Swell L. Preferential utilization of free cholesterol from high-density lipoproteins for biliary cholesterol secretion in man. *Science* 1978;200:62–4.

48. Melian EB, Plosker GL. Colesevelam. *Am J Cardiovasc Drugs* 2001;1:141–6; discussion 7–8.

49. Rifkind BM. Lipid Research Clinics Coronary Primary Prevention Trial: results and implications. *Am J Cardiol* 1984;54:30C-4C.

50. Insull W, Jr. Clinical utility of bile acid sequestrants in the treatment of dyslipidemia: a scientific review. *South Med J* 2006;99:257–73.

51. Ast M, Frishman WH. Bile acid sequestrants. *J Clin Pharmacol* 1990;30:99–106.

52. Sudhop T, Lütjohann D, von Bergmann K. Sterol transporters: targets of natural sterols and new lipid lowering drugs. *Pharmacol Ther* 2005;105:333–41.

53. Davies JP, Scott C, Oishi K, Liapis A, Ioannou YA. Inactivation of NPC1L1 causes multiple lipid transport defects and protects against diet-induced hypercholesterolemia. *J Biol Chem* 2005;280:12710–20.

54. Gupta EK, Ito MK. Ezetimibe: the first in a novel class of selective cholesterol-absorption inhibitors. *Heart Dis* 2002;4:399–409.

55. Bosner MS, Lange LG, Stenson WF, Ostlund RE Jr. Percent cholesterol absorption in normal women and men quantified with dual stable isotopic tracers and negative ion mass spectrometry. *J Lipid Res* 1999;40:302–8.

56. Kastelein JJ, Akdim F, Stroes ES, et al., and the ENHANCE Investigators: Simvastatin with or without ezetimibe in familialhypercholesterolemia. *N Engl J Med* 2008;358:1431–43.

57. Rossebø AB, Pedersen TR, Boman K, et al., for the SEAS Investigators. Intensive Lipid Lowering with Simvastatin and Ezetimibe in Aortic Stenosis. *N Engl J Med* 2008;359:1343–56.

58. Peto R, Emberson J, Landray M, et al. Analyses of cancer data from three ezetimibe trials. *N Engl J Med* 2008;359:1357–66.

59. Canner PL, Berge KG, Wenger NK, et al. Fifteen-year mortality in Coronary Drug Project patients: long-term benefit with niacin. *J Am Coll Cardiol* 1986;8:1245–55.

60. Carlson LA. Nicotinic acid: the broad-spectrum lipid drug. A 50th anniversary review. *J Intern Med* 2005;258:94–114.

61. Zhang Y, Schmidt RJ, Foxworthy P, et al. Niacin mediates lipolysis in adipose tissue through its G-protein coupled receptor HM74A. *Biochem Biophys Res Commun* 2005;334:729–32.

62. Ganji SH, Tavintharan S, Zhu D, Xing Y, Kamanna VS, Kashyap ML. Niacin noncompetitively inhibits DGAT2 but not DGAT1 activity in HepG2 cells. *J Lipid Res* 2004;45:1835–45.

63. Meyers CD, Kamanna VS, Kashyap ML. Niacin therapy in atherosclerosis. *Curr Opin Lipidol* 2004;15:659–65.

64. Jin FY, Kamanna VS, Kashyap ML. Niacin decreases removal of high-density lipoprotein apolipoprotein A-I but not cholesterol ester by Hep G2 cells. Implication for reverse cholesterol transport. *Arterioscler Thromb Vasc Biol* 1997;17:2020–8.

65. Carlson LA, Hamsten A, Asplund A. Pronounced lowering of serum levels of lipoprotein Lp(a) in hyperlipidaemic subjects treated with nicotinic acid. *J Intern Med* 1989;226:271–6.

66. Maciejewski-Lenoir D, Richman JG, Hakak Y, Gaidarov J, Behan DP, Connolly DT. Langerhans cells release prostaglandin D2 in response to nicotinic acid. *J Invest Dermatol* 2006;126:2637–46.

67. Lai E, De Lepeleire I, Crumley TM, et al. Suppression of niacin-induced vasodilation with an antagonist to prostaglandin D2 receptor subtype 1. *Clin Pharmacol Ther* 2007;81:849–57.

68. Guyton JR. Extended-release niacin for modifying the lipoprotein profile. *Expert Opin Pharmacother* 2004;5:1385–98.

69. Chang AM, Smith MJ, Galecki AT, Bloem CJ, Halter JB. Impaired beta-cell function in human aging: response to nicotinic acid-induced insulin resistance. *J Clin Endocrinol Metab* 2006;91:3303–9.

70. Canner PL, Fugerg CD, Terrin ML, McGovern ME. Benefits of niacin by glycemic status in patients with healed myocardial infarction (from the Coronary Drug Project). *Am J Cardiol* 2005;95:254–7.

71. Rubins HB, Robins SJ, Collins D, et al. Gemfibrozil for the secondary prevention of coronary heart disease in men with low levels of high-density lipoprotein cholesterol. Veterans Affairs High-Density Lipoprotein Cholesterol Intervention Trial Study Group. *N Engl J Med* 1999;341:410–18.

72. Keech A, Simes RJ, Barter P, et al.; FIELD Study Investigators. Effects of long-term fenofibrate therapy on cardiovascular events in 9795 people with type 2 diabetes mellitus (the FIELD study): randomised controlled trial. *Lancet* 2005;366: 1849–61.

73. Vu-Dac N, Schoonjans K, Kosykh V, et al. Fibrates increase human apolipoprotein A-II expression through activation of the peroxisome proliferator-activated receptor. *J Clin Invest* 1995;96:741–50.

74. Guérin M, Bruckert E, Dolphin PJ, Turpin G, Chapman MJ. Fenofibrate reduces plasma cholesteryl ester transfer from HDL to VLDL and normalizes the atherogenic, dense LDL profile in combined hyperlipidemia. *Arterioscler Thromb Vasc Biol* 1996;16: 763–72.

75. Yoshida H, Ishikawa T, Ayaori M, et al. Beneficial effect of gemfibrozil on the chemical composition and oxidative susceptibility of low density lipoprotein: a randomized, double-blind, placebo-controlled study. *Atherosclerosis* 1998;139: 179–87.

76. Zhao SP, Ye HJ, Zhou HN, Nie S, Li QZ. Gemfibrozil reduces release of tumor necrosis factor-alpha in peripheral blood mononuclear cells from healthy subjects and patients with coronary heart disease. *Clin Chim Acta* 2003;332:61–7.

77. de Maat MP, Knipscheer HC, Kastelein JJ, Kluft C. Modulation of plasma fibrinogen levels by ciprofibrate and gemfibrozil in primary hyperlipidaemia. *Thromb Haemost* 1997;77:75–9.

78. Shitara Y, Hirano M, Sato H, Sugiyama Y. Gemfibrozil and its glucuronide inhibit the organic anion transporting polypeptide 2 (OATP2/OATP1B1:SLC21A6)-mediated hepatic uptake and CYP2C8-mediated metabolism of cerivastatin: analysis of the mechanism of the clinically relevant drug-drug interaction between cerivastatin and gemfibrozil. *J Pharmacol Exp Ther* 2004;311:228–36.

79. Daviglus ML, Stamler J, Orencia AJ, et al. Fish consumption and the 30-year risk of fatal myocardial infarction. *N Engl J Med* 1997;336:1046–53.

80. Davidson MH. Mechanisms for the hypotriglyceridemic effect of marine omega-3 fatty acids. *Am J Cardiol* 2006;98(4A):27–33i.

81. Kris-Etherton PM, Harris WS, Appel LJ; American Heart Association Nutrition Committee. Fish consumption, fish oil, omega-3 fatty acids, and cardiovascular disease. *Circulation* 2002;106:2747–57.

82. Gotto AM, Pownall HJ (eds). *Manual of Lipid Disorders*. Baltimore: Williams & Wilkins, 1992.

Chapter 10

Obesity management and cardiovascular risk reduction

George A. Bray

Introduction

Let's begin with a brief description of the techniques that are available for the management of obesity. Obesity is the result of a long-term positive imbalance between energy intake and energy expenditure, which means that treatments can be focused on either energy intake or energy expenditure. Figure 10.1 is an energy balance diagram and serves as a basis for briefly reviewing therapeutic options [1].

Eating (energy intake) is a target for behavior therapy, drugs, and bariatric surgery for obesity. Physical activity and energy expenditure are targets for behavioral change and drugs, and patients who lose weight after bariatric surgery are often more physically active. When any of these therapeutic approaches is used consistently, weight loss is the expected result. In this chapter we will examine the consequences of this weight loss as they apply to the cardiovascular system. Since death from heart disease is the leading cause of death, weight loss might be expected both to benefit long-term survival and to have many intermediate effects on cardiovascular risk factors.

The metabolic syndrome has become one way of "bundling" a group of risk factors that together point toward the risk of diabetes or cardiovascular disease (CVD) [2]. There are several components that can be included in this syndrome. The Adult Treatment Panel criteria include central adiposity measured by waist circumference, an atherogenic dyslipidemia characterized by low HDL cholesterol and high triglycerides, impaired fasting glucose reflecting insulin resistance (as does the atherogenic dyslipidemia), and elevated blood pressure. When an individual has abnormalities in three of these five categories,

Metabolic Risk for Cardiovascular Disease, 1st edition. Edited by R. H. Eckel.
© 2011 American Heart Association. By Blackwell Publishing Ltd.

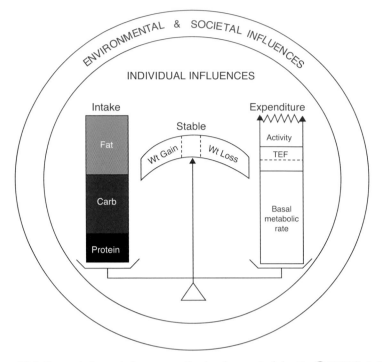

Figure 10.1 Energy balance: influences on the development of obesity. © 1998 G. A. Bray.

s/he is classified as having the metabolic syndrome [2]. In addition to these features, however, there are proinflammatory markers and procoagulant markers that are frequently abnormal in individuals with the metabolic syndrome. In the studies reviewed below, it will be clear that weight loss is associated with significant improvement in the metabolic syndrome and in the proinflammatory and procoagulant markers that are often present. To the extent that we are successful with weight loss it would be the ideal approach, since it will treat many of the features of the metabolic syndrome at one time [2].

One can view the consequences of obesity as resulting from either the mass of adipose tissue added to the body or from the metabolic consequences of enlarged fat deposits [3]. The "mass" effects of obesity depend on the specific location of the fat deposits. For the "metabolic" consequences, it is largely central and visceral fat that is important. Women have about 12% more body fat than men for any given BMI [4]. Yet women have fewer heart attacks and die, on average, at an older age than men. This implies that a significant proportion of the extra fat that women have is not "risky" fat in terms of CVD. Epidemiological studies show that fat on the hips and lower body may, in fact, be protective in terms of mortality risks [5]. Thus it is important to identify the "risky" fat and not to lump all fat depots into a single entity.

Benefits and potential risks of weight loss

Effect on mortality

There are two groups of studies that have examined weight loss and mortality. One group of observational studies suggests that weight loss is associated with increased mortality [6]. The limitation of these studies is that, in most cases, they cannot distinguish between intentional and unintentional weight loss. We have known since the time of Hippocrates, 2500 years ago, that unintentional weight loss is a bad prognostic sign for future health [7]. One approach to separating intentional and unintentional weight loss was taken by Allison and colleagues [8], who examined loss of lean body mass versus fat. When the weight loss was from lean body mass, there was an increased risk of mortality. In contrast, loss of body fat was associated with lowered risks of mortality [8].

The other approach to separating intentional and unintentional weight loss was to ask whether the weight loss was intentional. Documentation that intentional weight loss benefits mortality is scantier. In one study of intentional versus unintentional weight loss, Williamson and colleagues reported a 20% reduction in all-cause mortality among 15 069 women with health conditions who were monitored from 1959–60 to 1972. Most of the reduction in risk was related to decrease in cancer-related deaths. Mortality related to diabetes was reduced 30 to 40%. In women with no pre-existing illness ($n = 28,388$), intentional weight loss of 20 lb (9.1 kg) or more in the previous year was associated with a 25% reduction in all-cause mortality [9]. Using a different data set, Williamson and colleagues [10] carried out a prospective analysis of 12-year mortality among 4970 overweight individuals with diabetes, aged 40 to 64 years, enrolled in the American Cancer Society Prevention Study I. Intentional weight loss was reported by 34% of the cohort and resulted in a 25% decrease in total mortality and a 28% reduction in CVD and diabetes mortality. A weight loss of 20 to 29 lb (9.1 to 13.2 kg) was associated with the largest reductions in mortality. Similar results came from a follow-up of the National Health Interview Survey that included enough subjects to link 20 439 individuals to the National Death Index. In this group with a 9-year follow-up, those reporting intentional weight loss had a 24% lower overall mortality rate when compared to individuals not trying to lose weight [11,12]. A final large study in this category was conducted in the United Kingdom by Wanamethee and colleagues. Among individuals choosing to lose weight, the all-cause mortality was reduced 41%, but there was no association with intentional weight loss and death from cardiovascular causes [13].

Studies in the bariatric surgical literature suggest that voluntary, intentional weight loss is beneficial. In the follow-up of individuals who have had bariatric gastric bypass surgery, Flum and colleagues noted a modest overall survival benefit associated with the procedure, suggesting again that "intentional" weight loss can reduce mortality [14]. Two simultaneous publications have clearly established that intentional weight loss lowers mortality. The first, from the prospective matched-control study called the Swedish Obese Subjects study [15], found that mortality was reduced by 39% after an average follow-up of 10 years. The number of deaths from CVD was smaller, and although the study was too small for this effect to be statistically significant, with further follow-up it may turn out to be so. The second study, by Adams and colleagues [16], used Utah driver's licenses to match subjects by age and sex with patients who had received a gastric by-pass. In this study the risk of death from CVD was reduced, as were deaths from diabetes and cancer.

Intermediate risk factors

A considerable body of data documents that weight loss improves a number of the intermediate risk factors that predict disease [17–26]. In a systematic review of long-term weight loss studies and their applicability to clinical practice, Douketis and colleagues [19] found that dietary and lifestyle therapy provided < 5 kg weight loss after 2 to 4 years, and that pharmacological therapy could produce 5 to 10 kg weight loss over 1 to 2 years. Weight loss of ≥ 5% from baseline is not consistently associated with improvements in cardiovascular risk factors, and these benefits appear primarily in the individuals with concomitant cardiovascular risk factors.

Effects on morbidity

Hypertension and heart disease

One of the clearest examples of benefits from weight loss on cardiovascular risk factors comes from studies with hypertensive patients. Among these are the Trials of Hypertension Prevention (TOHP) [27,28] and the Trial of Nonpharmacologic Interventions in the Elderly (TONE) [29]. Individuals with high to normal blood pressure experienced a 21 to 34% decrease in the incidence of hypertension over an interval of 1.5 to 4 years with a modest weight loss of only 2 to 4%. Hypertensive individuals who maintained their weight loss following a weight loss intervention were able to maintain lower blood pressure compared to the individuals who regained weight, where blood pressure returned to baseline levels [30]. Among older people, a reduction in bodyweight by an average of 4% produced a 30% reduction in the combined incidence of CVD and hypertension. In the Premier study, over 800 people with borderline hypertension were enrolled into three groups: a control or advise-only group, a group who received an established behavioral intervention program, or a group who got both the behavioral intervention program along with the DASH diet [31,32]. The blood pressure was reduced by 3.7 to 4.3 mmHg in the two intervention groups compared to the advise-only group [31]. There was also a significant reduction in the prevalence of hypertension in the two treated groups. In a follow-up study, this group has shown that over 30 months subjects can retain about 50% of an initial weight loss, and still maintain the lower blood pressure [33].

In the Framingham cohort, the effect of weight loss on blood pressure was examined in middle-aged (30–49 years) and older (50–65 years) adults. After adjusting the confounding variables, they found that a 6.8% weight loss over 4 years was associated with a 21% to 29% decrease in risk of hypertension. After adjusting for cancer and cardiovascular risk, these percentages increased further, with middle-aged individuals reducing their risk of hypertension by 28% and older adults reducing their risk of hypertension by 37%. Thus a modest weight loss significantly reduced the risk of hypertension [34].

Several clinical trials have shown that weight loss can improve cardiovascular risk. The Stanford Coronary Risk Intervention Project may be the most famous of these [35]. It was a large, multi-community project in California. Using a multifactorial program of risk reduction that involved an intensive focus on re-ducing saturated fat and total fat, an increase in physical activity, and a modest 4% weight loss, the investigators showed that there was an approximately 40% reduction in probability of cardiac events and a slower rate of coronary artery stenosis. A second study in this group was the Lifestyle Heart Trial, which is a landmark in the diet–heart literature, because it shows that vigorous dietary intervention can reverse the risks of CVD [36,37]. A total of 48 individuals were recruited for this study, with half randomized to a very-low-fat diet as com-pared to the usual-care group. Over the course of 12 months, the treated group lost about 8% of their bodyweight and had a reduction in anginal symptoms, cardiac events, and coronary stenosis over the ensuing 5 years [36,37]. A graded reduction in cardiovascular risk was observed in still another study. A group of high-risk individuals aged 50 to 75 years were recruited. In those who suc-cessfully lost weight over a 6-month period, the odds ratio for coronary heart disease was 0.70 over the next 3 years [38]. Among those who gained weight, the cumulative CHD incidence was 18%, compared to 14% in those who gained weight or lost < 2 kg, but only 8% among those with at least a 7 kg weight loss.

In addition to the data showing improvement in cardiovascular outcomes with weight loss, there is evidence that weight loss improves the function of the heart [39]. It is possible to show a reduction in blood volume with a par-allel reduction in stroke volume. Cardiac output also falls, as does systemic arterial blood pressure. There is, however, little change in systemic arterial re-sistance after weight loss. Resting oxygen consumption declines as the size of the metabolic compartment is reduced. Possibly the most important change is the reduction in left ventricular mass. With obesity there is an eccentric hyper-trophy of the heart, which is reduced with weight loss. There may also be a decline in heart rate, a fall in the QT_c interval, and an increase in heart rate variability [39].

In addition to these positive effects there have also been important negative effects of some weight loss regimens on cardiac function. One of the early very low-calorie diet formulas contained a gelatin-based protein, and a number of deaths were reported [40]. These were thought to be due to an arrhythmia called torsades de pointes, due to prolongation of the QT_c interval. A second cardiac event following treatment of obesity occurred with fenfluramine and dexfenfluramine. In 1997, at the height of the use of fenfluramine/phentermine (the so-called fen/phen craze), Conley and colleagues reported 24 patients who developed aortic regurgitation while being treated with this combination [41]. The best estimates are that, with treatment for longer than 6 months, the prevalence of this problem may have been 20–30% among treated patients. In September 1997, fenfluramine and dexfenfluramine were withdrawn from the market.

Obstructive sleep apnea

In contrast to the relatively benign effects of excess weight on most components of respiratory function, overweight is often associated with sleep apnea which can be severe and may require clinical care [42]. This is a condition for which weight loss can be beneficial. Obstructive sleep apnea (OSA) is considerably more common in men than women and, as a group, these people are significantly taller than individuals without sleep apnea. An increased snoring index and increased maximal nocturnal sound intensity are characteristic. Nocturnal oxygen saturation is significantly reduced [43]. One interesting hypothesis is that the increased neck circumference and fat deposits in the pharyngeal area may lead to the OSA of overweight. A study of obese diabetics using polysomnography as the criterion showed that over 86% had sleep apnea with a mean apnea-hypopnea index of 20.5 ± 16.8 events/hour. A total of 30.5% of the participants had moderate sleep apnea ($15 \leq AHI < 30$), and 22.6% had the severe form ($AHI \geq 30$). Waist circumference was significantly related to the presence of OSA and severe sleep apnea was most likely in individuals with a higher BMI [44].

Sleep apnea benefits from weight loss. In twelve studies representing 342 patients that were identified for a meta-analysis, the pooled mean body mass index was reduced by $17.9 \, kg/m^2$ (from $55.3 \, kg/m^2$ to $37.7 \, kg/m^2$). The baseline apnea-hypopnea index of 54.7 events/hour was reduced by 38.2 events/hour to a final value of 15.8 events/hour. Although bariatric surgery significantly reduced the apnea-hypopnea index, the mean apnea-hypopnea index after surgical weight loss was still elevated and consistent with moderately severe OSA, suggesting that patients undergoing bariatric surgery should not expect a cure of OSA after surgical weight loss [45].

Dyslipidemia

The meta-analysis by Avenell and colleagues [46] suggests that weight loss has significant effects on lipid profiles and blood pressure, both important predictors of future CVD. Among various types of weight loss programs, there was a significant, but somewhat variable, effect on weight loss. In family-based intervention compared to a control group at 12 months ($n = 4$) weight loss was –2.96 kg (95% CI –5.31 to –0.60). With group versus individual therapy in four studies it was 1.59 kg (95% CI –1.81 to 5.00). When diet plus behavior therapy were compared to diet alone after 12 months in four studies, weight loss was –7.67 kg (95% CI –11.97 to –3.36). Finally, when diet and behavior therapy were compared against only a control group, the weight loss after 12 months was –7.21 kg (95% CI –8.68 to –5.75). With these weight losses, there was a reduction in blood pressure that averaged –4/–3 mmHg comparing systolic and diastolic blood pressure. Cholesterol and LDL cholesterol also declined by some 5 to 8 mg/dL and triglycerides fell by 18 mg/dL. In the meta-analysis of Avenell [46], the HDL cholesterol benefited at 12 months in two studies, with an increase of 0.10 nmol/L (95% CI 0.06 to 0.14) and triglycerides were lowered after 12 months by –0.18 nmol/L (95% CI –0.31 to –0.06). Thus some important risk factors for CVD are improved by weight loss.

Diabetes

Diabetes is a cardiovascular risk factor, and thus reduction in the incidence of diabetes would be expected to benefit cardiovascular outcomes. The risk of diabetes is reduced by modest weight loss [47–57]. This has now been reported in several prospective trials in patients with impaired glucose tolerance. The first report was by Pan and colleagues from China [47]. They showed a reduction in the incidence of new cases of diabetes by 31% with diet, by 46% with exercise, and by 42% with both after 6 years of follow-up. The next was the Finnish Diabetes Study [48–50]. Incidence of diabetes was reduced by 58% over 4 years with a 5.0% weight loss and increased exercise and improved diet [48]. This was followed by the US Diabetes Prevention Program (USDPP) which showed that, after 2.8 years of an intensive lifestyle program and an initial weight loss of 7% of bodyweight, the conversion rate was reduced by 58% compared to the placebo-treated control group [51–55,58]. The Japanese Diabetes Prevention Program (JaDPP) [56] and the Indian Diabetes Prevention Program (InDPP) [57] also reported reduced rates of conversion to diabetes of 57.4% over 4 years and 28.5% over 3 years, respectively.

The Diabetes Prevention Program participants also showed significant reductions in lipids and blood pressure in the intensive lifestyle group compared to the placebo group (Table 10.1). Similar reductions were seen in the Look AHEAD trial, which enrolled just over 5000 individuals with established diabetes and randomized them to placebo and intensive lifestyle treatment [59]. Those in the intensive lifestyle group also showed reductions in blood pressure and lipids after the first year of treatment, when weight loss was just over 8% in the treated group.

A number of weight loss medications also reduce the risk of developing diabetes.

Table 10.1 Changes in lipids and blood pressure with weight loss in the Diabetes Prevention Program and Look AHEAD trial

Variable	Diabetes Prevention Program		Look AHEAD Trial	
	Placebo	Lifestyle	Placebo	Lifestyle
Blood pressure (SBP/DBP)	−0.90/−089	−3.4/−3.6	−2.8/−1.8	−6.8/−3.0
Cholesterol (%)	−1.2%	−2.3%	–	–
LDL cholesterol	+1.3%	+0.7%	−4.6%	−5.0%
HDL cholesterol (mg/dL)	−0.1%	+1.9%	+3.2%	+7.8%
Triglycerides (mg/dL)	−11.9	−25.4	−14.6	30.3
Fibrinogen (% change 1 year)	0.6%	−2%	–	–
Tissue plasminogen activator	−5%	−20%	–	–
CRP: Males	0%	−30%	–	–
Females	0%	−20%		

Orlistat

Using data from the clinical trials of orlistat, Heymsfield and colleagues pooled information on 675 subjects from three of the 2-year studies in which glucose tolerance tests were available [60]. During treatment, 6.6% of the patients taking orlistat converted from a normal to an impaired glucose tolerance test, compared with 10.8% in the placebo-treated group. None of the orlistat-treated patients who originally had normal glucose tolerance developed diabetes, compared with 1.2% in the placebo-treated group. Of those who initially had normal glucose tolerance, 7.6% in the placebo group, but only 3% in the orlistat-treated group, developed diabetes. The effect of orlistat in preventing diabetes has been assessed in a 4-year study [61]. In this trial, weight was reduced by 2.8 kg (95% CI 1.1 to 4.5) compared to placebo, and the conversion rate of diabetes was reduced from 9% to 6% for a relative risk reduction of 37% (HR 0.63; 95% CI 0.46 to 0.86) [62]. The incidence of new cases of diabetes was also reduced from 10.9% to 5.2% ($P = 0.041$) during a 3-year period in which overweight patients were treated with orlistat and lifestyle or lifestyle alone [63]. A meta-analysis using the pooled data shows significant overall effects after one year of treatment on lipids and blood pressure with orlistat (Table 10.2).

Patients with diabetes treated with orlistat, 120 mg three times daily for 1 year, lost more weight than the placebo-treated group [64–66].

Table 10.2 A meta-analysis of the effects of orlistat on lipids and blood pressure

Change in cholesterol ($n = 7$ studies)	–0.34 mmol/L (95% CI –0.41 to –0.027) ($n = 7$ studies)
Change in LDL cholesterol ($n = 7$ studies)	–0.29 mmol/L (95% CI -0.34 to –0.24)
Change in HDL cholesterol ($n = 6$ studies)	–0.03 mmol/L (95% CI –0.05 to –0.01)
Change in triglycerides ($n = 6$ studies)	+0.03 mmol/L (95% CI –0.04 to 0.10)
Change in HbA1c ($n = 3$ studies)	–0.17% (95% CI –0.24 to –0.10 ($n = 3$ studies)
Change in systolic blood pressure ($n = 7$ studies)	–2.02 mm Hg (95% CI –2.87 to –1.17)
Change in diastolic blood pressure ($n = 7$ studies)	–1.64 mm Hg (95% CI –2.20 to –1.09)

Sibutramine

A number of studies have examined the effect of sibutramine in diabetic patients. In a 3-month (12-week) trial, patients with diabetes who were treated with 15 mg per day of sibutramine lost –2.4 kg (2.8%), compared with –0.1 kg (0.12%) in the placebo group [67]. In this study, hemoglobin A1c levels decreased 0.3% in the drug-treated group and remained stable in the placebo group. Fasting glucose values decreased 0.3 mg/dL in the drug-treated patients and increased 1.4 mg/dL in the placebo-treated group. In a 24-week trial, the dose of sibutramine was increased from 5 mg to 20 mg per day over 6 weeks [68]. Among those who completed the treatment, weight loss was –4.3 g (4.3%) in the sibutramine-treated patients, compared with –0.3 kg (0.3%) in placebo-treated patients. Hemoglobin A1c levels decreased 1.67% in the drug-treated group, compared with 0.53% in the placebo-treated group. These changes in glucose and hemoglobin A1c levels were expected from the amount of weight loss associated with drug treatment. In a 12-month multicenter, randomized placebo-controlled study [69], 194 patients with diabetes receiving metformin were assigned to placebo ($n = 64$), sibutramine 15 mg/d ($n = 68$), or sibutramine 20 mg/d ($n = 63$). At 12 months, weight loss in the 15 mg/d group was 5.5 ± 0.6 kg and in the 20 mg/d group it was 8.0 ± 0.9 kg, compared to 0.2 ± 0.5 kg in the placebo group. Glycemic control improved in parallel with weight loss. Sibutramine raised sitting diastolic blood pressure by more than 5 mmHg in 43% of those receiving 15 mg/d of sibutramine compared to 25% for the placebo group ($P < 0.05$). Pulse rate increased more than 10 beats/minute in 42% of those on sibutramine compared to 17% for those on placebo.

The 2-year trial by Redmon and colleagues [70] was a double-blind, randomized placebo-controlled trial that had a cross-over for the control group after the first year. The treatment group received sibutramine 10 mg/d for the entire 2 years. In addition they had a portion-controlled diet used for 7 days at the end of each 2 months. There was a significantly greater weight loss in the drug-treated group that reached –9.7 kg at 12 months, compared to –1.6 kg in the placebo-treated group. During the second year those receiving sibutramine continuously regained weight slowly, rising to a maximal loss of –6.3 kg at 24 months. In contrast, the group who received sibutramine during the second year weighed less at 24 months than those receiving sibutramine continuously (–6.3 kg in continuous treatment vs –9.7 kg for the cross-over group). There was an improvement in diabetic control associated with the weight loss.

A meta-analysis has been performed of eight studies in diabetic patients receiving sibutramine [71]. In the meta-analysis the changes in bodyweight, waist circumference, glucose, hemoglobin A1c, triglycerides, and HDL cholesterol favored sibutramine. The mean weight loss was –5.53 ± 2.2 for those treated with sibutramine and –0.90 ± 0.17 for the placebo-treated patients. There was no significant change in systolic blood pressure, but diastolic blood pressure was significantly higher in the sibutramine-treated patients [71]. In the meta-analysis by Norris and colleagues [72], the net weight loss over 12 to 26 weeks in four trials including 391 diabetics was –4.5 kg (95% CI –7.2 to –1.8).

As with other procedures for weight loss, patients treated with sibutramine experienced improvements in some lipid parameters. These are summarized in Table 10.3 from the meta-analysis of Avenell and colleagues [46]. There was

Table 10.3 A meta-analysis of effects of sibutramine on lipids and blood pressure

Change in cholesterol at 12 months ($n = 3$)	0.01 mmol/L (95% CI –0.15 to 0.18 mmol/L)
Change in LDL cholesterol at 12 months ($n = 2$)	–0.08 mmol/L (95% CI –0.23 to 0.07 mmol/L)
Change in HDL cholesterol at 12 months ($n = 2$)	0.10 mmol/L (95% CI 0.04 to 0.15 mmol/L)
Change in triglycerides at 12 months ($n = 4$)	–0.16 mmol/L (95% CI –0.26 to –0.05 mmol/L)
Change in SBP at 12 months ($n = 3$)	1.16 mmHg (95% CI –0.60 to 2.93 mmHg)
Change in DBP at 12 months ($n = 3$)	2.04 mmHg (95% CI 0.89 to 3.20 mmHg)

Adapted from Avenell et al. [46].

a small but significant rise in HDL cholesterol and a fall in triglycerides after 12 months. In contrast, cholesterol and LDL cholesterol showed no significant responses. There was no change in systolic blood pressure, but a small rise in diastolic blood pressure at the end of one year.

Bariatric surgery

Bariatric surgery has proven to be a very effective way to reverse the prevalence of diabetes and to reduce the incidence of new cases. Pories and colleagues were the first to note the marked effect on diabetes [73,74]. Although there were design issues with these retrospective studies, they showed an annual incidence of 4.5% in the control group contrasted with only 1% in the surgically operated group. The Swedish Obese Subjects study, a prospective controlled study, has also reported impressive data. After 2 years of follow-up the incidence of diabetes was 8% in the matched-control group and 1% in the surgical group. After 10 years the incidence of diabetes in the control group was 24%, compared to only 7% in the operated group. The incidence rate was related to the amount of weight lost. In the subgroup losing more than 12% of their initial bodyweight, there were no new cases, in contrast to 7% in those losing 2% and 9% in those gaining 4% [75]. At the other end, the rate of recovery from diabetes was 72% in the operated group and 21% in the control group. By 10 years the recovery rate was less, at 36% in the operated group and 13% in the control group [76]. This was reflected in the low odds ratio (OR) for diabetes (OR 0.10) and hyperinsulinemia (OR 0.10). In an unblended, randomized controlled trial Dixon and colleagues [77] enrolled 60 diabetic patients with a BMI between 30 and 40 kg/m^2 into either lap-band operation or a lifestyle program. At 2 years, the lap-band group had lost 20.7% of their bodyweight compared to 1.7% in the lifestyle group. The relative risk of remission from diabetes was 5.5 (95% CI 2.2 to 14.0) and was related to weight loss.

Metabolic syndrome

The data for improvement in metabolic syndrome come from studies with lifestyle intervention, with diet, and with medications. The Diabetes Prevention Program provides convincing evidence for this proposition [78]. A total of 1711 of the 3234 participants (53%) had the metabolic syndrome at randomization. This is comparable to the data for this age group provided by the National Center for Health Statistics [79]. The prevalence did not vary by gender or age groups (< 45; 45–60; > 60 years). However, ethnicity did affect the prevalence, which was lowest in Asians (41%) and highest in whites (57%).

Among African Americans, triglycerides were elevated in only 20.6%, compared with 47 to 53% for the Caucasian, Hispanic, Asian, and Native Americans. Among Native Americans, the prevalence of hypertension and impaired fasting glucose was lower than in the other groups. Approximately half of subjects with impaired glucose tolerance have the metabolic syndrome, with little difference by age, but differences by component. Lifestyle and metformin both reduced the incidence of metabolic syndrome, but lifestyle was more effective than metformin.

Several clinical trials with weight loss medications also show a reversal of the metabolic syndrome. The metabolic syndrome was present in about 50% of the subjects in several clinical trials with rimonabant. In the placebo groups after one year of treatment, the metabolic syndrome was still present in 53% of the subjects in the RIO Europe study [80], 51% of those in the RIO Lipids study [81], and 38% of those in the RIO North America study [82]. Substantial decreases occurred in the rimonabant-treated groups. For the RIO Europe and RIO Lipids groups, only 21% still had the metabolic syndrome, a 60% decrease. For the RIO North America group it was 7.9% – a decrease of almost 60% [80–82].

In a meta-analysis of pharmacological and lifestyle interventions to prevent or delay onset of type 2 diabetes, hazard ratios were reduced to 0.51 by lifestyle compared to standard treatment, the hazard ratio was reduced to HR –0.70 for oral diabetic medications versus control, to HR –0.44 by orlistat versus control, and to HR 0.32 for herbal preparations versus control [83].

Summary

This chapter has presented an energy balance concept for the development of obesity and viewed the risks from obesity as resulting from either excess weight or "metabolic" effects. Weight loss has been demonstrated to reduce the risk of future mortality and to improve an number of intermediate risk factors. Risks of hypertension, cardiovascular risk, obstructive sleep apnea, dyslipidemia and diabetes mellitus are all reduced by weight loss. Both orlistat and sibutramine have demonstrated benefits for many of these risk factors.

References

1. Bray GA. *Contemporary Diagnosis and Management of Obesity and the Metabolic Syndrome*, 3rd edn. Newtown, PA: Handbooks in Health Care, 2003.
2. Bray GA. *The Metabolic Syndrome and Obesity*, Totowa, NJ: Humana Press, 2007.
3. Bray GA. Medical consequences of obesity. *J Clin Endocrinol Metab* 2004;89:2583–9.
4. Gallagher D, Heymsfield SB, Heo M, Jebb SA, Murgatroyd PR, Sakamoto Y. Healthy percentage body fat ranges: an approach for developing guidelines based on body mass index. *Am J Clin Nutr* 2000;72:694–701.
5. Snijder MB, Dekker JM, Visser M, et al. Associations of hip and thigh circumferences independent of waist circumference with the incidence of type 2 diabetes: the Hoorn Study. *Am J Clin Nutr* 2003;77:1192–7.
6. Gregg, EW. The impact of voluntary weight loss on morbidity and mortality. In: Bray G, Bouchard C (eds) *Handbook of Obesity: Clinical Applications*, 3rd edn. New York: Informa Health Care, 2008, pp. 91–104.

7. Hippocrates. Oeuvres complètes d'Hippocrate: traduction nouvelle avec le texte grec en regard, collationné sur les manuscrits et toutes les éditions; accompagnée d'une introduction, . . . suivie d'une table générale des matières. Paris, J. B. Baillière, 1839.

8. Allison DB, Zhu SK, Plankey M, Faith MS, Heo M. Differential associations of body mass index and adiposity with all-cause mortality among men in the first and second National Health and Nutrition Examination Surveys (NHANES I and NHANES II) follow-up studies. *Int J Obes Relat Metab Disord* 2002;26:410–16.

9. Williamson DF, Pamuk E, Thun M, Flanders D, Byers T, Heath C. Prospective study of intentional weight loss and mortality in never-smoking overweight US white women aged 40–64 years. *Am J Epidemiol* 1995;141:1128–41. Erratum in: *Am J Epidemiol* 1995;142:369.

10. Williamson DF, Thompson TJ, Thun M, Flanders D, Pamuk E, Byers T. Intentional weight loss and mortality among overweight individuals with diabetes. *Diabetes Care* 2000;23:1499–504.

11. Gregg EW, Gerzoff RB, Thompson TJ, Williamson DF. Intentional weight loss and death in overweight and obese US adults 35 years of age and older. *Ann Intern Med* 2003;138:383–9.

12. Gregg EW, Gerzoff RB, Thompson TJ, Williamson DF. Trying to lose weight, losing weight, and 9-year mortality in overweight U.S. adults with diabetes. *Diabetes Care* 2004;27:657–62.

13. Wannamethee SG, Shaper AG, Lennon L. Reasons for intentional weight loss, unintentional weight loss, and mortality in older men. *Arch Intern Med* 2005;165:1035–40.

14. Flum DR, Salem L, Elrod JA, Dellinger EP, Cheadle A, Chan L. Early mortality among Medicare beneficiaries undergoing bariatric surgical procedures. *JAMA* 2005;294:1903–8.

15. Sjöström L, Narbro K, Sjöström CD, et al; Swedish Obese Subjects Study. Effects of bariatric surgery on mortality in Swedish obese subjects. *N Engl J Med* 2007;357:741–52.

16. Adams TD, Gress RE, Smith SC, et al. Long-term mortality after gastric bypass surgery. *N Engl J Med* 2007;357:753–61.

17. Obesity: preventing and managing the global epidemic. Report of a WHO consultation. World Health Organization *Tech Rep Ser* 2000;894:i-xii, 1–253.

18. Clinical Guidelines on the Identification, Evaluation, and Treatment of Overweight and Obesity in Adults – The Evidence Report. National Institutes of Health. *Obes Res* 1998;6 Suppl 2:51–209S.

19. Douketis JD, Macie C, Thabane L, Williamson DF. Systematic review of long-term weight loss studies in obese adults: clinical significance and applicability to clinical practice. *Int J Obes (Lond)* 2005;29:1153–67.

20. Hankey CR, Lean ME, Lowe GD, Rumley A, Woodward M. Effects of moderate weight loss on anginal symptoms and indices of coagulation and fibrinolysis in overweight patients with angina pectoris. *Eur J Clin Nutr* 2002;56:1039–45.

21. Aucott L, Poobalan A, Smith WC, Avenell A, Jung R, Broom J. Effects of weight loss in overweight/obese individuals and long-term hypertension outcomes: a systematic review. *Hypertension* 2005;45:1035–41.

22. Norris SL, Zhang X, Avenell A, et al. Long-term effectiveness of lifestyle and behavioral weight loss interventions in adults with type 2 diabetes: a meta-analysis. *Am J Med* 2004;117:762–74.

23. Esposito K, Pontillo A, Di Palo C, et al. Effect of weight loss and lifestyle changes on vascular inflammatory markers in obese women: a randomized trial. *JAMA* 2003;289:1799–804.

24. Ryan AS, Nicklas BJ. Reductions in plasma cytokine levels with weight loss improve insulin sensitivity in overweight and obese postmenopausal women. *Diabetes Care* 2004;27:1699–705.

25. Bishop NA, Guarente L. Genetic links between diet and lifespan: shared mechanisms from yeast to humans. *Nat Rev Genet* 2007;8:835–44.

26. Vasselli JR, Weindruch R, Heymsfield SB, et al. Intentional weight loss reduces mortality rate in a rodent model of dietary obesity. *Obes Res* 2005;13:693–702.

27. The effects of nonpharmacologic interventions on blood pressure of persons with high normal levels. Results of the Trials of Hypertension Prevention, Phase I. *JAMA* 1992;267:1213–20.

28. The Trials of Hypertension Prevention Collaborative Research Group. Effects of weight loss and sodium reduction intervention on blood pressure and hypertension incidence in overweight people with high-normal blood pressure. The Trials of Hypertension Prevention, phase II. *Arch Intern Med* 1997;157:657–67.

29. Whelton PK, Appel LJ, Espeland MA, et al. Sodium reduction and weight loss in the treatment of hypertension in older persons: a randomized controlled trial of nonpharmacologic interventions in the elderly (TONE). TONE Collaborative Research Group. *JAMA* 1998;279:839–46.

30. Stevens VJ, Obarzanek E, Cook NR, et al.; Trials for the Hypertension Prevention Research Group. Long-term weight loss and changes in blood pressure: results of the Trials of Hypertension Prevention, phase II. *Ann Intern Med* 2001;134:1–11.

31. Appel LJ, Champagne CM, Harsha DW, et al.; Writing Group of the PREMIER Collaborative Research Group. Effects of comprehensive lifestyle modification on blood pressure control: main results of the PREMIER clinical trial. *JAMA* 2003;289: 2083–93.

32. Elmer PJ, Obarzanek E, Vollmer WM, et al.; PREMIER Collaborative Research Group. Effects of comprehensive lifestyle modification on diet, weight, physical fitness, and blood pressure control: 18-month results of a randomized trial. *Ann Intern Med* 2006;144:485–95.

33. Svetkey LP, Stevens VJ, Brantley PJ, et al.; Weight Loss Maintenance Collaborative Research Group. Comparison of strategies for sustaining weight loss: the weight loss maintenance randomized controlled trial. *JAMA* 2008;299:1139–48.

34. Moore LL, Visioni AJ, Qureshi MM, Bradlee ML, Ellison RC, D'Agostino R. Weight loss in overweight adults and the long-term risk of hypertension: the Framingham study. *Arch Intern Med* 2005;165:1298–303.

35. Haskell WL, Alderman EL, Fair JM, et al. Effects of intensive multiple risk factor reduction on coronary atherosclerosis and clinical cardiac events in men and women with coronary artery disease. The Stanford Coronary Risk Intervention Project (SCRIP). *Circulation* 1994;89:975–90.

36. Ornish D. Can lifestyle changes reverse coronary heart disease? *World Rev Nutr Diet* 1993;72:38–48.

37. Ornish D, Scherwitz LW, Billings JH, et al. Intensive lifestyle changes for reversal of coronary heart disease. *JAMA* 1998;280:2001–7.

38. Eilat-Adar S, Eldar M, Goldbourt U. Association of intentional changes in body weight with coronary heart disease event rates in overweight subjects who have an additional coronary risk factor. *Am J Epidemiol* 2005;161:352–8.

39. Poirier P, Giles TD, Bray GA, et al.; American Heart Association; Obesity Committee of the Council on Nutrition, Physical Activity, and Metabolism. Obesity and cardiovascular disease: pathophysiology, evaluation, and effect of weight loss: an update of the 1997 American Heart Association Scientific Statement on Obesity and Heart Disease from the Obesity Committee of the Council on Nutrition, Physical Activity, and Metabolism. *Circulation* 2006;113:898–918.

40. Sours HE, Frattali VP, Brand CD, et al. Sudden death associated with very low calorie weight reduction regimens. *Am J Clin Nutr* 1981;34:453–61.

41. Connolly HM, Crary JL, McGoon MD, Hensrud DD, Edwards BS, Edwards WD, Schaff HV. Valvular heart disease associated with fenfluramine-phentermine. *N Engl J Med* 1997;337:581–8. Erratum in: *N Engl J Med* 1997;337:1783.

42. Strohl KP, Strobel RJ, Parisi RA. Obesity and pulmonary function. In: Bray GA, Bouchard C, James WP (eds) *Handbook of Obesity: Etiology and Pathophysiology*, 2nd edn. New York, Marcel Dekker, 2004; pp. 725–39.

43. Young T, Peppard PE, Taheri S. Excess weight and sleep-disordered breathing. *J Appl Physiol* 2005;99:1592–9.

44. Foster GD, Sanders MH, Millman R, Zammit G, Borradaile KE, Newman AB, Wadden TA, Kelley D, Wing RR, Sunyer FX, Darcey V, Kuna ST; Sleep AHEAD Research Group. Obstructive sleep apnea among obese patients with type 2 diabetes. *Diabetes Care* 2009;32:1017–19.

45. Greenburg DL, Lettieri CJ, Eliasson AH. Effects of surgical weight loss on measures of obstructive sleep apnea: a meta-analysis. *Am J Med* 2009;122:535–42.

46. Avenell A, Broom J, Brown TJ, et al. Systematic review of the long-term effects and economic consequences of treatments for obesity and implications for health improvement. *Health Technol Assess* 2004;8:iii–182.

47. Pan XR, Li GW, Hu YH, et al. Effects of diet and exercise in preventing NIDDM in people with impaired glucose tolerance. The Da Qing IGT and Diabetes Study. *Diabetes Care* 1997;20:537–44.

48. Tuomilehto J, Lindström J, Eriksson JG, et al.; Finnish Diabetes Prevention Study Group. Prevention of type 2 diabetes mellitus by changes in lifestyle among subjects with impaired glucose tolerance. *N Engl J Med* 2001;344:1343–50.

49. Laaksonen DE, Lindström J, Lakka TA, et al.; Finnish Diabetes Prevention Study. Physical activity in the prevention of type 2 diabetes: the Finnish Diabetes Prevention Study. *Diabetes* 2005;54:158–65.

50. Lindstrom J, Ilanne-Parikka P, Peltonen M, et al.; Finnish Diabetes Prevention Study Group. Sustained reduction in the incidence of type 2 diabetes by lifestyle intervention: follow-up of the Finnish Diabetes Prevention Study. *Lancet* 2006;368:1673–9.

51. The DPP Research Group. Design and methods for a clinical trial in the prevention of type 2 diabetes. *Diabetes Care* 1999;22:623–34.

52. The DPP Research Group. Baseline characteristics of the randomized cohort. *Diabetes Care* 2000;23:1619–29.

53. The DPP Research Group. Reduction in the incidence of type 2 diabetes with lifestyle intervention or metformin. *N Engl J Med* 2002;346:393–403.

54. *The DPP Research Group.* Effect of weight loss with lifestyle intervention on risk of diabetes. *Diabetes Care* 2006;29:2102–7.

55. The DPP Research Group. The influence of age on the effects of lifestyle modification and metformin in prevention of diabetes. *J Gerontol A Biol Sci Med Sci* 2006;61:1075–81.

56. Kosaka K, Noda M, Kuzuya T. Prevention of type 2 diabetes by lifestyle intervention: a Japanese trial in IGT males. *Diabetes Res Clin Pract* 2005;67:152–62.

57. Ramachandran A, Snehalatha C, Mary S, Mukesh B, Bhaskar AD, Vijay V; Indian Diabetes Prevention Programme (IDPP). The Indian Diabetes Prevention Programme shows that lifestyle modification and metformin prevent type 2 diabetes in Asian Indian subjects with impaired glucose tolerance (IDPP-1). *Diabetologia.* 2006;49:289–97.

58. Knowler WC, Barrett-Connor E, Fowler SE, et al.; Diabetes Prevention Program Research Group. Reduction in the incidence of type 2 diabetes with lifestyle intervention or metformin. *N Engl J Med* 2002;346:393–403.

59. Look AHEAD Research Group, Pi-Sunyer X, Blackburn G, Brancati FL, et al. Reduction in weight and cardiovascular disease risk factors in individuals with type 2 diabetes: one-year results of the look AHEAD trial. *Diabetes Care* 2007;30:1374–83.

60. Heymsfield SB, Segal KR, Hauptman J, et al. Effects of weight loss with orlistat on glucose tolerance and progression to type 2 diabetes in obese adults. *Arch Intern Med* 2000;160:1321–6.

61. Torgerson JS, Hauptman J, Boldrin MN, Sjöström L. XENical in the prevention of diabetes in obese subjects (XENDOS) study: a randomized study of orlistat as an adjunct to lifestyle changes for the prevention of type 2 diabetes in obese patients. *Diabetes Care* 2004;27:155–61. Erratum in: *Diabetes Care* 2004;27:856.

62. Padwal R, Majumdar SR, Johnson JA, Varney J, McAlister FA. A systematic review of drug therapy to delay or prevent type 2 diabetes. *Diabetes Care* 2005;28:736–44.

63. Richelsen B, Tonstad S, Rössner S, et al. Effect of orlistat on weight regain and cardiovascular risk factors following a very-low-energy diet in abdominally obese patients: a 3-year randomized, placebo-controlled study. *Diabetes Care* 2007;30:27–32.

64. Hollander PA, Elbein SC, Hirsch IB, et al. Role of orlistat in the treatment of obese patients with type 2 diabetes: a 1-year randomized double-blind study. *Diabetes Care* 1998;21:1288–94.

65. Kelley DE, Bray GA, Pi-Sunyer FX, et al. Clinical efficacy of orlistat therapy in overweight and obese patients with insulin-treated type 2 diabetes: a 1-year randomized controlled trial. *Diabetes Care* 2002;25:1033–41. Erratum in: *Diabetes Care* 2003;26:971.

66. Miles JM, Leiter L, Hollander P, et al. Effect of orlistat in overweight and obese patients with type 2 diabetes treated with metformin. *Diabetes Care* 2002;25:1123–8. Erratum in: *Diabetes Care* 2002;25:1671.

67. Finer N, Bloom SR, Frost GS, Banks LM, Griffiths J. Sibutramine is effective for weight loss and diabetic control in obesity with type 2 diabetes: a randomised, double-blind, placebo-controlled study. *Diabetes Obes Metab* 2000;2:105–12.

68. Fujioka K, Seaton TB, Rowe E, et al.; Sibutramine/Diabetes Clinical Study Group. Weight loss with sibutramine improves glycaemic control and other metabolic parameters in obese patients with type 2 diabetes mellitus. *Diabetes Obes Metab* 2000;2:175–87.

69. McNulty SJ, Ur E, Williams G; Multicenter Sibutramine Study Group. A randomized trial of sibutramine in the management of obese type 2 diabetic patients treated with metformin. *Diabetes Care* 2003;26:125–31.

70. Redmon JB, Reck KP, Raatz SK, et al. Two-year outcome of a combination of weight loss therapies for type 2 diabetes. *Diabetes Care* 2005;28:1311–15.
71. Vettor R, Serra R, Fabris R, Pagano C, Federspil G. Effect of sibutramine on weight management and metabolic control in type 2 diabetes: a meta-analysis of clinical studies. *Diabetes Care* 2005;28:942–9.
72. Norris SL, Zhang X, Avenell A, Gregg E, Schmid CH, Lau J. Long-term non-pharmacologic weight loss interventions for adults with prediabetes. *Cochrane Database Syst Rev* 2005; CD005270.
73. Pories WJ, Swanson MS, MacDonald KG, et al. Who would have thought it? An operation proves to be the most effective therapy for adult-onset diabetes mellitus. *Ann Surg* 1995;222:339–50; discussion 350–2.
74. Pories WJ, MacDonald KG Jr, Flickinger EG, et al. Is type II diabetes mellitus (NIDDM) a surgical disease? *Ann Surg* 1992;215:633–42; discussion 643.
75. Sjöström L. Surgical treatment of obesity: an overview and results from the SOS Study. In: Bray GA, Bouchard C (eds) *Handbook of Obesity: Clinical Applications*, 2nd edn. New York: Marcel Dekker, 2004; pp. 359–89.
76. Sjöström L, Lindroos AK, Peltonen M, et al.; Swedish Obese Subjects Study Scientific Group. Lifestyle, diabetes, and cardiovascular risk factors 10 years after bariatric surgery. *N Engl J Med* 2004;351:2683–93.
77. Dixon JB, O'Brien PE, Playfair J, et al. Adjustable gastric banding and conventional therapy for type 2 diabetes: a randomized controlled trial. *JAMA* 2008;299:316–23.
78. Orchard TJ, Temprosa M, Goldberg R, et al.; Diabetes Prevention Program Research Group. The effect of metformin and intensive lifestyle intervention on the metabolic syndrome: the Diabetes Prevention Program randomized trial. *Ann Intern Med* 2005;142:611–19.
79. Ford ES, Giles WH. A comparison of the prevalence of the metabolic syndrome using two proposed definitions. *Diabetes Care* 2003;26:575–81.
80. Van Gaal LF, Rissanen AM, Scheen AJ, Ziegler O, Rössner S; RIO-Europe Study Group. Effects of the cannabinoid-1 receptor blocker rimonabant on weight reduction and cardiovascular risk factors in overweight patients: 1-year experience from the RIO-Europe study. *Lance.* 2005;365:1389–97. Erratum in: *Lancet* 2005;366:370.
81. Després JP, Golay A, Sjöström L; Rimonabant in Obesity-Lipids Study Group. Effects of rimonabant on metabolic risk factors in overweight patients with dyslipidemia. *N Engl J Med* 2005;353:2121–34.
82. Pi-Sunyer FX, Aronne LJ, Heshmati HM, Devin J, Rosenstock J; RIO-North America Study Group. Effect of rimonabant, a cannabinoid-1 receptor blocker, on weight and cardiometabolic risk factors in overweight or obese patients: RIO-North America: a randomized controlled trial. *JAMA* 2006;295:761 75. Erratum in: *JAMA* 2006;295:1252.
83. Gillies CL, Abrams KR, Lambert PC, et al. Pharmacological and lifestyle interventions to prevent or delay type 2 diabetes in people with impaired glucose tolerance: systematic review and meta-analysis. *BMJ* 2007;334:299.

Chapter 11

Diabetes management and cardiovascular risk reduction

Jay S. Skyler

The chronic complications of diabetes include accelerated vascular disease, neurological deficits (diabetic neuropathy), and other organ-specific degenerative processes. The vascular disease is of two types: microangiopathy, a small blood vessel (capillary) disease specifically associated with diabetes, characterized by thickening of capillary basement membranes, and clinically manifested principally in the retina and kidney; and macroangiopathy, which is the accelerated frequency and severity of atherosclerotic disease of large blood vessels (arteries), clinically manifested principally in coronary arteries, cerebral vasculature, and peripheral vessels in the lower extremities.

Macrovascular disease is the major cause of death in patients with diabetes. Individuals with diabetes have a 2-fold to 6-fold increased risk of having a cardiovascular event compared to age-matched controls [1–3]. Heart failure is the most common cause of hospitalization for patients with diabetes, increased by 6-fold in men and 9-fold in women [4–6]. Although patients with diabetes have a higher prevalence of the traditional risk factors for coronary artery disease, these risk factors account for less than half of the excess mortality seen in this population. Thus, diabetes per se is an independent risk factor for the development of cardiovascular disease (CVD) [7]. In view of the increased cardiovascular risk in patients with diabetes, current recommendations are for aggressive control of all cardiovascular risk factors [8–11].

The evidence of the role of treatment of hyperglycemia and its impact on diabetic microvascular disease is unambiguous. Analyses from epidemiological studies demonstrate a significant relationship between prevailing level of glycemia and microvascular disease, particularly retinopathy [12,13]. More im-

Metabolic Risk for Cardiovascular Disease, 1st edition. Edited by R. H. Eckel.
© 2011 American Heart Association. By Blackwell Publishing Ltd.

portantly, randomized controlled clinical trials have demonstrated an unambiguous beneficial effect on microvascular disease of lowering glycemia (measured as HbA1c – A1c) to a level close to normal. This has been shown in patients both with type 1 [14,15] and type 2 diabetes [16,17]. Of note, this microvascular disease benefit has been seen principally with insulin, and to some extent sulfonylureas, but not with other classes of pharmacological agents. Whether the effects are of glycemic control per se or a consequence of increased circulating insulin levels cannot be distinguished.

In contrast, the role of treatment of hyperglycemia on macrovascular complications has been controversial. Epidemiological studies have shown a direct relationship between glycemic control and CVD [18–20]. This was also seen in an epidemiological analysis of the United Kingdom Prospective Diabetes Study (UKPDS) [21]. However, it should be noted that in UKPDS itself, although there was a 16% reduction in cardiovascular complications (combined fatal or nonfatal myocardial infarction and sudden death) in the intensive glycemic control arm, this difference was of borderline statistical significance ($P = 0.052$), and there was no suggestion of benefit on other CVD outcomes such as stroke [17]. Yet, in meta-analyses of older studies, including UKPDS, there seemed to be evidence of benefit of improved glycemic control [22,23]. Nonetheless, randomized trials evaluating the effects of improvement of glycemic control have not provided consistent evidence of effects of improved glycemic control on CVD outcomes in people with type 2 diabetes. On the other hand, in type 2 diabetes, there have been studies demonstrating that aggressive blood pressure control [24–26], lowering of LDL cholesterol [27–30], and use of aspirin therapy reduce CVD outcomes [31]. Moreover, the Steno Study used aggressive control of multiple risk factors in patients with type 2 diabetes and demonstrated a reduction in risk both of CVD outcomes and of mortality [32,33].

In the Diabetes Control and Complications Trial (DCCT) of type diabetes, a long-term follow-up study, the Epidemiology of Diabetes Interventions and Complications (EDIC), showed that subjects originally randomized to the intensive treatment group had a 42% reduction ($P = 0.02$) in CVD outcomes and a 57% reduction ($P = 0.02$) in the risk of non-fatal myocardial infarction, stroke, or CVD death compared to those originally randomized to the standard treatment group [34]. More recently, an analysis of the DCCT-EDIC cohort who had been followed up continuously for a mean of 18.5 years showed that cumulative incidence of CVD in those originally randomized to the intensive treatment group was 9% compared to 14% in those originally randomized to the standard treatment group [35].

Recently, several large, prospective, randomized controlled clinical trials were designed to explicitly examine the relationship of glycemic control and CVD outcomes in type 2 diabetes. These studies include the Action to Control Cardiovascular Risk in Diabetes (ACCORD) trial [36], the Action in Diabetes and Vascular Disease–Preterax and Diamicron Modified Release Controlled

Evaluation (ADVANCE) trial [37], and the Veterans Affairs Diabetes Trial (VADT) [38]. It should be noted that ADVANCE and VADT were completed, while ACCORD was terminated early (after a mean of only 3.5 years of follow-up) because of increased mortality in subjects randomized to a strategy of very intensive glycemic control with a target A1c of < 6%. In addition, during the same time frame, long-term follow-up from the UKPDS has become available [39].

ACCORD

ACCORD [36] used a double two-by-two factorial design in which all subjects (10 251) were randomly assigned to either intensive glycemic control (targeting A1c of < 6%) or standard glycemic control (targeting A1c of 7.0–7.9%), while some subjects (4733) participated in a blood pressure study in which they were randomly assigned to either intensive therapy (targeting systolic blood pressure < 120 mmHg) or standard therapy (targeting systolic blood pressure < 140 mmHg), and other subjects (5518) participated in a lipid control study in which they were randomly assigned to either fenofibrate or placebo while maintaining good control of low-density lipoprotein cholesterol with simvastatin. ACCORD participants had either history of a CVD event (age, 40 to 79 years) or significant CVD risk (age, 55 to 79 years with anatomical CVD, albuminuria, left ventricular hypertrophy, or at least two other CVD risk factors). At baseline, they were an average 62 years of age, had mean duration of diabetes of 10 years, with 35% already having had a CVD event.

The glycemic control component of ACCORD was explicitly testing the hypothesis that a therapeutic strategy designed to lower A1c to < 6.0% would reduce CVD event rates to a greater extent than a strategy that lowers and/or maintains A1c at 7.0–7.9%. To accomplish this, the treatment strategy in the intensive glycemic control group mandated that all subjects were started on at least two classes of glycemic control drugs. That strategy dictated that either doses be intensified or a new medication class added every month if A1c levels were > 6% *or* if either > 50% of premeal capillary glucose readings were > 100 mg/dL (5.6 mmol/L) *or* if > 50% of postmeal capillary glucose readings were > 140 mg/dL (7.8 mmol/L). Based on glucose readings, such change in therapy occurred *even if* A1c was < 6%. Regular automated electronic messaging, audits of achieved glycemia, and central feedback to sites were used to support glycemic intensification strategies in intensive subjects, and to remind investigators if a change in therapy should have occurred but had not. The ACCORD investigators noted that "the treatment approaches are experimental and not designed for current delivery in clinical practice." Thus, extraordinary effort was used in an attempt to achieve the very rigorous target of A1c < 6%. In doing so, compared with standard group participants, intensive group participants experienced more hypoglycemia (hypoglycemic episodes requiring

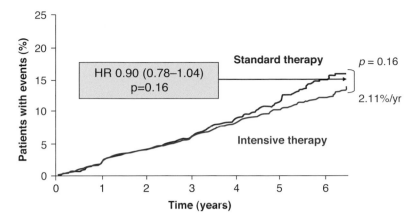

Figure 11.1 ACCORD: Treatment effect on primary outcome (cumulative incidence of non-fatal MI, non-fatal stroke, and CVD death). Redrawn from ACCORD Study Group [36] with permission, Copyright © [2008] Massachusetts Medical Society. All rights reserved.

medical assistance were 3.1% per year vs. 1.0% per year), more weight gain (a 9-fold increase in weight gain and a doubling of the likelihood of gaining > 10 kg), and more fluid retention. Median A1c levels of 6.4% and 7.5% were achieved in the two groups, with maximal separation between the arms achieved within one year.

The primary outcome was a composite of non-fatal myocardial infarction, non-fatal stroke, or death from cardiovascular causes. During follow-up, this primary outcome occurred in 352 patients in the intensive therapy group versus 371 in the standard therapy group (hazard ratio, 0.90; 95% confidence interval [CI], 0.78 to 1.04; $P = 0.16$) (Figure 11.1) [36]. Thus, there was a trend towards beneficial effect on the primary outcome, in spite of the fact that the study was terminated early after a mean of only 3.5 years, and in spite of the observed event rate (2.3% per year) being less than expected (2.9% per year). The reduced event rate likely was in part due to other risk factors being treated aggressively and equally in both groups (statin use in 88% with mean LDL cholesterol at study end of 91 mg/dL (2.35 mmol/L), mean blood pressure at study end of 122/67 mmHg, antiplatelet therapy use by 76% of subjects, and less than 10% of subjects being smokers). In a prespecified subgroup analysis, subjects without a previous CVD event had a beneficial effect of intensive therapy ($P = 0.04$). In another subgroup analysis, subjects who had a baseline A1c < 8% also had a beneficial effect of intensive therapy ($P = 0.03$). These findings suggest that ACCORD may ultimately have shown beneficial effects overall, had early termination not occurred.

Unfortunately, as noted, there was increased (all-cause) mortality in the intensive therapy group as compared to the standard therapy group (1.41% per

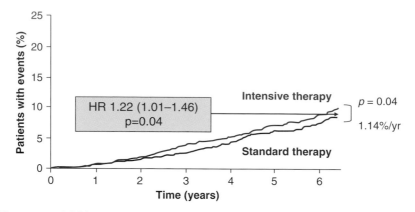

Figure 11.2 ACCORD: Treatment effect on all-cause mortality. Redrawn from ACCORD Study Group [36] with permission, Copyright © [2008] Massachusetts Medical Society.

year vs 1.14% per year; 257 vs. 203 deaths over a mean 3.5 years of follow-up; hazard ratio, 1.22; 95% CI, 1.01 to 1.46; $P = 0.04$) (Figure 11.2) [36].

A subsequent analysis found that symptomatic, severe hypoglycemia – manifest as either blood glucose concentration of less than 50 mg/dL (2.8 mmol/L) or symptoms that resolved with treatment and that required either the assistance of another person or medical assistance – was associated with an increased risk of death within each study arm. Perhaps somewhat surprisingly, however, the risk of death was lower in the intensive arm than in the standard arm among participants experiencing hypoglycemia, suggesting that severe hypoglycemia does not appear to account for the mortality difference in the two study arms [40].

There were significantly increased risks for hypoglycemia among women, African-Americans, those with less than a high school education, older participants, and those already using insulin before randomization. Surprisingly, those having greater initial declines of A1c had a reduced risk of hypoglycemia in both treatment groups, and the risk of hypoglycemia requiring medical assistance increased with higher A1c levels [41].

There were three baseline characteristics associated with increased mortality: self-reported history of neuropathy, higher baseline A1c (> 8.5%), and aspirin use [42]. Interestingly, however, during the course of the study, excess mortality risk with intensive strategy versus standard strategy occurred at A1c levels above 7% and there was a steady increase of risk with A1c levels from 6 to 9% in the intensive strategy group [43]. Further, the excess mortality risk with intensive strategy versus standard strategy occurred when intensive participants failed to reduce their A1c in the first year of treatment [43]. A steady increase of risk of CVD death was also noted with increase of A1c levels from 6 to 9% in the intensive strategy group, whereas the standard strategy group had a U-shaped curve relating A1c and CVD death [44]. In the intensive strategy group, the risk of myocardial infarction paralleled that of increased CVD death, i.e. a steady increase of risk with increase of A1c levels from 6 to 9%, while in the standard group the risk of myocardial infarction had a flat relationship with A1c level [44]. Epidemiological analyses of the whole population showed that a 1% higher average A1c was associated with 18–23% greater risk of all-cause mortality, CV mortality, myocardial infarction, and stroke [44].

Given all of this about the ACCORD glycemic control study, my interpretation is that it is wrong to conclude that lower A1c was responsible for increased death. Rather, the extreme measures taken to lower A1c were associated with increased mortality in those who failed to respond to interventions that attempted to lower A1c, and that beneficial effects of intervention were seen in those who had no previous CVD event and were likely earlier in the course of their disease (lower baseline A1c and less neuropathy). It is unfortunate that the ACCORD glycemic control study was terminated early, as there was a trend for overall CVD reduction that failed to attain statistical significance in part because of the shortened duration of the study.

The ACCORD blood pressure [45] and lipid [46] studies did continue to completion, with a mean follow-up of 4.7 years. These studies included 4733 and 5518 subjects, respectively.

As noted above, the ACCORD blood pressure study targeted systolic blood pressure < 120 mmHg in the intensive therapy group and < 140 mmHg in the standard therapy group. In fact, the mean systolic blood pressure achieved was 119.3 mmHg in the intensive therapy group and 133.5 mmHg in the standard therapy group [45]. As in the glycemic control component of ACCORD, the primary outcome was a composite of non-fatal myocardial infarction, non-fatal stroke, or death from cardiovascular causes. During follow-up, this primary outcome occurred in 1.87% of patients in the intensive therapy group and 2.09% of patients in the standard therapy group (hazard ratio 0.88; 95% CI, 0.73 to 1.06; $P = 0.20$). The annual rates of (all-cause) mortality were 1.28% and 1.19% in the two groups (hazard ratio, 1.07; 95% CI, 0.85 to 1.35; $P = 0.55$). Thus, there was no difference either in the primary composite outcome or in mortality between the two groups. On the other hand, the annual rate of stroke, a pre-specified secondary outcome, was significantly reduced in the intensive group (0.32%) versus that seen in the standard group (0.53%) (hazard ratio, 0.59; 95% CI, 0.39 to 0.89; $P = 0.01$). However, the intensive therapy group had a higher rate of serious adverse events attributed to antihypertensive treatment (3.3%) than that seen in the standard therapy group (1.3%) ($P < 0.001$). These events included hypotension, syncope, bradycardia or arrhythmia, as well as higher rates of hypokalemia and elevations in serum creatinine level. The authors concluded that "the results provide no evidence that the strategy of intensive blood-pressure control reduces the rate of a composite of major cardiovascular events in such patients." My interpretation is that this is an overly conservative conclusion. The separation of blood pressure between the two groups was only 14.2 mmHg, with the standard therapy group achieving a quite respectable 133.5 mmHg, close to the recommended target of 130 mmHg [9,10]. The AC-CORD authors acknowledge "it was not the intent of this trial to test the (recommended) blood-pressure goal of 130 mmHg." Rather, ACCORD tested goals of < 140 mmHg versus < 120 mmHg, a 20 mmHg difference. Although a case can be made that a strategy aiming at < 120 mmHg is not supported by the data, it still seems to this observer that the recommended blood pressure goal of 130 mmHg should be sustained. This is particularly the case in that ACCORD did show a reduction in the risk for stroke.

As noted above, the ACCORD lipid control study randomly assigned subjects to either fenofibrate or placebo while maintaining good control of low-density lipoprotein cholesterol with simvastatin. Baseline lipids in the ACCORD lipid study were: mean total cholesterol 175.2 ± 37.3 mg/dL, mean LDL cholesterol 100.6 ± 30.7 mg/dL, mean HDL cholesterol 38.1 ± 7.8 mg/dL, and median triglycerides 162 mg/dL (intraquartile range 113–229) [46]. At the exit visit, the mean LDL cholesterol level was 81.1 mg/dL in the fenofibrate group and 80.0 mg/dL in the placebo group ($P = 0.16$), the mean HDL cholesterol level was 41.2 mg/dL in the fenofibrate group and 40.5 mg/dL in the placebo group ($P = 0.01$), and the median triglyceride was 122 mg/dL in the fenofibrate group and 144 mg/dL in the placebo group ($P < 0.0001$) [46]. The primary outcome was a composite of non-fatal myocardial infarction, non-fatal stroke, or death from cardiovascular causes. During follow-up, this primary outcome occurred in 2.2% in the fenofibrate group and 2.4% in the placebo group (hazard ratio 0.92; 95% CI, 0.79 to 1.08; $P = 0.32$). The annual rates of (all-cause) mortality were 1.5% and 1.6% in the two groups (hazard ratio, 0.91; 95% CI, 0.75 to 1.10; $P = 0.33$). Thus, there was no difference in either in the primary composite outcome nor in mortality between the two groups. Prespecified subgroup analyses did suggest heterogeneity in treatment effect according to gender, with a benefit for men and possible harm for women ($P = 0.01$ for interaction). The authors concluded that the results do not support the routine use of combination therapy with fenofibrate and simvastatin, rather than statin therapy alone, in the majority of high-risk patients with type 2 diabetes. There also was a suggestion of effect according to baseline lipid levels: patients with both the highest triglyceride levels and the lowest HDL cholesterol levels appeared to benefit from fenofibrate, although this did not quite reach statistical significance ($P = 0.057$). It should be appreciated, that although there were statistically significant differences in the triglyceride and HDL cholesterol levels achieved in the two groups, the triglycerides remained only modestly altered in the placebo group (median 144 mg/dL) and the difference in HDL cholesterol was trivial (41.2 versus 40.5 mg/dL). Whether a drug with greater effect on raising HDL cholesterol (e.g., niacin) would have proven to have incremental effect versus statin alone was not tested.

ADVANCE

ADVANCE [37] used a two-by-two factorial design in which subjects (11 140) were randomly assigned to either intensive glycemic control (initially with the sulfonylurea gliclizide and additional medications as needed with a target A1c < 6.5%) or to standard glycemic control (initially with any medication except gliclizide with target A1c according to "local guidelines") and to a blood pressure study in which they were randomly assigned to receive therapy with either perindopril and indapamide or matching placebo. Median A1c levels of 6.5% and 7.3% were achieved in the two glycemic arms, although maximal separation between the arms took several years to achieve.

The primary outcome of ADVANCE was a composite of major macrovascular events (death from cardiovascular causes, non-fatal myocardial infarction, or non-fatal stroke) and major microvascular events (new or worsening nephropathy or retinopathy), assessed both jointly and separately [37]. After a median of 5 years of follow-up, the combined primary outcome occurred less in the intensive therapy group than in the standard therapy group [18.1% vs. 20.0%; hazard ratio, 0.90; 95% CI, 0.82 to 0.98; $P = 0.01$), as did major microvascular events (9.4% vs. 10.9%; hazard ratio, 0.86; 95% CI, 0.77 to 0.97; $P = 0.01$), primarily because of a reduction in the incidence of nephropathy, with no significant effect on retinopathy. There were no significant effects of glycemic control on major macrovascular events (hazard ratio, 0.94; 95% CI, 0.84 to 1.06; $P = 0.32$) (Figure 11.3), death from cardiovascular causes (hazard ratio, 0.88; 95% CI, 0.74 to 1.04; $P = 0.12$), or death from any cause.

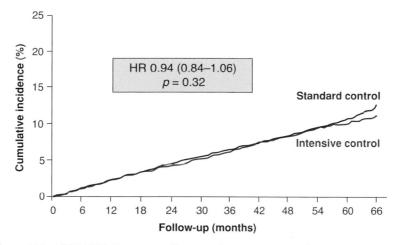

Figure 11.3 ADVANCE: Treatment effect on primary macrovascular outcome (cumulative incidence of non-fatal MI, non-fatal stroke, and CVD death). Redrawn from ADVANCE Collaborative Group [37] with permission, Copyright © [2008] Massachusetts Medical Society. All rights reserved.

The observed macrovascular event rate (2.2% per year) was less than expected (3.0% per year), although use of other drugs that favorably impact CVD risk was lower in ADVANCE (statin use in 47% with mean LDL cholesterol at study end of 102 mg/dL (2.63 mmol/L), mean blood pressure at study end of 136/74 mmHg, antiplatelet therapy use by 62% of subjects, and 8% of subjects smokers). ADVANCE specifically enrolled subjects with relatively high risk of CVD, with 32% having had a previous CVD event. (Enrollment criteria required that subjects be at least 55 years of age at study entry and have a history of major macrovascular or microvascular disease or at least one other risk factor for vascular disease.) In a prespecified subgroup analysis, subjects without a previous CVD event had a beneficial effect of intensive therapy (risk reduction 14%, 95% CI, 4 to 23) not seen in those with a previous CVD event (risk reduction 4%, 95% CI, –10 to 16). Interestingly, in another subgroup analysis, beneficial effects were seen only among subjects not treated with statins.

My interpretation is that ADVANCE had but minimal difference in attained A1c between treatment arms, thus limiting its ability to detect an effect on CVD outcomes. Apparently, microvascular (renal) outcomes require less lowering of A1c than do CVD outcomes, and thus these were beneficially impacted. In subgroup analyses, beneficial effects of intervention were seen in those who had no previous CVD event and were likely earlier in the course of their disease.

The blood pressure component was reported separately [47]. In this component of ADVANCE, 11 140 subjects with a mean blood pressure at baseline of 145/81 mmHg were randomized to add to ongoing therapy either a fixed combination of perindopril and indapamide or matching placebo. Compared to placebo, the intervention group achieved a lowering of blood pressure of 5.6/2.2 mmHg. After a mean of 4.3 years of follow-up, the combined primary outcome occurred less in the intervention group than the placebo group (15·5% versus 16·8%; hazard ratio, 0.91; 95% CI, 0.83 to1.00, $P = 0.04$). The separate reductions in macrovascular and microvascular events were similar but were not independently significant. The relative risk of death from cardiovascular disease was reduced by 18% ($P = 0.03$) and death from any cause was reduced by 14% ($P = 0.03$).

The ADVANCE investigators have examined the magnitude and independence of the effects of blood pressure lowering and intensive glucose control in their cohort [48]. There was no interaction between the effects of blood pressure lowering and intensive glucose control for any of the prespecified clinical outcomes. The separate effects of the two interventions for renal outcomes and death appeared to be additive [48].

VADT

VADT [38] was a smaller, simpler study in which subjects (1791) were randomly assigned to either intensive glycemic control (target A1c < 6.0%) or to standard

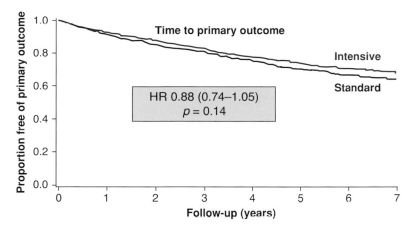

Figure 11.4 VADT: Treatment effect on primary outcome (survival curve for non-fatal MI, non-fatal stroke, CVD death, hospitalization for CHF, and revascularization). Redrawn from Duckworth et al. [38] with permission, Copyright © [2009] Massachusetts Medical Society. All rights reserved.

glycemic control (target A1c at least 1.5% higher than the intensive group). Median A1c levels of 6.9% and 8.4% were achieved in the two groups, within the first year of the study.

The primary outcome of the VADT was a composite of CVD events (death from cardiovascular causes, non-fatal myocardial infarction, non-fatal stroke, revascularization, hospitalization for heart failure, and amputation for ischemia). After a median of 6 years of follow-up, the primary outcome was not significantly lower in the intensive therapy group than in the standard therapy group (hazard ratio, 0.88; 95% CI 0.74 to 1.05; $P-0.14$) (Figure 11.4). Although there were more CVD deaths in the intensive therapy group than in the standard therapy group (36 vs. 29; sudden deaths 11 vs. 4), the difference was not statistically significant.

The observed macrovascular event rate (5.6% per year) was less than expected (6.7% per year). Other risk factors were treated aggressively and equally in both groups (statin use in 84% with mean LDL cholesterol at study end of 75 mg/dL or 1.94 mmol/L, mean blood pressure at study end of 127/69 mmHg, antiplatelet therapy use by 93% of subjects, and 17% of subjects smokers). VADT specifically enrolled subjects with relatively high risk of CVD, with 40% having had a previous CVD event. In a post-hoc subgroup analysis, it was suggested in the intensive glycemic control arm, subjects with less than approximately 10 years' duration of diabetes at randomization had a CVD benefit while those with longer duration of disease had a neutral or adverse effect. Another post-hoc analysis suggested that severe hypoglycemia within the past 90 days was a predictor both of the primary outcome and of CVD mortality.

In terms of microvascular disease, VADT found that progression from normal to either microalbuminuria or macroalbuminuria ($P = 0.03$) and progression from either normal or microalbuminuria to macroalbuminuria ($P = 0.04$) favor intensive treatment. Any progression of albuminuria was statistically significant ($P < 0.01$); 13.8% of the patients in the standard therapy group, as compared with 9.1% of patients in the intensive therapy group, had worsening albuminuria [49].

A substudy investigated the hypothesis that baseline calcified coronary atherosclerosis may determine CVD events in response to intensive glycemic control within VADT [50]. Baseline coronary atherosclerosis was assessed by coronary artery calcium (CAC) measured by computed tomography. In the substudy there were 89 cardiovascular events among 301 participants during a median follow-up duration of 5.2 years. There was a progressive diminution of benefit with increasing CAC. Subgroup analyses were also conducted for clinically relevant CAC categories, and found that for the subgroup with CAC scores over 100, 11 of 62 individuals had events, while only 1 of 52 individuals with CAC of 100 or less suffered an event. Most interestingly, for those with CAC scores over 100 the hazard ratio for intensive treatment was 0.74 (95% CI 0.46 to 1.20; $P = 0.21$), while for the subgroup with CAC of 100 or less, the corresponding hazard ratio was 0.08 (95% CI 0.008 to 0.77; $P = 0.03$), with event rates of 39 and 4 per 1000 person-years, respectively. These data are consistent with the notion that intensive glycemic control reduces cardiovascular events in those with less extensive calcified coronary atherosclerosis.

It appears to me that one of the most important outcomes from VADT is the substudy of CAC, which showed that intervention reduces CVD events in those with less extensive disease. This is consistent with the subgroup analyses from ACCORD and ADVANCE, in which beneficial effects of intervention were seen in those who had no previous CVD event and were likely earlier in the course of their disease.

UKPDS

In UKPDS, of 5102 patients with newly diagnosed type 2 diabetes, 4209 were randomly assigned to receive either conventional therapy (dietary restriction) or intensive therapy (either sulfonylurea or insulin or, in overweight patients, metformin) for glucose control [17]. After the study was reported in 1998, 3277 patients were asked to attend annual UKPDS clinics for an additional 5 years of post-trial monitoring, but no attempts were made to maintain their previously assigned therapies. In years 6 to 10 post-trial, patients were assessed further through questionnaires. Long-term follow-up of the UKPDS, including those 10 years of post-trial monitoring, has now been reported, so that median overall follow-up was 17.0 years (range 16 to 30 years) [39]. It is important to note that all subjects in the UKPDS were recruited at the time of diagnosis of

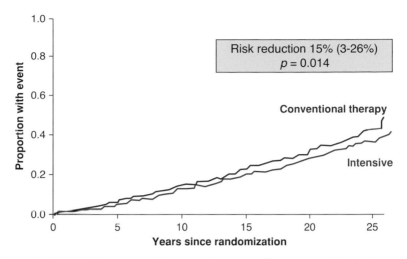

Figure 11.5 UKPDS: Long-term follow-up of treatment effect on cumulative incidence of myocardial infarction. Redrawn from Holman et al. [39] with permission, Copyright © [2009] Massachusetts Medical Society. All rights reserved.

diabetes, thus they were treated from the earliest possible time in the course of the disease. Although, as noted above, in the original UKPDS report, the hazard ratio for myocardial infarction just missed reaching statistical significance for a beneficial effect of improved glycemic control (hazard ratio 0.84, $P = 0.52$), with post-trial monitoring during which glycemic control was equivalent in both groups, a clear beneficial effect of glycemic control emerged for myocardial infarction (hazard ratio 0.85, 95% CI 0.74 to 0.97; $P = 0.01$) (Figure 11.5). Beneficial effects on diabetes-related death (hazard ratio 0.83, 95% CI 0.73 to 0.96; $P = 0.01$) and all-cause mortality (hazard ratio 0.87, 95% CI 0.69 to 0.96; $P = 0.007$) also emerged, while the beneficial effects on microvascular disease and on "any diabetes related endpoint" were sustained. Intriguingly, although metformin use (in a very small subset of obese subjects) never resulted in significant difference in glycemic control [51], its earlier demonstrated beneficial effects on myocardial infarction, diabetes-related death, and all-cause mortality also were sustained. Also sustained was the absence of an effect of metformin on microvascular outcomes [39]. The fact that metformin did not impact glycemic control or microvascular outcomes, but did reduce myocardial infarction, diabetes-related death, and all-cause mortality, suggests that the beneficial effects on these outcomes may be a consequence of an impact on something other than glycemia.

In my view, the lessons from UKPDS are that early glycemic control is important, and that long-term observation may be necessary in order to observe the effects of glycemia on CVD outcomes.

Like ACCORD and ADVANCE, UKPDS also had embedded in it a blood pressure study, dubbed the Hypertension in Diabetes Study (HDS) [52]. This component of UKPDS included 1148 hypertensive patients with type 2 diabetes (mean age 56, mean blood pressure at entry 160/94 mmHg) randomized 2:1 to either "tight control" or "less tight control" of blood pressure. Median follow-up was 8.4 years. Mean blood pressure during follow-up was significantly reduced in the "tight control" group (144/82 mmHg) compared to the "less tight control" group (154/87 mmHg) ($P < 0.0001$), but the blood pressure levels in both groups were higher than current targets. Nonetheless, in the "tight control" group, there were reductions in risk of "diabetes related end points," deaths related to diabetes, strokes, and microvascular end points [52]. A subsequent epidemiological analysis showed that for each 10 mmHg decrease in mean systolic blood pressure there were reductions in risk of each of these outcomes, with no threshold of risk observed [53]. This analysis also suggested the lowest risk was in those with systolic blood pressure less than 120 mmHg [53]. Moreover, when glycemia and blood pressure were examined together in a combined analysis, the risk of complications was found to be associated independently and additively with hyperglycemia and hypertension [54]. This led the authors to conclude that intensive treatment of both these risk factors is required to minimize the incidence of complications [54]. Yet, in contrast to the long-term effects of glycemic control [39], the benefits of previously improved blood pressure control were not sustained when between-group differences in blood pressure were lost during long-term follow-up [55].

PROactive

The PROactive (PROspective pioglitAzone Clinical Trial In macroVascular Events) study [56] is mentioned here because it is included in several of the meta-analyses discussed below. It was a secondary intervention trial as patients had to have evidence of extensive macrovascular disease before recruitment, defined by one or more of the following: myocardial infarction, stroke, percutaneous coronary intervention, or coronary artery bypass surgery at least 6 months before entry, acute coronary syndrome at least 3 months before entry, or objective evidence of coronary artery disease or obstructive arterial disease in the leg. It was not a study of glycemic control per se, but rather a study of pioglitazone (versus placebo) in addition to previous diabetes therapy. However, since it was a study of 5238 patients with type 2 diabetes, and since the pioglitazone group had better glycemic control than the placebo group (0.5% greater A1c decrement with pioglitazone), and since it assessed CVD outcomes, it has been included in several meta-analyses to be discussed. The primary endpoint was the composite of all-cause mortality, non-fatal myocardial infarction (including silent myocardial infarction), stroke, acute coronary syndrome, endovascular or surgical intervention in the coronary or leg arteries, and amputation above the ankle. This endpoint did not achieve statistical significance (hazard ratio 0.90; 95% CI, 0.80 to1.02; $P = 0.095$). However, a beneficial effect was seen in the "principal" secondary endpoint, which was the composite of all-cause mortality, non-fatal myocardial infarction, and stroke (hazard ratio 0.84, 0.72 to0.98; $P = 0.027$).

Meta-analyses

Since the publication of ACCORD, ADVANCE, and VADT, there have been six meta-analyses [57–62] – including one conducted by the collected authors of ACCORD, ADVANCE, VADT, and UKPDS [62]. These have all included ADVANCE, ACCORD, VADT, and the original UKPDS study, while three have also included PROactive [57,59,61].

One meta-analysis, by Ma et al. [60], also included three other smaller studies, Kumamoto, Steno-2, and an earlier VA Pilot Study. That analysis divided the studies into those that achieved an A1c of less than 7.0% (ADVANCE, ACCORD, VADT) versus those that achieved an A1c of 7.0–7.9% (UKPDS, Kumamoto, Steno-2, VA Pilot Study). That analysis found no benefits of intensive glycemic control on macrovascular and microvascular complications ($P > 0.1$), but a higher rate of severe hypoglycemia ($P < 0.00001$) in the intensive control group when the target A1c level was $< 7.0\%$; but when the target A1c was 7.0 7.9%, the intensive control group showed benefits on the reduction of microvascular events ($P < 0.05$) without increasing risk of severe hypoglycemia ($P = 0.74$), but no influence on macrovascular complications ($P > 0.1$). That is not surprising in that ADVANCE, ACCORD, and VADT did not show benefit on CVD outcomes.

The other five meta-analyses, with or without inclusion of PROactive, have found that collectively there is beneficial effect on CVD outcomes of intensive therapy (Figure 11.6) and that there is not increased mortality (Figure 11.7) [62]. The meta-analysis by the collected authors of ACCORD, ADVANCE, VADT, and UKPDS also confirmed the finding that the benefit is confined to those without pre-existing CVD (Figure 11.8) [62]. That meta-analysis is particularly important since it had access to the individual primary outcome data from the trials [62].

As noted, all three of the new studies ACCORD, ADVANCE, VADT – failed to demonstrate a beneficial effect on CVD events in the total cohort studied. Yet, interestingly, as noted, in prespecified subgroup analyses in both ACCORD and ADVANCE, as well as a post-hoc analysis in VADT, there was a beneficial effect on CVD events in subjects who were earlier in the disease course, without previous CVD events. This was confirmed in the meta-analysis by Turnbull et al. [62]. To this writer, these are crucial observations, as it may very well be

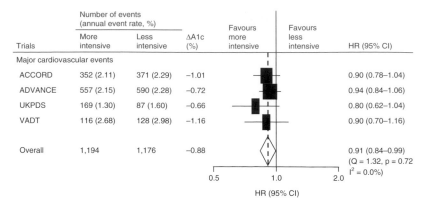

Figure 11.6 Meta-analysis of ACCORD, ADVANCE, VADT, and UKPDS studies examining treatment effects on major cardiovascular events. Redrawn with kind permission from Springer Science+Business Media: Turnbull FM, Abraira C, Anderson RJ, et al. Intensive glucose control and macrovascular outcomes in type 2 diabetes. *Diabetologia* 2009;52:2288–98.

that improvement of glycemic control does not have the potential for reversing disease in damaged vessels. It is ironic that in the design of CVD clinical trials investigators often seek to enroll individuals with clearly established disease as they will have a higher CVD event rate going forward, thus reducing the sample size and/or the duration of follow-up needed to answer the question. Yet, these may be the very individuals who should be excluded. In fact, a recent FDA *Guidance* for development of diabetes drugs recommends that phase 3

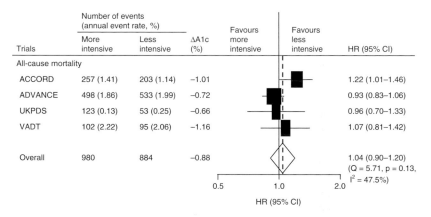

Figure 11.7 Meta-analysis of ACCORD, ADVANCE, VADT, and UKPDS studies examining treatment effects on all-cause mortality. Redrawn with kind permission from Springer Science+Business Media: Turnbull FM, Abraira C, Anderson RJ, et al. Intensive glucose control and macrovascular outcomes in type 2 diabetes. *Diabetologia* 2009;52:2288–98.

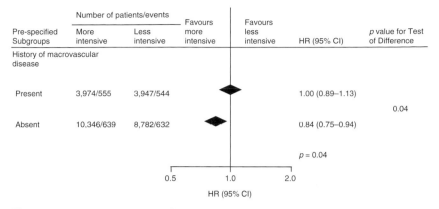

Figure 11.8 Sub-group analysis for major CVD events in subjects with and without a previous history of macrovascular disease. Redrawn with kind permission from Springer Science+Business Media: Turnbull FM, Abraira C, Anderson RJ, et al. Intensive glucose control and macrovascular outcomes in type 2 diabetes. *Diabetologia* 2009;52:2288–98.

programs enroll patients at *increased* cardiovascular risk ("for example, enrolling elderly patients, those with prior cardiovascular disease and risk factors, those with longstanding diabetes, and those with renal impairment increases the likelihood that a sufficient number of cardiovascular events will occur and improves generalizability of results") [63,64]. Although the guidance calls for evaluation of whether a given treatment increases cardiovascular risk and does not ask pharmaceutical companies to show a cardiovascular benefit, given the data reviewed herein, this may not be the wisest approach.

Regarding sample size and trial duration, it is important to note that in many trials of CVD risk in diabetes the curves defining event rates do not diverge until periods much longer than the duration of follow-up in ADVANCE and VADT, let alone the markedly abbreviated follow-up in ACCORD [17,33,34, 39,56]. Longer duration of follow-up might very well have demonstrated an unambiguous beneficial effect in the entire studied cohorts, rather than only in the subgroup analyses. This was certainly the case for the UKPDS extended follow-up, which demonstrated that early intervention has beneficial effects on outcome. It is my bias that future studies of glycemic control and CVD events should be designed as primary prevention studies and confined to subjects without a previous CVD event. Admittedly, this may require larger sample sizes and longer duration of follow-up, but the question could be better answered. Unfortunately, the level of glycemic control achieved in UKPDS was not as aggressive as that in the more recent studies, leaving unclear the degree of glycemic control which should be sought.

Another factor influences the sample size and study duration equation. The observed event rates in all three new studies were less than the expected event rates, as noted in the trial summaries above. This may be a consequence of other CVD risk factors being treated aggressively and effectively, including statin usage, blood pressure control, antiplatelet therapy, and smoking cessation. With all of these interventions being used, the incremental beneficial effect of glycemic control may be obscured, unless a very large and long trial is conducted. The aggressive use of these other interventions is quite appropriate. Indeed, in both ADVANCE [37] and PROactive [56], in subgroup analyses the beneficial effect of glycemic intervention was confined to those not using statins.

ACCORD was terminated early because of an increased death rate in the intensive glycemic control group. It must not have been easy for the Data Safety and Monitoring Board (DSMB) to make that decision. Indeed, there were 54 more deaths in the intensive control group than in the standard group. However, given that there were a large number of subjects enrolled, and 3.5 years of follow-up, the death rates in the two groups were 14 per 1000 per year versus 11 per 1000 per year. With an emerging trend favoring intensive therapy for the primary study outcome, and the study question extraordinarily important, some might question whether a difference in death rate of 3 per 1000 per year warranted early termination. The DSMB chose the cautious approach, which is clearly safer for trial participants, but leaves us with a critical unanswered question.

One thing is clear: in patients with diabetes, comprehensive care involves treatment of all modifiable CVD risk factors. These should be treated aggressively, including statin usage, blood pressure control, antiplatelet therapy, and smoking cessation.

In type 1 diabetes, results from DCCT for both microvascular endpoints and CVD have demonstrated the benefits of intensive glycemic control. In type 2 diabetes, glycemic control also decreases microvascular disease risk. Thus, glycemic goals for most patients should remain unchanged, i.e., targeting an A1c of < 7%. Lower A1c should be sought in pregnant women, and would be quite acceptable if relatively easily achieved without provoking significant hypoglycemia, particularly in patients with shorter duration of type 2 diabetes and without established CVD. Higher A1c targets would seem acceptable for patients with hypoglycemia unawareness and/or known history of severe hypoglycemia, established CVD, and for older frail patients [11,65].

References

1. Hu FB, Stampfer MJ, Solomon CG, et al. The impact of diabetes mellitus on mortality from all causes and coronary heart disease in women: 20 years of follow-up. *Arch Intern Med* 2001;161:1717–23.
2. Fox CS, Coady S, Sorlie PD, et al. Trends in cardiovascular complications of diabetes. *JAMA* 2004;292:2495–9.
3. Fox C, Coady S, Sorlie P, et al. Increasing cardiovascular disease burden due to diabetes mellitus: the Framingham Heart Study. *Circulation* 2007;115:1544–50.

4. Bell DSH. Heart failure: the frequent, forgotten, and often fatal complication of diabetes. *Diabetes Care* 2003;26:2433–41.
5. Nichols GA, Gullion CM, Koro CE, Ephross SA, Brown JB. The incidence of congestive heart failure in type 2 diabetes: an update. *Diabetes Care* 2004;27:1879–84.
6. Baliga V, Sapsford R. Review article: Diabetes mellitus and heart failure – an overview of epidemiology and management. *Diabetes Vasc Dis Res* 2009;6:164–71.
7. Stamler J, Vaccaro O, Neaton JD, Wentworth D. Diabetes, other risk factors, and 12-year cardiovascular mortality for men screened in the Multiple Risk Factor Intervention Trial. *Diabetes Care* 1993;16:434–44.
8. Eckel RH, Kahn R, Robertson RM, Rizza RA. Preventing Cardiovascular Disease and Diabetes. A Call to Action from the American Diabetes Association and the American Heart Association. *Circulation* 2006;113:2943–6.
9. Rydén L, Standl E, Bartnik M, et al.; Task Force on Diabetes and Cardiovascular Diseases of the European Society of Cardiology (ESC); European Association for the Study of Diabetes (EASD). Guidelines on diabetes, pre-diabetes, and cardiovascular diseases: executive summary. The Task Force on Diabetes and Cardiovascular Diseases of the European Society of Cardiology (ESC) and of the European Association for the Study of Diabetes (EASD). *Eur Heart J* 2007;28:88–136.
10. Buse JB, Ginsberg HN, Bakris GL, et al., American Heart Association, American Diabetes Association. Primary prevention of cardiovascular diseases in people with diabetes mellitus: a scientific statement from the American Heart Association and the American Diabetes Association. *Diabetes Care* 2007;30:162–72 and *Circulation* 2007;115:114–26.
11. Skyler JS, Bergenstal R, Bonow RO, et al. Intensive Glycemic Control and the Prevention of Cardiovascular Events: Implications of the ACCORD, ADVANCE, and VADT Diabetes Trials. A Position Statement of the American Diabetes Association and A Scientific Statement of the American College of Cardiology Foundation and the American Heart Association. *Diabetes Care* 2009;32:187–92, *Circulation* 2009: 119; 351–7, and *J Am Coll Cardiol* 2009: 53: 298–304.
12. Klein R, Klein BEK, Moss SE, Cruickshanks KJ. Relationship of hyperglycemia to the long-term incidence and progression of diabetic retinopathy. *Arch Intern Med* 1994;154:2169–78.
13. Klein R. Hyperglycemia and microvascular and macrovascular disease in diabetes. *Diabetes Care* 1995;18:258–68.
14. DCCT. The effect of intensive treatment of diabetes on the development and progression of long-term complications in insulin-dependent diabetes mellitus. The Diabetes Control and Complications Trial Research Group. *N Engl J Med* 1993;329:977–86.
15. Reichard P, Bengt-Nilsson B-Y, Rosenqvist U. The effect of long-term intensified insulin treatment on the development of microvascular complications of diabetes mellitus. *N Engl J Med* 1993;329:304–9.
16. Ohkubo Y, Kishikawa H, Araki E, et al. Intensive insulin therapy prevents the progression of diabetic microvascular complications in Japanese patients with non-insulin-dependent diabetes mellitus: a randomized prospective 6-year study. *Diabetes Res Clin Pract* 1995;28:103–17.
17. UK Prospective Diabetes Study (UKPDS) Group. Intensive blood-glucose control with sulphonylureas or insulin compared with conventional treatment and risk of complications in patients with type 2 diabetes (UKPDS 33). *Lancet* 1998;352:837–53.

18. Fuller JH, Shipley MJ, Rose G, Jarrett RJ, Keen H. Mortality from coronary heart disease and stroke in relation to degree of glycaemia: the Whitehall study. *BMJ* 1983;287:867–70.

19. Standl E, Balletshofer B, Dahl B, et al. Predictors of 10-year macrovascular and overall mortality in patients with NIDDM: the Munich General Practitioner Project. *Diabetologia* 1996;39:1540–5.

20. Khaw KT, Wareham N, Bingham S, Luben R, Welch A, Day N. Association of hemoglobin A1c with cardiovascular disease and mortality in adults: the European prospective investigation into cancer in Norfolk. *Ann Intern Med* 2004;141:413–20.

21. Stratton IM, Adler AI, Neil HA, et al. Association of glycaemia with macrovascular and microvascular complications of type 2 diabetes (UKPDS 35): prospective observational study. *BMJ* 2000;321:405–12.

22. Selvin E, Marinopoulos S, Berkenblit G, et al. Meta-analysis: glycosylated hemoglobin and cardiovascular disease in diabetes mellitus. *Ann Intern Med* 2004;141:421–31.

23. Stettler C, Allemann S, Jüni P, et al. Glycemic control and macrovascular disease in types 1 and 2 diabetes mellitus: meta-analysis of randomized trials. *Am Heart J* 2006;152:27–38.

24. Hansson L, Zanchetti A, Carruthers SG, et al.; HOT Study Group. Effects of intensive blood-pressure lowering and low-dose aspirin in patients with hypertension: principal results of the Hypertension Optimal Treatment (HOT) randomised trial. *Lancet* 1998;351:1755–62.

25. Heart Outcomes Prevention Evaluation (HOPE) Study Investigators. Effects of ramipril on cardiovascular and microvascular outcomes in people with diabetes mellitus: results of the HOPE study and MICRO-HOPE substudy. *Lancet* 2000;355:253–9.

26. Turnbull F, Neal B, Algert C, et al.; Blood Pressure Lowering Treatment Trialists' Collaboration. Effects of different blood pressure-lowering regimens on major cardiovascular events in individuals with and without diabetes mellitus: results of prospectively designed overviews of randomized trials. *Arch Intern Med* 2005;165:1410–19.

27. Pyrälä K, Pedersen TR, Kjekshus J, Faergeman O, Olsson AG, Thorgeirsson G. Cholesterol lowering with simvastatin improves prognosis of diabetic patients with coronary heart disease. A subgroup analysis of the Scandinavian Simvastatin Survival Study (4S). *Diabetes Care* 1997;20:614–20.

28. Goldberg RB, Mellies MJ, Sacks FM, et al. Cardiovascular events and their reduction with pravastatin in diabetic and glucoseintolerant myocardial infarction survivors with average cholesterol levels: subgroup analyses in the cholesterol and recurrent events (CARE) trial. The Care Investigators. *Circulation* 1998;98:2513–19.

29. Heart Protection Study Collaborative Group. MRC/BHF Heart Protection Study of cholesterol-lowering with simvastatin in 5963 people with diabetes: a randomised placebocontrolled trial. *Lancet* 2003;361:2005–16.

30. Colhoun HM, Betteridge DJ, Durrington PN, et al.; CARDS Investigators. Primary prevention of cardiovascular disease with atorvastatin in type 2 diabetes in the Collaborative Atorvastatin Diabetes Study (CARDS): multicentre randomized placebo controlled trial. *Lancet* 2004;364:685–96.

31. Antithrombotic Trialists' (ATT) Collaboration, Baigent C, Blackwell L, Collins R, et al. Aspirin in the primary and secondary prevention of vascular disease: collaborative meta-analysis of individual participant data from randomised trials. *Lancet* 2009;373:1849–60.

32. Gaede P, Vedel P, Larsen N, Jensen GVH, Parving HH, Pedersen O. Multifactorial intervention and cardiovascular disease in patients with type 2 diabetes. *N Engl J Med* 2003;348:383–93.

33. Gaede P, Lund-Andersen H, Parving H-H, Pedersen O: Effect of a multifactorial intervention on mortality in type 2 diabetes. *N Engl J Med* 2008;358:580–91.

34. Nathan DM, Cleary PA, Backlund JY, et al. Intensive diabetes treatment and cardiovascular disease in patients with type 1 diabetes. *N Engl J Med* 2005;353:2643–53.

35. Diabetes Control and Complications Trial/Epidemiology of Diabetes Interventions and Complications (DCCT/EDIC) Research Group, Nathan DM, Zinman B, Cleary PA, et al. Modern-Day Clinical Course of Type 1 Diabetes Mellitus After 30 Years' Duration: The Diabetes Control and Complications Trial/Epidemiology of Diabetes Interventions and Complications and Pittsburgh Epidemiology of Diabetes Complications Experience (1983–2005). *Arch Intern Med* 2009;169:1307–16.

36. Action to Control Cardiovascular Risk in Diabetes Study Group, Gerstein HC, Miller ME, Byington RP, et al. Effects of intensive glucose lowering in type 2 diabetes. *N Engl J Med* 2008;358:2545–59.

37. The ADVANCE Collaborative Group, Patel A, MacMahon S, Chalmers J, et al. Intensive blood glucose control and vascular outcomes in patients with type 2 diabetes. *N Engl J Med* 2008;358:2560–72.

38. Duckworth W, Abraira C, Moritz T, et al.; VADT Investigators. Glucose control and vascular complications in veterans with type 2 diabetes. *N Engl J Med* 2009;360:129–39. Erratum in: *N Engl J Med* 2009;361:1024–25, 1028.

39. Holman RR, Paul SK, Bethel MA, Matthews DR, Neil HA. 10-year follow-up of intensive glucose control in type 2 diabetes. *N Engl J Med* 2008;359:1577–89.

40. Bonds DE, Miller ME, Bergenstal RM, et al. The association between symptomatic, severe hypoglycaemia and mortality in type 2 diabetes: retrospective epidemiological analysis of the ACCORD study. *BMJ* 2010;340:b4909.

41. Miller ME, Bonds DE, Gerstein HC, et al.; ACCORD Investigators. The effects of baseline characteristics, glycaemia treatment approach, and glycated haemoglobin concentration on the risk of severe hypoglycaemia: post hoc epidemiological analysis of the ACCORD study. *BMJ*. 2010;340:b5444.

42. Calles-Escandón J, Lovato LC, Simons-Morton DG, et al. Effect of intensive compared with standard glycemia treatment strategies on mortality by baseline subgroup characteristics: The ACCORD trial. *Diabetes Care* 2010;33:721–7.

43. Riddle MC, Ambrosius WT, Brillon DJ, et al. for the ACCORD Investigators. Epidemiologic relationships between A1c and all-cause mortality during a median 3.4-year follow-up of glycemic treatment in the ACCORD Trial. *Diabetes Care* 2010;33:983–90.

44. Riddle MC. Update on ACCORD. International Diabetes Federation, Montreal, Thursday 22 October 2009.

45. The ACCORD Study Group. Effects of intensive blood-pressure control in type 2 diabetes mellitus. *N Engl J Med* 2010; March 14 [Epub ahead of print].

46. The ACCORD Study Group. Effects of combination lipid therapy in type 2 diabetes mellitus. *N Engl J Med* 2010; March 14 [Epub ahead of print].

47. Patel A; ADVANCE Collaborative Group, MacMahon S, Chalmers J, Neal B, et al. Effects of a fixed combination of perindopril and indapamide on macrovascular and microvascular outcomes in patients with type 2 diabetes mellitus (the ADVANCE trial): a randomised controlled trial. *Lancet* 2007;370:829–40.

48. Zoungas S, de Galan BE, Ninomiya T, et al., on behalf of the ADVANCE Collaborative Group. Combined Effects of Routine Blood Pressure Lowering and Intensive Glucose Control on Macrovascular and Microvascular Outcomes in Patients With Type 2 Diabetes: New results from the ADVANCE trial. *Diabetes Care* 2009;32:2068–74.

49. Moritz T, Duckworth W, Abraira C. Veterans Affairs Diabetes Trial – Corrections. *N Engl J Med* 2009;361:1024–5.

50. Reaven PD, Moritz TE, Schwenke DC, et al., for the Veterans Affairs Diabetes Trial. Intensive Glucose-Lowering Therapy Reduces Cardiovascular Disease Events in Veterans Affairs Diabetes Trial Participants With Lower Calcified Coronary Atherosclerosis. *Diabetes* 2009;58:2642–8.

51. UK Prospective Diabetes Study (UKPDS) Group. Effect of intensive blood-glucose control with metformin on complications in overweight patients with type 2 diabetes (UKPDS 34). *Lancet* 1998;352:854–65.

52. UK Prospective Diabetes Study Group. Tight blood pressure control and risk of macrovascular and microvascular complications in type 2 diabetes: UKPDS 38. *BMJ* 1998;317:703–13.

53. Adler AI, Stratton IM, Neil HA, et al. Association of systolic blood pressure with macrovascular and microvascular complications of type 2 diabetes (UKPDS 36): prospective observational study. *BMJ* 2000;321:412–19.

54. Stratton IM, Cull CA, Adler AI, Matthews DR, Neil HA, Holman RR. Additive effects of glycaemia and blood pressure exposure on risk of complications in type 2 diabetes: a prospective observational study (UKPDS 75). *Diabetologia* 2006;49:1761–9.

55. Holman RR, Paul SK, Bethel MA, Neil HA, Matthews DR. Long-term follow-up after tight control of blood pressure in type 2 diabetes. *N Engl J Med* 2008;359:1565–76.

56. Dormandy JA, Charbonnel B, Eckland DJ, et al.; PROactive investigators. Secondary prevention of macrovascular events in patients with type 2 diabetes in the PROactive Study (PROspective pioglitAzone Clinical Trial In macroVascular Events): a randomised controlled trial. *Lancet* 2005;366:1279–89.

57. Ray KK, Seshasai SR, Wijesuriya S, et al. Effect of intensive control of glucose on cardiovascular outcomes and death in patients with diabetes mellitus: a meta-analysis of randomised controlled trials. *Lancet* 2009;373:1765–72.

58. Kelly TN, Bazzano LA, Fonseca VA, Thethi TK, Reynolds K, He J. Systematic Review: Glucose control and cardiovascular disease in type 2 diabetes. *Ann Intern Med* 2009;151:394–403.

59. Mannucci E, Monami M, Lamanna C, Gori F, Marchionni N. Prevention of cardiovascular disease through glycemic control in type 2 diabetes: a meta-analysis of randomized clinical trials. *Nutr Metab Cardiovasc Dis* 2009;19:604–12.

60. Ma J, Yang W, Fang N, Zhu W, Wei M. The association between intensive glycemic control and vascular complications in type 2 diabetes mellitus: a meta-analysis. *Nutr Metab Cardiovasc Dis* 2009;19:596–603.

61. Tkác I. Effect of intensive glycemic control on cardiovascular outcomes and all-cause mortality in type 2 diabetes: overview and metaanalysis of five trials. *Diabetes Res Clin Pract* 2009;86(Suppl 1): S57–62.

62. Turnbull FM, Abraira C, Anderson RJ, et al. Intensive glucose control and macrovascular outcomes in type 2 diabetes. *Diabetologia* 2009;52:2288–98.
63. Joffe HV, Parks MH, Temple R. Impact of cardiovascular outcomes on the development and approval of medications for the treatment of diabetes mellitus. *Rev Endocr Metab Disord* 2010;11:21–30.
64. Guidance for industry: Diabetes mellitus – evaluating cardiovascular risk in new antidiabetic therapies to treat type 2 diabetes. In: *Guidances (drugs)*. United States Food and Drug Administration. 2008. http://www.fda.gov/downloads/Drugs/GuidanceComplianceRegulatoryInformation/Guidances/ucm071627.pdf.
65. American Diabetes Association. Standards of Medical Care in Diabetes – 2010. *Diabetes Care* 2010;33:S11–61.

Chapter 12

A healthy lifestyle and cardiovascular risk reduction

Arne V. Astrup

There is robust evidence to support the argument that a substantial proportion of the cardiovascular disease (CVD) seen today can be prevented by a generally healthier lifestyle in the population as a whole, and by targeting lifestyle change and medical management of cardiovascular risk factors in high-risk individuals. Prevention does not mean that CVD and death can be avoided, but rather that the onset of disease can be postponed and life expectancy prolonged. With the exception of smoking cessation, preventive lifestyle intervention will probably not save money on a societal level, as people will live longer and require medical care for other illnesses, and extended social support [1]. According to Kahn et al. [2] effective prevention in the US population could potentially reduce the incidence of myocardial infarction by > 60%, reduce the incidence of stroke by ~ 30%, and increase life expectancy by an average of 1.3 years.

European studies have found that population-wide, best-practice interventions have the potential to reduce coronary heart disease mortality by 57%, and for primary prevention the corresponding reductions would be 75–85% [3]. This analysis did not, however, include the effect of weight reduction in the overweight section of the population.

Effective medical management of high-risk individuals by aspirin, lipid and blood pressure lowering drugs, and by management of dysglycemia and obesity are dealt with in other chapters of this book. The present chapter will focus on smoking, impaired sleep, physical activity, and intake of *trans* fatty acids.

The most effective way to reduce the risk for CVD is to maintain a healthy lifestyle. Stampfer et al. defined subjects at low risk among adult women as those who were non-smokers, had a BMI below 25 kg/m^2, consumed an average of

Metabolic Risk for Cardiovascular Disease, 1st edition. Edited by R. H. Eckel.
© 2011 American Heart Association. By Blackwell Publishing Ltd.

half a unit of alcohol per day, engaged in moderate-to-vigorous physical activity for at least 30 min per day, and had a diet moderately high in cereal fiber, marine n-3 fatty acids, and folate, with a high ratio of polyunsaturated to saturated fat, and low in *trans* fat and glycemic load [4]. They found that only 3% of the US population complied with this lifestyle, but they had a relative risk of coronary events of only 0.17 as compared with all women not achieving a healthy lifestyle, and that 82% of coronary events could be attributed to lack of adherence to this healthy lifestyle.

Generally the advice for reducing the risk for CVD can be summarized by the following elements [5].

Eat a healthy, balanced diet

Habitual diet should be low in industrially produced *trans* and saturated fats, added sugar and salt, and contain plenty of fruit and vegetables (at least 4.5 cups or more a day), whole grain, high-fiber products, and oily fish. Fish such as herrings, kippers, mackerel, pilchards or sardines, salmon, and trout contain oils that can reduce the risk of thrombosis in the context of a healthy eating pattern and energy balance. Other foods that have a beneficial impact on CVD risk are beans, peas, lentils, and oats, because they contain soluble fiber.

Be more physically active

Regular aerobic (cardiovascular) exercise, for at least 30 minutes a day for a total of at least 150 minutes a week, has a beneficial impact on several CVD risk factors, and also helps to maintain a healthy bodyweight.

Keep to a healthy weight

Overweight and obesity, and in particular abdominal fat distribution, increase the risk of CVD, and weight reduction has been shown to decrease incidence and cardiovascular mortality in severely obese subjects. Obese individuals are known to be capable of losing weight, but weight maintenance is more problematic, so prevention of weight gain is a primary focus.

Give up smoking

For smokers, giving up will reduce the risk of developing coronary heart disease by 50%. Smoking causes the majority of cases of coronary thrombosis in people under the age of 50.

Reduce your alcohol consumption

Small amounts of alcohol may help to reduce CVD. However, excessive alcohol consumption increases blood pressure and risk of stroke, among several other health risks, and it is therefore advisable that individuals abide by public health recommendations regarding alcohol consumption. Health guidelines in the United Kingdom recommend that men consume no more than three to four units of alcohol a day, and that women do not exceed two to three units. Binge drinking should be avoided. The American Heart Association diet and lifestyle recommendations say that alcohol consumption should be kept in moderation (no more than one drink for women and no more than two drinks for men per day).

Keep your blood pressure under control

Eating a healthy diet that is low in saturated fat, and high in fruit, vegetables, and low-fat and fat-free dairy products, and exercising regularly can help achieve a normal blood pressure. In addition, avoiding smoking and excessive alcohol consumption assists in maintaining a normal blood pressure. For those who require medication, adherence to medications and long-term medical follow-up may be necessary to reach and maintain the desired blood pressure goal.

Keep your diabetes under control

Individuals with diabetes have a greater risk of developing CVD. The risk of developing type 2 diabetes can be reduced dramatically by maintain a healthy bodyweight, being physically active, and eating a healthy diet.

Take any medication that is prescribed

For patients who have CVD, medication may relieve symptoms and reduce the risk for further progression.

Multifactor interventions

For clinicians and their patients, the total reduction in risk for CVD achieved by a healthy lifestyle is more relevant than addressing each of the lifestyle components individually. However, the flip side of the coin in these studies is that the contribution of each of the components remains uncertain. Regarding the primary prevention of CVD, larger intervention studies are obviously required to demonstrate a risk reduction, but observational epidemiological studies have suggested that dramatic health gains can be achieved. An analysis by Asaria et al. [6] found that 13.8 million deaths could be prevented over 10 years if measures to reduce tobacco and salt exposure were implemented. About three out of four deaths averted would be from cardiovascular diseases [6]. Hu et al. found that the incidence of coronary disease declined by 31% from 1981 to 1992, while the proportion of smokers declined by 41%, the proportion of postmenopausal women using HRT increased by 175%, and the prevalence of overweight increased by 38%. These factors could explain a 21% decline in the incidence of coronary disease, representing 68% of the overall decline. The reduction in smoking could account for a 13% decline in the incidence, improved diet could account for a 16% decline; and increase in HRT could explain a further 9% decline. However, the increase in overweight could account for an 8% increase in incidence in coronary disease [7].

Major benefits could also be achieved from secondary prevention of CVD. Ornish et al. [8] showed that intensive lifestyle changes (fat-reduced diet, aerobic exercise, stress management training, smoking cessation, group psychosocial support) for 5 years produced greater regression of coronary atherosclerosis and fewer cardiac events than in a control group [1,2]. An effect of comprehensive cardiac rehabilitation sessions was recently assessed in the randomized controlled GOSPEL trial in post-myocardial infarction patients, comparing a long-term, reinforced, multifactorial educational and behavioral intervention with usual care, including supervised aerobic exercise and lifestyle modification consisting of risk factor counseling about a Mediterranean diet, smoking cessation, and stress management [9]. The targets of the intervention strategy were smoking cessation, adoption of a healthy Mediterranean diet, increase in physical activity up to at least 3 hours per week at 60% to 75% of the mean maximum heart rate, and maintenance of BMI at $< 25 \, kg/m^2$ and blood pressure of $< 140/85 \, mmHg$. After 3 years of observation there were only small improvements in most of the lifestyle variables, and these did not significantly reduce the primary endpoint [9], though several secondary endpoints were decreased: cardiovascular mortality plus non-fatal myocardial infarction and stroke (3.2% vs 4.8%; HR, 0.67), cardiac death plus non-fatal myocardial infarction (2.5% vs 4.0%; HR, 0.64), and non-fatal myocardial infarction (1.4% vs 2.7%; HR, 0.52). The intervention group still had plenty of room for further improvement in lifestyle, such as smoking cessation and weight gain prevention, and this emphasizes the potential for health benefits that can be achieved even in patients with established CVD.

The importance of dietary modification is not entirely clear. A systematic review and meta-analysis of trials aiming at reducing total fat and saturated fat included 27 studies (40 intervention arms, 30 901 person-years) [10]. The analysis found no significant effect on total mortality (RR 0.98, 95% CI 0.86 to 1.12), a trend toward protection from cardiovascular mortality (RR: 0.91, CI 0.77 to 1.07), and protection from cardiovascular events (RR: 0.84, CI 0.72 to 0.99). Interventions lasting more than 2 years showed significant reductions in the rate of cardiovascular events and a trend toward reduction in total mortality. Increasing the amount of n-3 fatty acids in the diet seems to increase the effect on CVD [1,2,11].

Smoking

A smoke-free environment is an important part of a healthy lifestyle. The first major epidemiological study showing a strong correlation between smoking and CVD was published around 1960, and although observational studies could not provide definitive evidence that tobacco smoke is responsible for increased coronary risk, it prompted the first anti-smoking measures by the US Surgeon General in his 1964 report. Smoking is a highly addictive habit, and despite major reductions in smoking prevalence in most Western countries over the last 50 years, tobacco use continues to grow in global importance as a leading preventable cause of CVD. Tobacco smoking exerts both prothrombotic and atherogenic effects, and it increases the risk of acute myocardial infarction, sudden cardiac death, stroke, aortic aneurysm, and peripheral vascular disease [12]. It has been found that even low-level exposure (e.g., passive smoking) increases the risk of acute myocardial infarction. Fortunately, smoking cessation and avoidance of passive smoking rapidly reduces this risk. A major problem with smoking cessation is that the majority of smokers experience a weight gain when they stop smoking which, in many cases, leads to taking up the habit again. It has been estimated that more people in the USA die from obesity-related complications than from tobacco. Only a small proportion of the weight gain observed in the population can be attributed to smoking cessation [13], but the observation emphasizes the need to include advice on prevention of weight gain in the package of smoking cessation tools.

Proven cost-effective and safe cessation interventions already exist, such as physician advice, counseling, and nicotine replacement therapy. These should be offered on a routine basis to all smokers. This is especially important for those individuals at risk for CVD, and for patients with established or even acute CVD. Clinicians need to play an active role in supporting patients to completely stop smoking.

Physical inactivity

Regular physical activity is an important part of a healthy lifestyle, and sedentary behavior can account for a substantial risk for CVD. Individuals who regularly undertake physical activity have a decreased risk of obesity, heart disease, hypertension, diabetes, and premature mortality. Systematic reviews and meta-analyses have consistently found that physical activity is associated with a marked decrease in cardiovascular and all-cause mortality in both men and women, even after adjusting for other relevant risk factors.

Nocon et al. recently reported a meta-analysis including 33 studies with 883 372 participants, with follow-up ranging from 4 years to over 20 years [14]. Physical activity was associated with a risk reduction of 35% in cardiovascular mortality (95% CI, 30–40%). All-cause mortality was reduced by 33% (28–37%). Oguma et al. examined the dose–response relationship in women based on a meta-analysis of 30 studies and found, when studies were combined according to relative levels of physical activity, that the risk reduction showed a dose–response relationship for coronary heart disease (CHD) (RR = 1, 0.78, 0.53,

0.61, respectively, for studies with four physical activity levels, $n = 5$) and for stroke (RR = 1, 0.73, 0.68) [15]. For overall CVD the reduction was also substantial (RR = 1, 0.82, 0.78) [15]. When studies were combined by absolute walking amount, even 1 hour of walking per week was associated with reduced risk of CVD outcome.

However, the time engaged in physical activity is probably too simplistic a measure to allow definitive conclusions regarding optimal physical activity for improving health. Fitness level and physical activity are interrelated, but it has been found that being unfit is a risk factor distinct from inactivity, and is in itself worthy of screening and intervention. Recommendations for physical activity should not be formulated on the basis of fitness studies because this may inappropriately demote the status of physical fitness as a risk factor while exaggerating the public health benefits of moderate amounts of physical activity [16]. Analyses from the Health Professionals' Follow-up Study of the importance of levels of leisure-time physical activity for incidence of CHD found that total physical activity, running, weight training, and rowing were each inversely associated with risk of CHD. Men who ran for an hour or more per week had a 42% risk reduction (RR, 0.58; 95% CI, 0.44–0.77) compared with men who did not run [17]. Men who trained with weights for 30 minutes or more per week had a 23% risk reduction and those who rowed for 1 hour or more per week had an 18% risk reduction compared to those who did not undertake these activities. Average exercise intensity was also associated with reduced CHD risk, independent of the total volume of physical activity. Half an hour or more of brisk walking per day was associated with an 18% risk reduction, but walking pace was associated with reduced CHD risk independent of the number of walking hours. These results show that various activities can be used, and that exercise intensity and fitness should be considered as well as the amount of time spent on exercise activities when calculating the health benefits of physical activity.

With an increasing proportion of the population being either overweight or obese, the question has been raised whether physical activity can eliminate the adverse health effect of obesity. In a recent meta-analysis of observational studies Blair and Brodney concluded that: (i) regular physical activity clearly attenuates many of the health risks associated with overweight or obesity; (ii) physical activity appears to not only attenuate the health risks of overweight and obesity, but active obese individuals actually have lower morbidity and mortality than normal weight individuals who are sedentary; and (iii) inactivity and low cardiorespiratory fitness are as important as overweight and obesity as mortality predictors [18]. Notably, their findings were entirely based on observational studies, and randomized clinical trials addressing these questions should be undertaken. Patients with established CVD will benefit from more exercise and increasing fitness, and the risk of sudden death induced by exercise is negligible compared with the benefits.

In order to reduce the ill health caused by physical inactivity. The 2009 federal guidelines recommend that all adults avoid inactivity and do at least 150 minutes a week of moderate intensity, or 75 minutes a week of vigorous intensity aerobic physical activity or an equivalent amount [19]. Recently, the CDC analyzed data from the Behavioral Risk Factor Surveillance System (BRFSS) and found that from 2001 to 2005 the prevalence of regular physical activity increased 8.6% among women overall (from 43.0% to 46.7%) and 3.5% among men (from 48.0% to 49.7%) [19]. These figures may reflect some over-reporting bias, but they suggest that efforts to increase the proportion of individuals complying with the recommendations are increasing. However, they also demonstrate that the majority of the adult population does not meet the recommendations for physical activity, and there is obviously potential for further reductions in the incidence of CVD by activating the sedentary section of the population. State and local public health agencies, and other public health stakeholders, should continue to implement evidence-based, culturally appropriate initiatives to further increase physical activity and fitness levels in all adults.

Sleep

Sleep of sufficient duration and quality is inherent as part of a healthy lifestyle, and too little high-quality sleep promotes CVD through a disrupted appetite control, and through effects on metabolism that increase the risk of type 2 diabetes. Too little sleep has become a common health problem in Western societies. The average duration of sleep has decreased approximately 1 hour compared to 30 years ago [20], with more severely impaired sleep seen in certain individuals and/or groups. Sleep loss, widespread in modern societies, is an under-recognized public health problem that has a cumulative effect on physical and mental health. Epidemiological studies support the hypothesis that there are links between impaired sleep and overweight, especially in the young [21–23]. A number of intervention studies also imply that disturbed sleep has an impact on numerous physiological functions, such as appetite-regulating hormones, substrate metabolism, and blood pressure [23–27]. In addition, numerous reports have found too little or impaired sleep to be a risk factor for mental distress, depression, anxiety, obesity, hypertension, diabetes, high cholesterol levels, and premature CVD death [2]. Though confounding by other adverse health behaviors such as cigarette smoking, physical inactivity, and heavy drinking may be important, there is accumulating evidence that too little and impaired sleep per se increase risk of CVD, partly directly and partly through weight gain and insulin resistance [2]. Recently, King et al. [28] found a robust association between objectively measured sleep duration and 5-year incidence of coronary artery calcification, a subclinical predictor of future CHD events. They found that 1 hour more sleep decreased the estimated odds of calcification incidence by 33%. The magnitude of the observed effect was similar to that of other important CVD risk factors (e.g., one additional hour of sleep reduced risk similarly to a reduction of 16.5 mmHg in systolic blood pressure) [28].

Recent intervention studies have provided a mechanistic explanation for the deleterious effects of sleep deprivation on health. These physiological data suggest that short-term partial sleep restriction leads to striking alterations in metabolic and endocrine functions, such as insulin resistance, increased sympathetic tone, elevated levels of cortisol and proinflammatory cytokines, and decreased leptin and increased ghrelin levels [23]. Furthermore, abnormal sleep–wake patterns probably alter intracellular circadian clocks, which may potentiate disrupted metabolism [29]. Chronic lack of sleep is stressful and biologically demanding and must be avoided if good health is a goal.

There seems to be good reason to question patients about sleep duration and sleep quality, and to recommend efforts to ensure that they get sufficient amounts of high-quality sleep. The optimal sleep duration for adults appears to be 7–8 hours. Sleep of longer duration is a strong risk factor for increased mortality [30], but it is unclear whether the association is confounded by other adverse health behaviors. More than 7.5 hours of sleep may increase the risk of cerebrovascular deaths, both in women and men [31]. It is not clear why sleep exceeding 7.5 hours should be associated with excess mortality, and the observation has not been confirmed by all studies. Long sleep duration may not be a causal factor for the increased mortality in itself, and sleep apnea may be an underlying confounding factor.

It should be kept in mind that there are still research questions to be answered, and there is obviously a need for randomized controlled trials to demonstrate that improved sleep duration and quality can reduce risk for CVD. However, there is no risk in taking a pragmatic approach and encouraging a good night's sleep as an adjunct to other health measures. Sleep is a modifiable risk factor and the benefit of increasing sleep duration in at-risk individuals outweighs the harms.

Dietary issues

A reduction of CVD can be achieved by modifying the diet to affect risk factors such as body weight and the components of the metabolic syndrome (LDL cholesterol, postprandial triglycerides, blood pressure, and so on). The effect of nutrition is covered by Chapter 4 and dietary recommendations are summarized above. The only dietary consideration addressed in the present chapter is the role of industrially produced *trans* fatty acids.

Trans fatty acids and cardiovascular disease

It is paradoxical that for over 50 years health authorities have advised consumers to replace butter with margarines, and to use spreads and hard vegetable margarines to improve health, and in particular to reduce the risk of CVD. We now know that the public would have been better off had they ignored this advice and continued to use butter because hard margarines and spreads contain large amounts of industrially produced *trans* fatty acids, which seem to be the most harmful single dietary component in terms of raising the risk for CVD. Fatty acids of *trans* configuration come from two different sources: from industrially produced partially hydrogenated fat (IP-TFA) used in frying oils, margarines, spreads, and bakery products, and from ruminant fat in dairy and meat products (RP-TFA) [32]. The first source may contain up to 60% of the fatty acids in *trans* form, whereas the content in ruminant fat does not generally exceed 6%. In Western Europe, including Scandinavia, the average daily intake of IP-TFA has decreased during the last two decades due to societal pressure and a legislative ban, whereas the intake of RP-TFA has remained fairly stable [33]. Despite this decrease, in many countries it is still possible to consume more than 20 grams of IP-TFA in a single meal consisting of some popular foods, even though average intake of IP-TFA in these countries is low [33,34]. Subgroups of the populations may therefore, on average, consume more than 5 grams IP-TFA per day. This level of consumption is not usually possible for RP-TFA. A daily intake of 5 grams TFA (primarily IP-TFA) is associated with a 29% increased risk of CHD [35]. Such an association is not found for daily intakes of RP-TFA of up to 4 grams. In a worldwide study of the IP-TFA content in fast foods, biscuits, and snacks, contents of IP-TFA of up to 50% of the fat in some products were found, enabling consumers to ingest 36 grams of IP-TFA in a single meal in the USA [34]. A daily intake of 5 grams of *trans* fat, corresponding to 2% of energy intake, is associated with an approximately 30% increase in CHD risk [35].

Does *trans* fat promote obesity and the metabolic syndrome?

Observational studies have found that a high intake of IP-TFA increases the risk of weight gain and gain in abdominal fatness more than other fat sources [36]. Although unaccounted residual confounding cannot be ruled out, other research indicates that the relationship is causal. Firstly, IP-TFA serves as a ligand for the PPAR-g system and can exert a biological effect that promotes abdominal obesity [35]. Secondly, a recently reported long-term randomized trial in monkeys found robust evidence that IP-TFA induces weight gain and abdominal obesity [37]. For 6 years the monkeys were fed two different isocaloric, Western-style diets containing either 8% of calories from *trans* fat or the same amount of fat calories as *cis*-monounsaturated fat. After 6 years the IP-TFA-fed monkeys had gained 7.2% in bodyweight, compared to a 1.8% increase in bodyweight in monkeys fed *cis*-monounsaturated fats. CT scans showed that the monkeys on the *trans*-fat diet had deposited 30% more abdominal fat than the monkeys on the *cis*-monounsaturated fat diet [34]. Taken together these studies suggest that IP-TFA may be obesity promoting, and that it particularly facilitates the deposition of harmful abdominal fat [38]. These findings can help to explain why high intakes of IP-TFA may increase the risk of type 2 diabetes [39].

The high amount of IP-TFA in popular foods, the evidence of a more harmful effect on health of IP-TFA than of RP-TFA, and the feasibility of eliminating IP-TFA from foods without side effects for the population, suggests that a selective elimination of IP-TFA from our food is a low hanging fruit in the quest for a more healthy diet for subgroups of the population. The American Heart Association recommends in an overall healthy diet to keep *trans* fat intake to less than 1% of energy.

Summary

On a population level epidemiological studies suggest that a healthy lifestyle with no tobacco smoking, avoidance of excessive alcohol consumption, adequate sleep and regular physical activity, an ideal body weight, and a healthy diet, can reduce the risk for cardiovascular disease up to 85–95%. Adequate treatment of risk factors would add ∼221 million life-years and 244 million quality-adjusted life-years to the US adult population, or an average of 1.3 years of life expectancy for all adults. To achieve this, intensive management targeting the individual, as well as major changes in the toxic environment that tends to maintain unhealthy habits, is required.

References

1. Gaziano TA, Galea G, Reddy KS. Scaling up interventions for chronic disease prevention: the evidence. *Lancet* 2007;370:1939–46.
2. Kahn R, Robertson RM, Smith R, Eddy D. The impact of prevention on reducing the burden of cardiovascular disease. *Diabetes Care* 2008;31:1686–96.
3. Kivimäki M, Shipley MJ, Ferrie JE, et al. Best-practice interventions to reduce socioeconomic inequalities of coronary heart disease mortality in UK: a prospective occupational cohort study. *Lancet* 2008;372:1648–54.
4. Stampfer M, Hu FB, Manson JE, Rimm EB, Willett WC. Primary prevention of coronary heart disease in women through diet and lifestyle. *N Engl J Med* 2000;343:16–22.
5. NHS Choices content: Preventing heart disease. http://www.nhs.uk/Conditions/Coronary-heart-disease/Pages/Prevention.aspx?url=Pages/What-is-it.aspx, accessed on 9 March 2009.
6. Asaria P, Chisholm D, Mathers C, Ezzati M, Beaglehole R. Chronic disease prevention: health effects and financial costs of strategies to reduce salt intake and control tobacco use. *Lancet* 2007;370:2044–53.
7. Hu FB, Stampfer MJ, Manson JE, et al. Trends in the incidence of coronary heart disease and changes in diet and lifestyle in women. *N Engl J Med* 2000;343:530–7.
8. Ornish D, Scherwitz LW, Billings JH, et al. Intensive lifestyle changes for reversal of coronary heart disease. *JAMA* 1998;280:2001–7.
9. Giannuzzi P, Temporelli PL, Marchioli R, et al., for the GOSPEL Investigators. Global secondary prevention strategies to limit event recurrence after myocardial infarction

results of the GOSPEL study, a multicenter, randomized controlled trial from the Italian Cardiac Rehabilitation Network. *Arch Intern Med* 2008;168:2194–204.

10. Hooper L, Summerbell CD, Higgins JPT, et al. Reduced or modified dietary fat for preventing cardiovascular disease. *Cochrane Database Syst Rev* 2001;(3):CD002137. DOI: 10.1002/14651858.CD002137.

11. Gissi-HF Investigators, Tavazzi L, Maggioni AP, Marchioli R, et al. Effect of n-3 polyunsaturated fatty acids in patients with chronic heart failure (the GISSI-HF trial): a randomised, double-blind, placebo-controlled trial. *Lancet* 2008;372:1223–30.

12. Bullen C. Impact of tobacco smoking and smoking cessation on cardiovascular risk and disease. *Expert Rev Cardiovasc Ther* 2008;6:883–95.

13. Flegal KM, Troiano RP, Pamuk ER, Kuczmarski RJ, Campbell SM. The influence of smoking cessation on the prevalence of overweight in the United States. *N Engl J Med* 1995;333; 1165–70.

14. Nocon M, Hiemann T, Müller-Riemenschneider F, Thalau F, Roll S, Willich SN. Association of physical activity with all-cause and cardiovascular mortality: a systematic review and meta-analysis. *Eur J Cardiovasc Prev Rehabil* 2008;15:239–46.

15. Oguma Y, Shinoda-Tagawa T. Physical activity decreases cardiovascular disease risk in women: review and meta-analysis. *Am J Prev Med* 2004;26:407–18.

16. Williams PT. Physical fitness and activity as separate heart disease risk factors: a meta-analysis. *Med Sci Sports Exerc* 2001;33:754–61.

17. Tanasescu M, Leitzmann MF, Rimm EB, Willett WC, Stampfer MJ, Hu FB. Exercise type and intensity in relation to coronary heart disease in men. *JAMA* 2002;288:1994–2000.

18. Blair SN, Brodney S. Effects of physical inactivity and obesity on morbidity and mortality: current evidence and research issues. *Med Sci Sports Exerc* 1999;31(suppl 11):S646–62.

19. www.health.gov/paguidelines. Published 2009.

20. Ayas NT, White DP, Al-Delaimy WK, et al. A prospective study of self-reported sleep duration and incident diabetes in women. *Diabetes Care* 2003;26:380–4.

21. Chaput JP, Brunet M, Tremblay A. Relationship between short sleeping hours and childhood overweight/obesity: results from the 'Quebec en Forme' Project. *Int J Obes* 2006;30:1080–5.

22. Reilly JJ, Armstrong J, Dorosty AR, et al., for the Avon Longitudinal Study of Parents and Children Study Team. Early life risk factors for obesity in childhood: cohort study. *BMJ* 2005;330:1357–63.

23. Taheri S, Lin L, Austin D, Young T, Mignot E. Short sleep duration is associated with reduced leptin, elevated ghrelin, and increased body mass index. *PLoS Med* 2004;1:e62.

24. Mullington JM, Haack M, Toth M, Serrador JM, Meier-Ewert HK. Cardiovascular, inflammatory, and metabolic consequences of sleep deprivation. *Prog Cardiovasc Dis* 2009;51:294–302.

25. Lusardi P, Mugellini A, Preti P, Zoppi A, Derosa G, Fogari R. Effects of a restricted sleep regimen on ambulatory blood pressure monitoring in normotensive subjects. *Am J Hypertens* 1996;9:503–5.

26. Lusardi P, Zoppi A, Preti P, Pesce RM, Piazza E, Fogari R. Effects of insufficient sleep on blood pressure in hypertensive patients: a 24-h study. *Am J Hypertens* 1999;12; 63–8.

27. Spiegel K, Leproult R, L'hermite-Baleriaux M, Copinschi G, Penev PD, Van CE. Leptin levels are dependent on sleep duration: relationships with sympathovagal balance, carbohydrate regulation, cortisol, and thyrotropin. *J Clin Endocrinol Metab* 2004;89:5762–71.

28. King CR, Knutson KL, Rathouz PJ, Sidney S, Liu K, Lauderdale DS. Short sleep duration and incident coronary artery calcification. *JAMA* 2008;300:2859–66.

29. Knutson KL, Spiegel K, Penev P, Van Cauter E. The metabolic consequences of sleep deprivation. *Sleep Med Rev* 2007;11:163–78.

30. Al Lawati NM, Patel SR, Ayas NT. Epidemiology, risk factors, and consequences of obstructive sleep apnea and short sleep duration. *Prog Cardiovasc Dis* 2009;51:285–93.

31. Kripke DF, Garfinkel L, Wingard DL, Klauber MR, Marler MR. Mortality associated with sleep duration and insomnia. *Arch Gen Psychiatry* 2002;59:131–6.

32. Stender S, Dyerberg J, Bysted A, Leth T, Astrup A. A trans world journey. *Atheroscl Suppl* 2006;7:47–52.

33. Stender S, Astrup Λ, Dyerberg J. Ruminant and industrially produced trans fatty acids: health aspects. *Food Nutr Res* 2008;52– Epub 2008 Mar 12, doi: 10.3402/fnr.v52i0.1651.

34. Mozaffarian D, Katan MB, Ascherio A, Stampfer MJ, Willett WC. Trans fatty acids and cardiovascular disease. *N Engl J Med* 2006;354:1601–13.

35. Stender S, Dyerberg J, Astrup A. High levels of industrially produced trans fat in popular fast foods. *N Engl J Med* 2006;354:1650–2.

36. Koh-Banerjee P, Chu NF, Spiegelman D, et al. Prospective study of the association of changes in dietary intake, physical activity, alcohol consumption, and smoking with 9-y gain in waist circumference among 16 587 US men. *Am J Clin Nutr* 2003;78:719–27.

37. Kavanagh K, Jones KL, Sawyer J, et al. Trans fat diet induces abdominal obesity and changes in insulin sensitivity in monkeys. *Obesity* 2007;15:1675–84.

38. Stender S, Dyerberg J, Astrup A. Fast food: unfriendly and unhealthy. *Int J Obes* 2007;31:887–90.

39. Salmeron J, Hu FB, Manson JE, et al. Dietary fat intake and risk of type 2 diabetes in women. *Am J Clin Nutr* 2001;73:1019–26.

Index

Note: Italicized *f* and *t* refer to figures and tables.

(Author Disclosure Table)

Working group member	Employment	Research grant	Other research support	Speakers bureau/honoraria	Expert witness	Ownership interest	Consultant/advisory board	Other
Astrup	None	PhD project/Arla Foods[+]	None	None	None	None	Arla Foods/Almond AB*, Unilever*, Global Dairy Platform*	None
Bray	None	None	None	None	None	None	Amylin Pharmaceuticals*, Orexigen Pharmaceuticals*	None
Eckel	University of Colorado	Diadexus,[+] Glaxco Smith Kline[+]	None	Vindico,* Metobolic Health Inst[a]	None	None	GTC Nutrition[+], Pfizer*	Cardiometobolic Health Congress[+]
Farmer	Baylor College of Medicine	None	None	None	None	None	Merck, Pfizer*	
Gerstein	McMaster University	Sanofi-Aventis[+], GSK[+]	None	Sanofi-Aventis*, GSK*, Lily*, Merck*, Roche*	None	None	Sanofi-Aventis[+], GSK[+], Minimal-Medtronic*, AstraZeneca*	Novo Nordisk[+]
Gotto	Weill Cornell Medical College	None	None	None	None	Aegerion Pharmaceuticals[+], Arisaph Pharmaceuticals[+]	DuPont*, KOWA[+], Merck[+], Merck/Schering Plough[+], Novartis*, Reliant Pharmaceuticals*	None

Working group member	Employment	Research grant	Other research support	Speakers bureau/ honoraria	Expert witness	Ownership interest	Consultant/ advisory board	Other
Haskell	Stanford University	None	None	None	None	None	None	None
Kahn	VA Puget Sound Health Care System	None	None	None	None	None	None	None
Kraus	Duke University Medical Center	None	None	None	None	None	None	None
Lichtenstein	Jean Mayer USDA HNRCA at Tufts University	None	None	None	None	None	None	None
Poirier	Institut de cardiologie et de pneumologie	None	None	None	None	None	None	None
Sacks	Harvard University and Brigham & Women's Hospital, Boston	ISIS[+], R3i Foundation[+]	None	MediMedia*	Pfizer*	None	Genzyme*, Aegerion* ,Merck*, ISIS* , AstraZeneca , Lilly* , Abbott* WebMD* , Solvay*, SherborneGibbs*, RealCME*, Roche*, Guidepoint* , JMP*	R3i Foundation[+], Metabolic Syndrome Institute[+]

Skyler	University of Miami	None	Sanofi-Aventis+, GSK+	None	Nove-Nordisk+, Eli Lilly & Co+, Glaxo-Smith Kline*, Servier*	None	Amylin Pharmaceuticals+, MannKind Corp+	Sanofi-Aventis+	Board of Directors – Amylin Pharmaceuticals+
Smith	University of North Carolina	None	None	None	None	None	None	None	None
Taylor	Stanford Medical Center	None	None	None	None	None	None	None	None
Trockel	Stanford University	None	None	None	None	None	None	None	None
Utzschneider	Veterans Affairs	None	None	None	None	None	None	None	None
Wang	Austin Heart	None	None	None	Abbott*	None	None	None	None
Wilson	Emory University	None	Sanofi-Aventis+, GSK+	None	Sanofi-Aventis*, GSK*	None	None	Merck*	None

*Modest
+Significant

This represents the relationships of writing group members that may be perceived as actual or reasonably perceived conflicts of interest as reported on the Disclosure Questionnaire which all writing group members are required to complete and submit. A relationship is considered to be "Significant" if (a) the person receives $10,000 or more during any 12 month period, or 5% or more of the person's gross income; or (b) the person owns 5% or more of the voting stock or share of the entity, or owns $10,000 or more of the fair market value of the entity. A relationship is considered to be "Modest" if it is less than "Significant" under the preceding definition.